Deformity Correction in Total Knee Arthroplasty

Arun B. Mullaji • Gautam M. Shetty

Deformity Correction in Total Knee Arthroplasty

Springer

Arun B. Mullaji, FRCS Ed, MCh Orth, MS Orth
Consultant Joint Replacement Surgeon
Department of Orthopaedic Surgery
Breach Candy Hospital
Mumbai, Maharashtra, India

Gautam M. Shetty, MS Orth
Consultant Arthritis Care and Joint Replacement Surgery
Asian Orthopedic Institute
Asian Heart Institute and Research Center
Mumbai, Maharashtra, India

ISBN 978-1-4939-0565-2 ISBN 978-1-4939-0566-9 (eBook)
DOI 10.1007/978-1-4939-0566-9
Springer New York Heidelberg Dordrecht London

Library of Congress Control Number: 2014939034

Printed on acid-free paper

Springer is part of Springer Science+Business Media (www.springer.com)

To Shati, Nini, Mom and Dad

Arun B. Mullaji

To Priyanka. Thank you for everything
To my Parents for their inspiration, guidance and patience
To all my teachers

Gautam M. Shetty

Foreword

It is my pleasure and honour to write the Foreword for this book, *Deformity Correction in Total Knee Arthroplasty*, written by Drs. Arun Mullaji and Gautam Shetty. I have long admired their surgical expertise in the management of patients with severe angular deformity.

In 12 chapters, this book gives comprehensive and practical instruction to surgeons in the management of varus and valgus deformity, contracture and hyperextension, stiffness and instability and rotational and extra-articular deformity.

The text begins with advice regarding preoperative planning and ends with postoperative pain management and rehabilitation. Each chapter, when appropriate, includes the application of computer navigation techniques.

This book is clearly written, well illustrated, practical and comprehensive. The technical tips provided are numerous and indispensable to any surgeon who treats patients with the severest of angular deformities and instabilities.

I congratulate the authors on their profound contribution to the field of total knee arthroplasty.

Boston, MA, USA — Richard D. Scott, MD

Preface

With rapid advancement in technology and materials in total knee arthroplasty (TKA), long-term survival and function of the total knee are now more and more dependent on restoring accurate limb alignment, precise component position and optimum soft-tissue balance. Furthermore, a large number of early revisions in TKA are related to causes such as malalignment, malposition and instability.

Correct technique is the key to ensuring optimum function and long-term survival of the knee. This is all the more crucial and challenging to achieve in arthritic knees with severe and complex deformities. Many patients in the developing world present for TKA after years of neglect of their knee arthritis. The number of TKAs being performed in these nations is escalating in exponential fashion. Hence, correction of severe knee deformities forms an important part of TKA for orthopaedic surgeons working in these regions and also those in developed nations occasionally treating such patients.

This book outlines the basic principles of deformity correction in total knee arthroplasty with a special focus on severe and complex deformities. Starting with the initial key step of preoperative planning, this volume goes on to specifically describe how to deal with different types of deformities encountered in patients who undergo TKA. This book is more of a "how-to-do" manual, replete with specific tips on deformity correction in primary TKA rather than an exhaustive presentation on TKA. It does not deal with general issues related to TKA such as anatomy, kinematics, complications and revision surgery which are well covered in standard texts. With a focussed approach to the basic purpose and premise of this book, we have steered clear of controversial debates commonly encountered in TKA. However, with the experience of nearly 10,000 TKAs (including over 3,000 computer-assisted TKAs) behind us, we have distilled the lessons we have learnt with the use of both conventional surgery and computer navigation in TKA to further refine our technique. Hence, several chapters in this book have a concluding section describing the technique of deformity correction using computer navigation.

This book is aimed at orthopaedic surgeons and joint replacement surgeons who need to understand the principles of deformity correction especially in arthritic knees with severe and complex deformities before embarking on TKA (whether conventional or computer assisted) and will be useful in fine-tuning their planning and surgical technique.

We are grateful to Dr. Richard Scott, MD, a teacher, researcher and pioneer in the art and science of joint replacement surgery, for writing the foreword.

We thank Dr. Fahad Shaikh, DNB Orth (fellow in Joint Replacement Surgery, Breach Candy Hospital, Mumbai, India), for helping us obtain clinical and radiographic images of patients. We thank Dr. Vipul Chavda, BPT, MPT (Sports Medicine), Consultant Physical Therapist, Prakruti Sports Science & Physiotherapy Clinic Pvt. Ltd., Mumbai, India for providing clinical images for the Postoperative Rehabilitation section of Chapter 12. We also would like to thank the associate editor Kristopher Spring and the developmental editor Kevin Wright for their invaluable assistance in the preparation and publication of this book.

Mumbai, India Arun B. Mullaji
Mumbai, India Gautam M. Shetty

Authors

Arun B. Mullaji, FRCS Ed,
MCh Orth, MS Orth,
Consultant Joint Replacement Surgeon,
Department of Orthopaedic Surgery,
Breach Candy Hospital,
Mumbai,
India

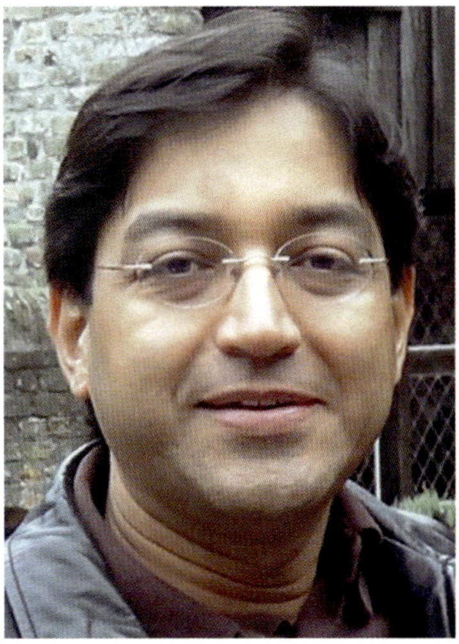

Gautam M. Shetty, MS Orth
Consultant Asian Orthopedic Institute,
Asian Heart Institute
and Research Center,
Mumbai,
India

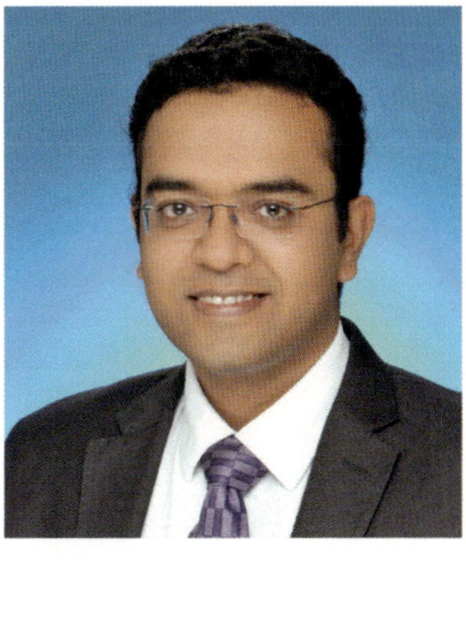

Contents

Part I

Preoperative Planning and Basic Technique of Total Knee Arthroplasty

Preoperative Planning

1

Introduction

Preoperative planning is paramount before undertaking any surgical procedure. This cannot be overemphasised for a procedure like total knee arthroplasty (TKA) where the goals include accurate restoration of limb alignment, optimum soft-tissue balancing and achieving a satisfactory range of motion (ROM). The use of computer navigation during TKA does not diminish the role of preoperative planning. The first important step in preoperative planning is proper selection of the patient and a thorough physical examination. This step gives important clues regarding patient complaints and disability and the expectation which a patient may have from the procedure. Physical examination may reveal clues as to what to expect during surgery in terms of pathoanatomic changes in the arthritic joint and how to plan for it during surgery. Imaging using plain radiographs helps in confirming the extent of knee arthritis and severity of deformity and is useful for planning the procedure. This chapter elaborates on physical examination and imaging for a patient who is to undergo TKA.

The Patient

Studies have shown that patient demographics are changing and increasingly younger, heavier, and more active patients with higher expectations are coming up for total knee arthroplasty (TKA) [1–3]. Patient satisfaction regarding TKA is primarily based on postoperative pain, ROM and functional ability and absence of complications related to TKA. An initial assessment of the patient should address issues related to patient's expectations and apprehensions regarding the surgical procedure. Studies have shown that patients with high somatisation and depression scores preoperatively continue to remain dissatisfied with the outcome of joint replacement despite lack of clinical or radiographic reasons for it [4–6]. Although the presence of psychological disorder is not a contraindication for surgical intervention, these issues need to be considered by the surgeon. With simultaneous bilateral TKAs, issues that frequently concern patients are whether the procedure will be more painful, the postoperative functional recovery slower and if they have to be dependent on others for their daily activity after surgery compared to staged bilateral TKAs (SBTKAs) or unilateral TKAs. An uneventful postoperative recovery and the risk of complications after SBTKA are also major concerns with patients. The authors in a prospective study conducted at their centre found that pain, function and complication rates in patients who underwent simultaneous bilateral computer-assisted TKA were comparable to those who underwent unilateral TKA [7]. Hence, the surgeon needs to address these issues before surgery so that patients can take an informed decision.

A.B. Mullaji, G.M. Shetty, *Deformity Correction in Total Knee Arthroplasty*,
DOI 10.1007/978-1-4939-0566-9_1, © Springer Science+Business Media New York 2014

Physical Examination

Before examining the knee, an assessment of gait and functional disability of the patient is invaluable. An abnormal gait with severe waddling or knee instability may be one of the features in patients with arthritic knee pain. Evidence of lateral thrust of the tibia or knee hyperextension during gait may indicate severe laxity or incompetence of the lateral collateral ligaments and posterior capsule, respectively (Fig. 1.1). Patients walking with severe intoeing or outtoeing may indicate a torsional abnormality in the limb.

Examination of the knee per se includes noting the type and degree of knee deformity, joint range of motion, instability, patellar tracking and condition of the skin over the knee joint. A combination of severe flexion or hyperextension deformity along with varus or valgus deformity adds to the complexity of the surgical technique (Fig. 1.1). Knees with severe instability or recurvatum deformity entail minimal bony resection and the possibility of using constrained prosthesis. The presence of knee recurvatum should alert the surgeon about the possibility of a neurological condition. This should be investigated and documented whenever necessary. Severe knee stiffness or severe flexion deformity indicates the need for a thorough posterior clearance or release with more liberal bone cuts to correct the deformity. In cases with severe stiffness or flexion deformity, quadriceps function may be difficult to assess, and any weakness will be revealed only after the TKA. Hence, such patients may require prolonged aggressive physiotherapy with or without splints (e.g. push-knee splint) postoperatively. Apart from the knee, a thorough examination of the entire lower limb is also warranted. Abnormal torsion of the tibia using the two malleoli as landmarks helps in deciding the rotational position of the tibial tray during TKA. Abnormal torsion in the tibia needs to be taken into account while determining rotational placement of the tibial component, or a mobile-bearing design may have to be used in order to avoid femoral and tibial rotational mismatch and postoperative gait abnormalities. Examination of the hindfoot similarly should be part of patient assessment. Both varus and valgus knees may be commonly associated with hindfoot valgus (Fig. 1.1). This tends to persist even after accurately correcting the knee deformity and influences the weight-bearing axis [8]. Hence, in cases with severe flat feet and hindfoot valgus, a medial arch support may be needed

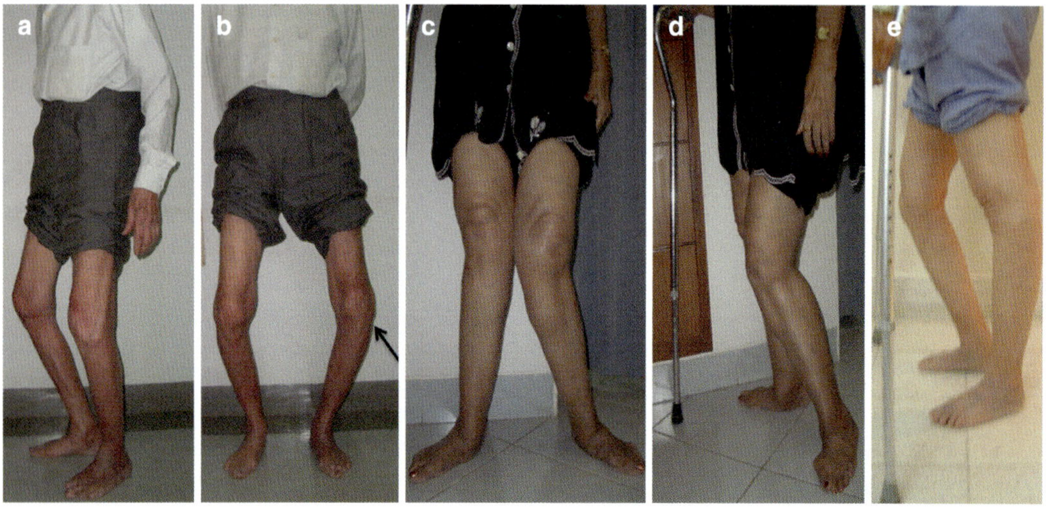

Fig. 1.1 Clinical photographs of various types of deformities encountered in knee arthritis. (**a**) Patient has a combination of severe bilateral varus and fixed flexion deformities of the knees. (**b**) Note the lateral subluxation of the tibia on the *left side* (*arrow*) on weight bearing indicating overstretched lateral soft-tissue structures. (**c**, **d**) Patient has a combination of valgus and fixed flexion deformity of the knee. The patient also has severe bilateral flatfeet and hindfoot valgus. (**e**) An uncommon recurvatum deformity of the knee

after surgery in order to improve the stance and gait of the patient. Proximally, the hip needs to be examined to rule out any hip pathology which may contribute to referred pain in the knee.

A fixed external rotation deformity of the hip especially in the very obese may lead to technical difficulties during the surgical procedure. Apart from these, a general assessment of peripheral limb circulation and neurological assessment and an assessment of the lumbar spine are important as any pathology related to these regions may have an effect on the postoperative functional and pain outcome of TKA. In fact it has been shown that nearly half the dissatisfied patients with an otherwise satisfactory TKA actually have symptoms related to the spine [9].

The condition of the contralateral limb and knee and that of the other joints as well as overall general physical condition of the patient needs to be assessed as these also influence postoperative satisfaction [9]. Overloading of the contralateral knee may predispose it to accelerated degenerative changes, while presence of fixed flexion or varus deformity may require compensatory footwear to correct limb length. Severe deformities may require bilateral TKAs to be performed.

Imaging

Plain Radiographs

Patients being considered for total knee arthroplasty (TKA) need to be investigated primarily using plain radiographs (either conventional or digital) such as the weight-bearing full-length hip-to-ankle radiograph, weight-bearing anteroposterior view and lateral and skyline views of the knee. These radiographs help in assessing the type and extent of knee deformity, the degree of joint space loss and bone loss, the amount of lateral or medial laxity, the distribution and amount of osteophytes and loose bodies, the presence of extra-articular deformities or pathologies and the general bone quality in the patient. Preoperative radiographs are also invaluable in planning the procedure and determining the technical difficulty that the surgeon may encounter.

Weight-Bearing Full-Length Hip-to-Ankle Radiograph

Controversy surrounds the use of weight-bearing hip-to-ankle radiographs in planning TKA. The use of these radiographs in cases with extra-articular deformities is generally accepted. Although their use in uncomplicated cases has been disputed [10–12], several reports have advocated their use routinely [13–16]. The authors obtain a weight-bearing long hip-to-ankle radiograph in all cases for TKA routinely not only to rule out extra-articular pathologies or deformities but also since most of the planning and radiographic assessment such as degree of deformity, plane of bone resection, amount of joint laxity and position of the femoral and tibial components in the coronal plane are done with respect to the mechanical axes of the femur and tibia. The following angles and radiographic features can be determined with this radiograph:

Frontal or Coronal Alignment – Relying on standard knee anteroposterior radiographs may grossly underestimate the knee deformity when compared to long hip-to-ankle radiographs especially in cases with severe coronal bowing of the femur (Fig. 1.2) which is common in patients with knee osteoarthritis [16–18]. The long hip-to-ankle radiograph helps in accurate estimation of preoperative knee deformity measured as the hip-knee-ankle (HKA) angle. This is defined as the angle between the mechanical axis of the femur (centre of the femoral head to the centre of the knee) and mechanical axis of the tibia (centre of the knee to the centre of the tibial plafond).

Distal Femoral Resection – The distal femoral valgus correction angle (VCA) decides the valgus angle at which the distal femur needs to be cut in the coronal plane in order to align the femoral component perpendicular to the mechanical axis of the femur. This is calculated as the angle between the mechanical axis of the femur and the distal anatomic axis of the femur (Fig. 1.3). Although the VCA is commonly believed to be between 5° and 7°, a recent study by the authors involving 503 arthritic limbs has shown wide variation in its value among patients with knee arthritis [18]. It may vary between 2.6° and 11.4° with 56 % of the limbs having a VCA outside the

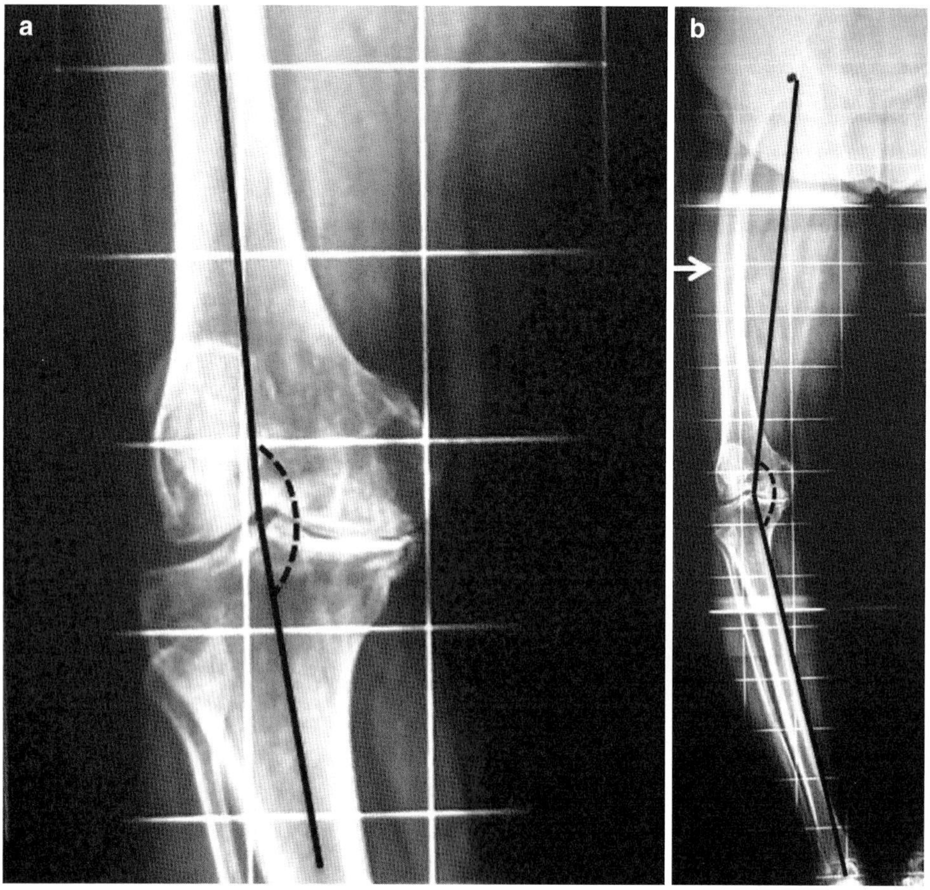

Fig. 1.2 Short films can be misleading! (**a**) A standing anteroposterior knee radiograph shows 4° varus deformity of the knee when calculated using the anatomic axes (femorotibial angle or FTA). (**b**) Weight-bearing long hip-to-ankle radiograph of the same patient shows that the deformity is approximately 20° when calculated using the mechanical axes (hip-knee-ankle or HKA angle). Note the extra-articular deformity caused by severe coronal bowing of the femur (*arrow*)

5–7° range [18]. The percentage of limbs with VCA >7° was significantly more in varus knees and with VCA <5° more in valgus knees. Preoperative deformity showed significant correlation with VCA. The VCA can also be affected by excessive coronal bowing of the femoral shaft or variation in the femoral neck shaft angle. Excessive coxa vara and lateral femoral bowing both increase the VCA, and excessive coxa valga and medial femoral bowing have the reverse effect [18]. During conventional TKA, extremes of VCA will render use of an intramedullary femoral guide rod difficult due to distortion of the femoral canal and may lead to error in placement of the distal femoral cutting block. Hence, in these cases, a shorter guide rod needs to be used, and owing to such great variability among limbs, the VCA should be selected in each limb based on measurements done on preoperative long films. Although extremes of VCA or extra-articular deformity are irrelevant when placing the femoral component in computer-assisted TKA (as the software uses only the centre of the femoral head and centre of distal femur to plan the distal cut), these findings on the long weight-bearing radiograph may indicate the need for extensive soft-tissue releases for restoration of limb alignment and optimum gap balancing during TKA irrespective of the technique used (Fig. 1.4). When knee varus is associated with minimal osteophytes and

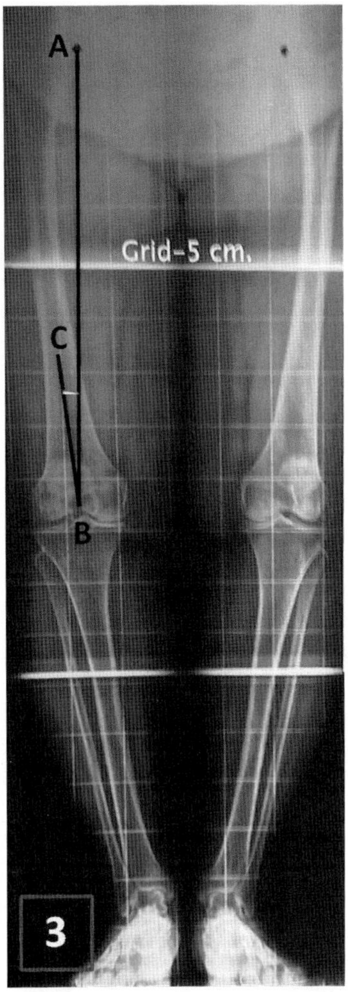

Fig. 1.3 Distal femoral valgus correction angle (VCA). Distal femoral valgus correction angle (VCA) decides the valgus angle at which the distal femur needs to be cut in order to align the femoral component at 90° to the mechanical axis of the femur. This is calculated as the angle (angle ABC) between the mechanical axis of the femur (line AB) and the distal anatomic axis of the femur (line CB)

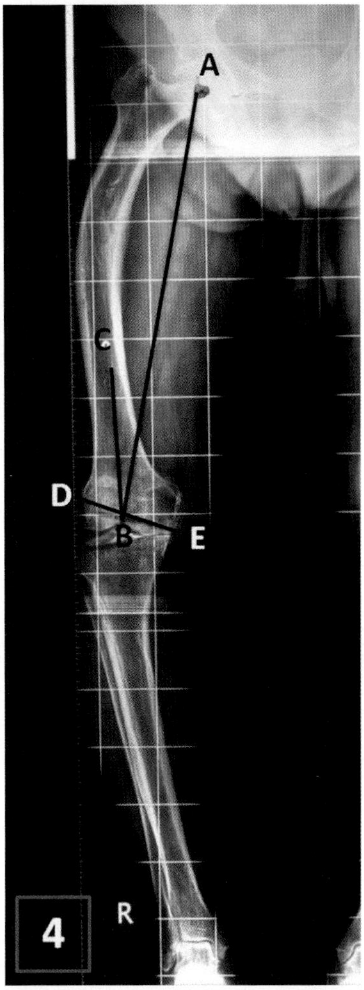

Fig. 1.4 Extreme of distal femoral valgus correction angle (VCA). A case of extreme distal femoral valgus correction angle (angle ABC) of 17° due to a malunited femoral fracture. The distal femoral cut (line DE) drawn perpendicular to the mechanical axis of femur (line AB) endangers the femoral attachment of lateral collateral ligament. Hence, a corrective osteotomy of the extra-articular deformity is warranted

a high VCA due to excessive femoral bowing, extensive soft-tissue release may have to be combined with a sliding medial condylar osteotomy during TKA [19].

Preoperative Joint Divergence Angle (JDA) – Varus knee deformities are associated with tight medial and lax lateral and soft-tissue structures. A fair indication of these soft-tissue changes can be obtained on a weight-bearing full-length radiograph. The proposed distal femoral and proximal tibial cuts are drawn perpendicular to the mechanical axes of the femur and the tibia. The angle formed by the proposed tibial and femoral resections (preoperative JDA) will give a fair estimation of the site (medial or lateral) and degree of soft-tissue contracture and the extent of soft-tissue release that may be required. Similarly, it will also give a fair estimation of the degree of laxity in the opposite compartment and how much bone resection may be required.

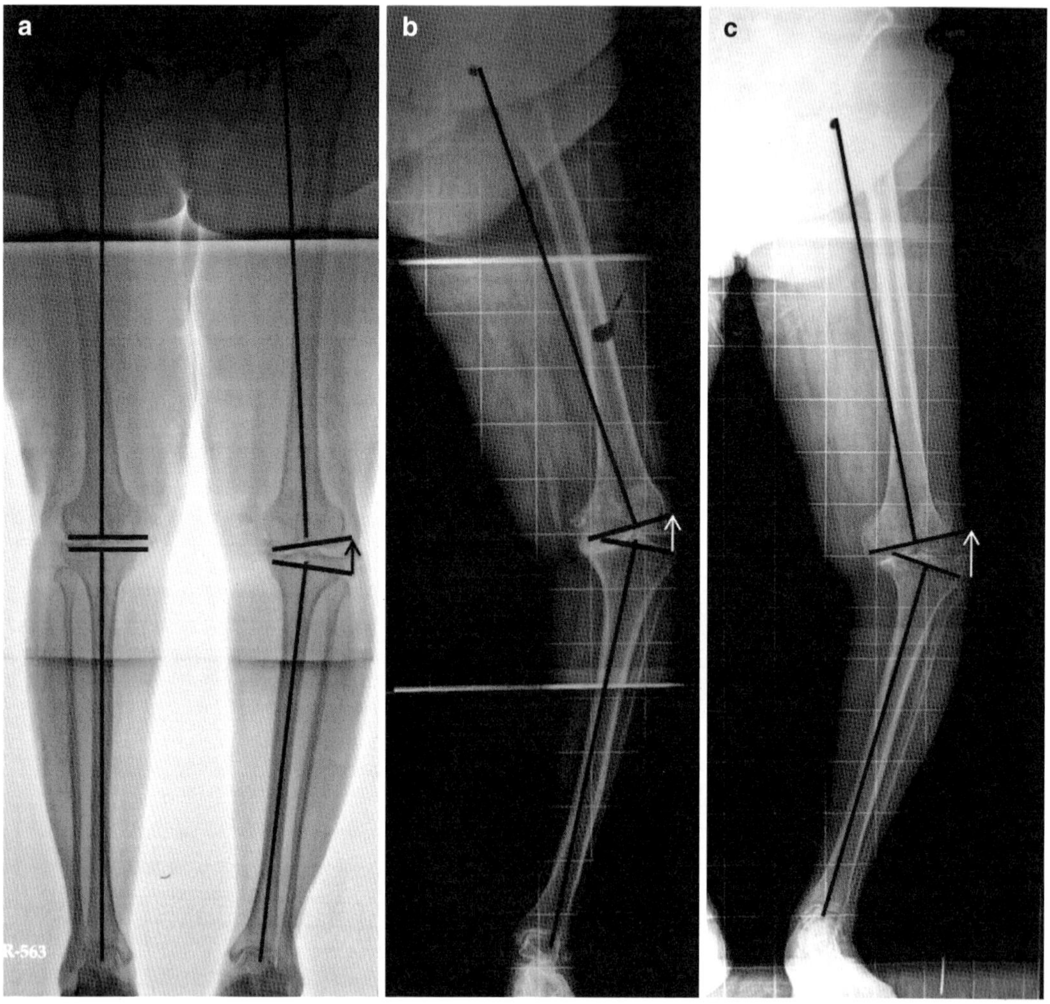

Fig. 1.5 Preoperative joint divergence angle (JDA). (**a**) Mild varus deformity on the *right side* where the distal femoral and proximal tibial resection planes are parallel to each other (JDA almost zero) implying that minimal medial soft tissue is needed for gap balancing; on the *left side* with moderate varus deformity, the lateral side shows moderate laxity (*arrow*). (**b**) An example of severe lateral laxity due to severe varus deformity. This case will require substantial medial release in order to balance it with the lateral side especially due to the associated femoral shaft bowing present. (**c**) Here the lateral laxity is very severe with associated lateral subluxation of the tibia despite the degree of varus deformity being lesser than in patient (**b**) creating a large JDA

Lesser the angle or more parallel the lines, lesser will be the amount of release required for correction (Fig. 1.5a, b). Similarly greater the angle or more divergent the lines, greater will be the amount of release required and more conservative the bone cuts (Fig. 1.5c).

Extra-Articular Deformities or Implant In Situ – A full-length radiograph will also reveal any extra-articular deformity (EAD) in the limb, hip pathology, prior trauma/surgery, associated stress fractures or an implant in situ. Excessive coronal bowing of the femur is a common cause of extra-articular deformity in arthritic knees undergoing TKA [16, 17]. Mullaji et al. [16] have reported that up to 20 % of varus arthritic knees have significant femoral bowing in the coronal plane in Asian patients. Stress fractures although uncommon are an important cause of extra-articular deformity [20]. Depending on the type seen on preoperative radiographs, TKA may have to be combined with long tibial stem extenders, metal augments or corrective osteotomies [20]. Similarly, in the tibia, extra-articular deformity due to malunited or ununited fractures, stress fractures, post-high tibial osteotomy or excessive tibial bowing may be present. Although most of these cases of knee arthritis with extra-articular deformities can be managed by extensive intra-articular soft-tissue releases, a corrective osteotomy may be rarely required [17]. This is discussed in detail in Chap. 8 on EADs.

The presence of implants will warrant the need to use computer navigation which will bypass the hardware or extramedullary cutting guides as use of intramedullary jigs may not be possible (Fig. 1.6a). However, in some cases where the implant may be close to the knee joint, they may have to be removed before implantation of the prosthesis especially the tibial component (Fig. 1.6b). We have shown that navigation is useful in cases of altered hip centre [21].

What to Look for in a Weight-Bearing Long Hip-to-Ankle Radiograph?

- Degree of limb malalignment or deformity based on hip-knee-ankle (HKA) angle.
- Distal femoral valgus correction angle (VCA) – the greater the angle, the greater the need for an extensive soft-tissue release with or without an osteotomy.
- Extra-articular deformity – is a corrective osteotomy required?
- Stress fractures, prior trauma.
- Prior surgery with implant in situ and hip pathology.

Weight-Bearing Knee Anteroposterior (AP) Radiograph

The knee AP view is probably the most commonly used radiograph for diagnosis of knee arthritis and planning for TKA. It is important

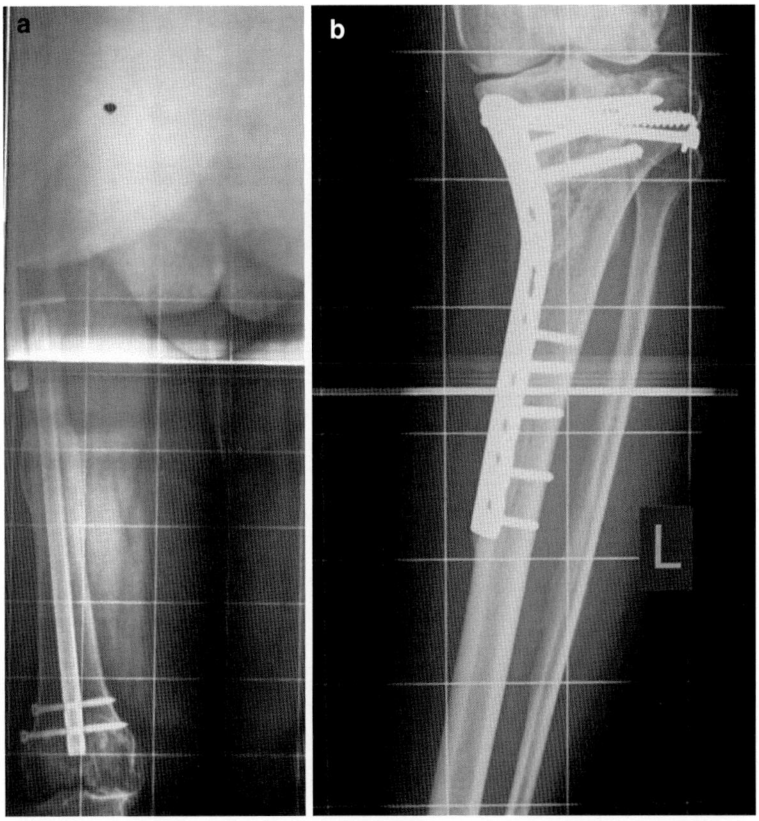

Fig. 1.6 Implant in situ. (**a**) A case with intramedullary nail in the femur which will not interfere during CAS TKA. (**b**) A case with proximal tibial plating with a malunited fracture. Implant needs to be removed and a corrective osteotomy may be required

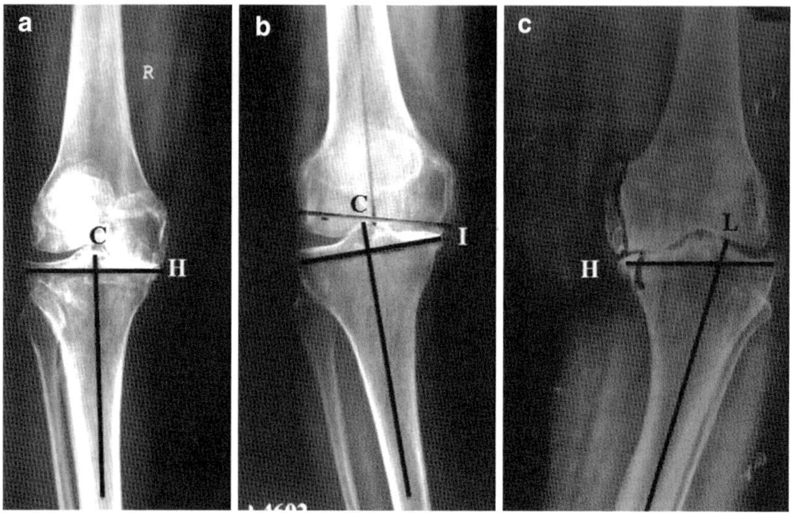

Fig. 1.7 Centre of putative tibial base. (**a**) Proximal end of the tibial medullary axis passing through the centre of the tibial spine (*C*) with a horizontal tibial articular surface (*H*). (**b**) Proximal end of the tibial medullary axis passing through the centre of the tibial spine with an inclined tibial articular surface (*I*). (**c**) Proximal end of the tibial medullary axis passing lateral to the tibial spine (*L*) with a horizontal tibial articular surface indicating proximal tibia vara

that the knee AP view is obtained while the patient is weight-bearing as a supine view may underestimate the degree of arthritis, deformity and instability. This view allows a closer look at the knee in the coronal plane and is an important part of the preoperative planning process for TKA. As previously mentioned, although this view may underestimate the degree of knee deformity and will not show extra-articular bony deformity, it is invaluable in assessing certain features around the knee joint which gives an idea of what to expect during TKA.

Tibial and Femoral Resection – Tibial and femoral resections are performed perpendicular to their respective mechanical axes. Traditionally, the amount of tibial resection is primarily based on the actual thickness of the thinnest tibial component. If the composite thickness is 8 mm, then generally 8 mm of the less affected tibial plateau should be resected. However, both tibial and femoral resections need to be conservative in cases with severe bone loss, severe lateral or medial laxity in varus or valgus, recurvatum deformity and in knees with gross instability. More than usual distal femur may have to be occasionally resected in knees with fixed flexion deformity to achieve correction. By marking out these resections, the surgeon can get a good idea of the amount of bone being resected, and if the relative thickness of the medial and lateral tibial plateau and distal femur condyles matches the preoperative markings.

Centre of Putative Tibial Tray – In most cases this point on a knee AP radiograph is the proximal end of the tibial medullary axis and is also noted during registration in CAS (Fig. 1.7a, b). However, in varus knees with proximal tibia vara or other extra-articular deformities, the proximal end of the tibial medullary axis may lie lateral or medial to the tibial spines (Fig. 1.7c). In such limbs this lateral or medial point should be marked on x-rays and also for registering the tibial centre point instead of the midpoint of the tibial spines. This will ensure central placement of the stem of the tibial tray which is especially important when a tibial stem extender is being used. This is also the case in post-high tibial osteotomy (HTO) knees where the registration point may be medial or lateral, and using this point will centralise the tibial component without the need for an offset stem. Lateralisation of the tibial centre registration point, commonly seen in limbs

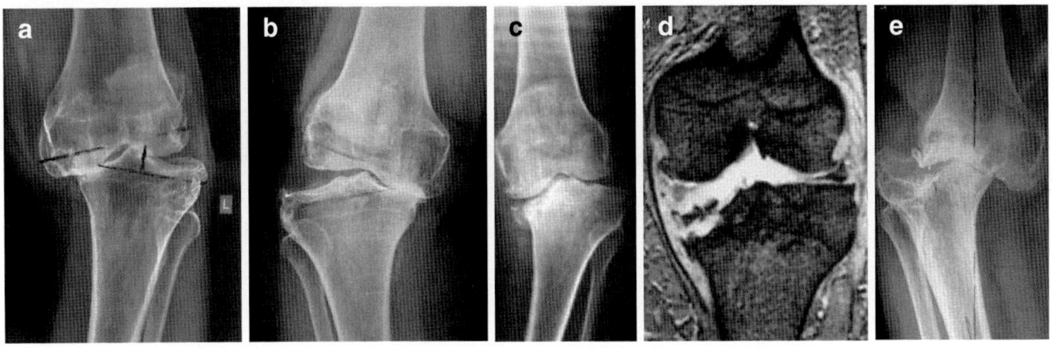

Fig. 1.8 Grades of bone defects. (**a**) Moderate medial tibial bone loss with moderate lateral laxity. This can be tackled with bone cement. (**b**) Moderate medial tibial bone loss with severe lateral laxity. Tibial cut needs to be minimised in view of severe lateral laxity and hence the bone defect may require bone grafting. (**c**) Severe medial tibial bone loss with severe lateral laxity. (**d**) The true extent of bone defect in patient (**c**) can be seen on the MRI. Minimal bone cuts and severe lateral laxity in this case will leave a substantial bone defect which may need a metal augment. (**e**) Severe lateral femoral condyle bone defect which will need a lateral distal femoral augment with a femoral stem

with tibia vara, indicates that the tibial tray may have to be lateralised and the soft-tissue release may have to be combined with a reduction osteotomy in order to achieve correction of malalignment and medio-lateral balance. This is significant in a case where metaphyseal tibia vara may be the main cause of knee varus deformity (Fig. 1.7c).

Osteophytes – Medial or lateral tibial and femoral osteophytes are commonly seen in knee arthritis especially in severe cases where they may be abundant. The presence of osteophytes indicates that their excision will offer a certain degree of correction and correspondingly less soft-tissue release may have to be performed. Similarly in cases of mild to moderate knee deformity but with significant lateral laxity or with extra-articular deformity where osteophytes may be minimal or absent, extensive soft-tissue release may be required in order to correct deformity and balance the medio-lateral gaps.

Bone Defect – Severe varus or valgus knees may be associated with medial or lateral tibial and femoral bone loss. These bone defects usually occur in long-standing severe knee arthritis. However, bone loss may be substantial in knees associated with intra-articular stress fractures. Depending on the severity, bone defects may be dealt with using cement, bone graft or metal augments. Large bone defects may be reduced in size during surgery by taking a thicker tibial bone cut and lateralisation of the tibial tray with a reduction osteotomy. The subsequent bone defect may be filled with bone cement (Fig. 1.8a). However, the amount of tibial cut may have to be minimised in cases with severe instability or recurvatum deformity. In such cases the bone defect may have to be filled with bone grafts (Fig. 1.8b). Cases with substantial bone defect need to be treated with metal augments (Fig. 1.8c, d). Rarely, severe bone loss may be seen in the femoral condyles where a metal augment and femoral stem may have to be used (Fig. 1.8e)

What to Look for in a Weight-Bearing Knee AP Radiograph?

- Relative amounts of medial and lateral tibial and femoral resections
- Centre of the putative tibial tray, especially if a longer stem is to be used
- Osteophytes (especially posterior femoral, medial femoral and tibial)
- Bone defects

Knee Lateral Radiograph

Lateral knee radiograph gives a clear sagittal picture of the knee joint. This view gives a fair estimation of the posterior osteophytes, joint line and patellar position and tibial slope.

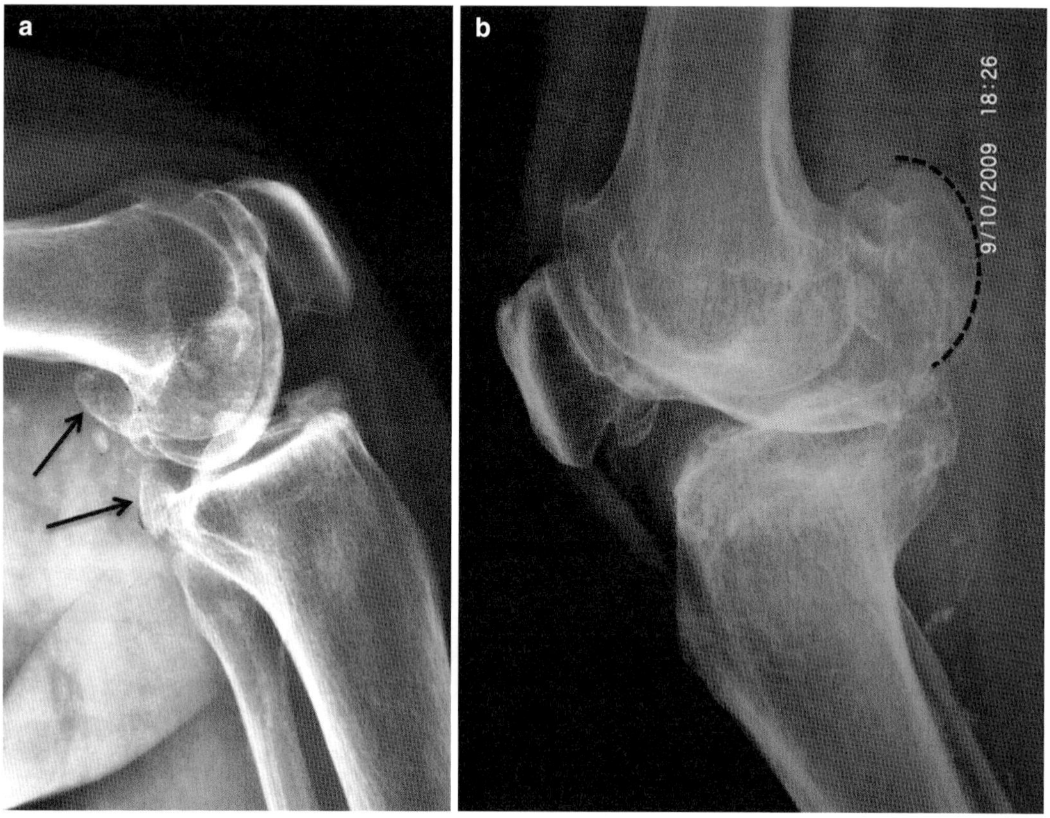

Fig. 1.9 Posterior osteophytes. (**a**) Numerous osteophytes on the posterior aspect of the femur and tibia (*arrows*). (**b**) A single large posterior femoral osteophyte covering the entire posterior surface of the femoral condyle. This needs to be removed prior to registration to avoid error

Osteophytes – Posterior osteophytes are commonly seen in knee arthritis and are the most common cause of a fixed flexion deformity in an arthritic knee. Ensuring complete excision of these posterior osteophytes helps in achieving substantial correction of a fixed flexion deformity and reducing the need for an extensive soft-tissue release and additional bone resection. These osteophytes need to be removed prior to assessing the extension gap. Rarely these osteophytes may grow large to cover the entire posterior condyle of the femur (Fig. 1.9). Femoral registration prior to removal of such osteophytes may cause error and result in the computer suggesting an oversized femoral component.

Joint Line and Patella Height – Preoperative alteration of patellar height and joint line is occasionally seen with patella baja and is often seen in knees with a prior high tibial osteotomy. This can be measured on the lateral radiograph using the tip of the fibular head as reference (Fig. 1.10). If there is significant alteration of the joint line, achieving flexion-extension gap balance and accurate sizing and placement of femoral component is crucial during TKA. Conservative bone cuts and proper gap balancing may help in avoiding the use of a thicker insert which may further elevate the joint line.

Tibial Slope – The tibial slope may be altered in knees with severe bone defects and in post-HTO knees. This should be noted in the preoperative lateral knee radiograph so that angle of tibial slope may be correspondingly adjusted during surgery.

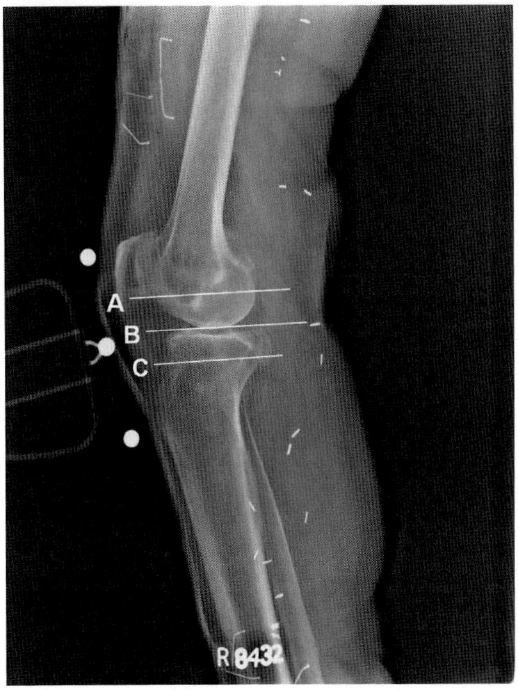

Fig. 1.10 Joint line and patellar height. Distance AB, patellar height; Distance BC, joint line

What to Look for in a Knee Lateral Radiograph?
Posterior osteophytes
Joint line and patellar height
Tibial slope

Preoperative Templating for Component Size
Similar to total hip arthroplasty, preoperative templating on radiographs is an option in TKA to determine femoral and tibial component size. Aslam et al. [22] in a retrospective study using manual templating on radiographs reported that 49 % of the femoral components and 67 % of the tibial components were correctly templated to the exact size with fair to moderate agreement between templated size and actual implant size. Hence, they concluded that templating for TKA is prone to error and can only be used as an approximate guide. However, Peek et al. [23] in a retrospective study using digital templating reported better reliability with 71 % of the femoral components and 60 % of the tibial components correctly templated to the exact size. They concluded that digital templating with a calibrating device can be useful for preoperative planning of total knee arthroplasty. The authors do not perform preoperative templating for component size. The gap-balancing technique used by us relies on medio-lateral and flexion-extension gap balance to determine the tibial and femoral component size. However, we do make sure that extremes of component sizes are made available during surgery when such a situation is anticipated based on the built of the patient and the skeletal built on radiographs. Hence, a tall well-built male patient may be expected to have a larger than usual femoral and tibial component size.

Computed Tomography (CT) Scan

This investigation is rarely indicated as part of the preoperative evaluation in TKA. It may be performed to assess any torsional abnormalities in the femur or tibia due to malunited fractures or osteotomies.

Magnetic Resonance Imaging (MRI)

An MRI scan may be required rarely in ankylosed knees to assess the condition of the quadriceps muscle and patellar tendon. It may also be done to confirm the diagnosis of an impending stress fracture [20] which may not be obvious on plain radiographs (Fig. 1.11). It may also be useful in cases with an intra-articular stress fracture to delineate the size of bone defect and the vascularity of an ununited fragment. It is helpful in patients being considered for unicompartmental arthroplasty – those with involvement of other compartments would be more suitable for a TKA.

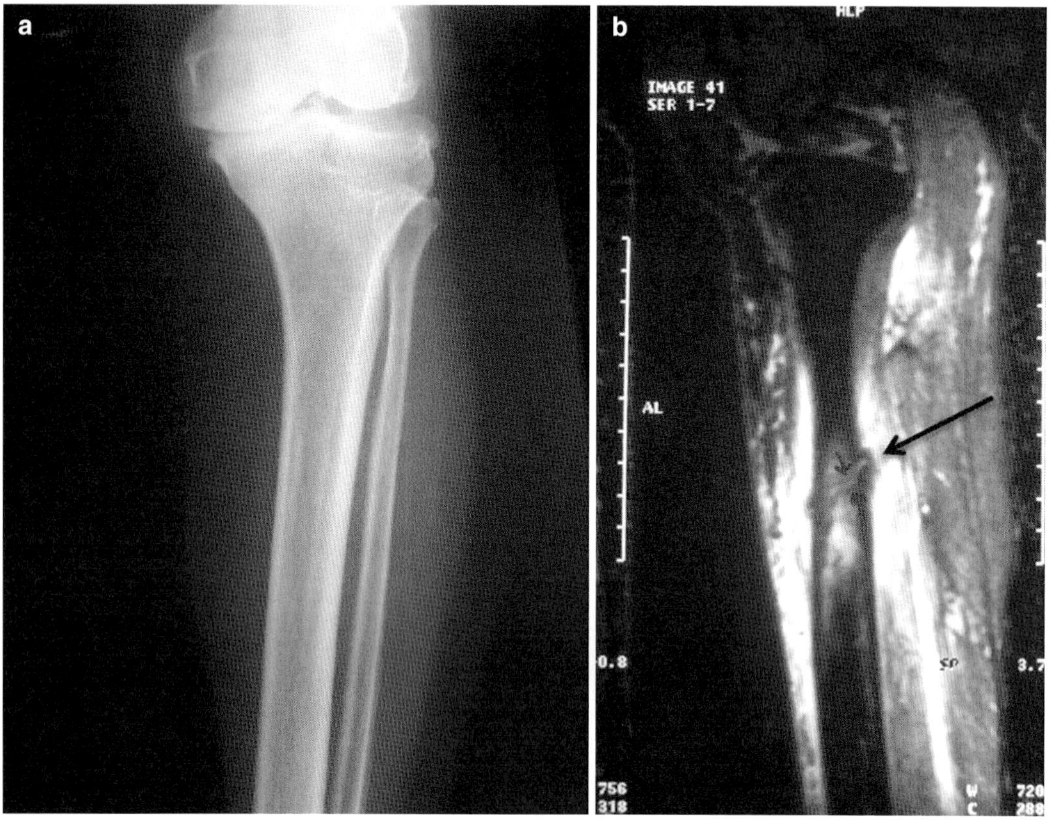

Fig. 1.11 MRI to detect stress fracture. (**a**) Plain radiograph is normal, whereas (**b**) the MRI shows an impending stress fracture (*arrow*)

Electromyography and Nerve Conduction Studies (EMG-NCV)

An EMG-NCV study of the lower limb may need to be done in cases with long-standing fixed flexion deformity to determine the status of the quadriceps and hamstring muscles and in cases with knee recurvatum deformity to rule out neurological causes. It may also be performed in chronic uncontrolled diabetics with neuropathy and in patients with chronic low back pain and radiculopathy to document the extent of neuromuscular involvement as their symptoms due to the underlying condition may persist even after TKA.

Selection of Implants

The authors use a cruciate-substituting design during TKA in all their patients. The rationale behind this is that a majority of arthritic knees, especially the ones with severe deformities, show significant degeneration of the posterior cruciate ligament (PCL) [24, 25]. Hence, in this situation the PCL cannot be relied on to achieve gap balancing and is best substituted. Hence, the authors have elaborated here only on variations of cruciate-substituting designs.

Design

The two primary designs commonly used in primary TKA are a fixed-bearing or a mobile-bearing design. The decision to use either one is primarily based on the surgeon. Several studies have reported on the benefits of using a mobile-bearing design in terms of improved wear resistance and postoperative function such as knee flexion [26, 27]. However, the authors primarily use a fixed-bearing design in most of their patients and have specific indications for a mobile-bearing knee. First, an active patient who wants and expects to perform activities involving high flexion of the knee such as sitting cross-legged on the floor or squatting postoperatively may benefit from a mobile-bearing design due to a certain degree of extra rotation that the implant may provide when knee is placed in the cross-legged position [28]. Second, in cases with rotational deformities of the tibia, a mobile-bearing design may mitigate and compensate for the rotational mismatch between the tibia and the implant position. However, the surgeon needs to be aware that an optimally balanced knee is an absolute prerequisite to the use of a mobile-bearing design. Any compromise on this aspect will result in complications such as instability and bearing "spin-out" with the use of a mobile-bearing design. Hence, the authors feel that a surgeon should use a mobile-bearing design only when one has achieved optimum soft-tissue balance, especially in flexion.

On the tibial side in fixed-bearing designs, the surgeon has two options – a modular design and an all-polyethylene monoblock design. Modern all-polyethylene tibial components have shown comparable results in mid- to long-term follow-up studies and offer several advantages [29]. These include lower cost, avoidance of locking-mechanism issues and backside wear and increased poly-thickness after identical bone resections. However, there are certain disadvantages with this tibial design which include lack of modularity which restricts intraoperative options and during early revision TKAs when a liner exchange is indicated [29]. The authors use an all-polyethylene tibial component whenever the bone quality is found to be good and the knee well balanced and well aligned intraoperatively. A metal-backed tibia is used when the bone quality is poor, patient is heavy, additional components such as a stem or augment needs to be used and if the balance is suboptimal with lateral laxity.

Recently an added dimension to the femoral component design has been the "high-flexion" feature. Although advocates of this design have reported benefits in terms of improved flexion, the reported literature is not very convincing on this. Recent reports have also shown increased incidence of early loosening of the femoral components with these high-flexion designs [30, 31]. The authors have not used this design in their patients since there does not seem to be any significant improvement in function and the risks in terms of early revision seem to far outweigh the benefits.

Constraint

Most knees undergoing primary TKA can be managed using prostheses with the least constraint, i.e. either a cruciate-retaining or a cruciate-substituting design. Rarely is a more constrained design or hinge prosthesis needed. A proper clinical and radiographic evaluation will indicate the need of a constrained implant during TKA. A constrained design (such as the TC3) may be indicated in cases where the opposite collateral may be excessively lax (i.e. the medial collateral in valgus knees and the lateral collateral in varus knees) and the knee unstable (Fig. 1.12). A hinge design may be rarely indicated when the knee is grossly unstable, and ligament balancing may not be possible due to soft-tissue incompetence (Fig. 1.12).

Extras

Additional components may sometimes be required while using a regular cruciate-substituting (CS) design. These include the following.

Long Stem Extenders: Tibial stem extenders may be required in cases with large tibial bone defects where bone graft or metal augments are used in order to provide additional stability to the tibial component. It may also be used when a corrective tibial osteotomy is anticipated or in cases with acute or impending stress fracture. Long femoral stem extenders are rarely used to supplement fixation when a distal metal augment is used for severe femoral bone loss or to stabilise a distal femoral corrective osteotomy.

Augments/Wedges: Metal augments may be used in knees with substantial bone loss in profound arthritic deformities especially when associated with an intra-articular stress fracture.

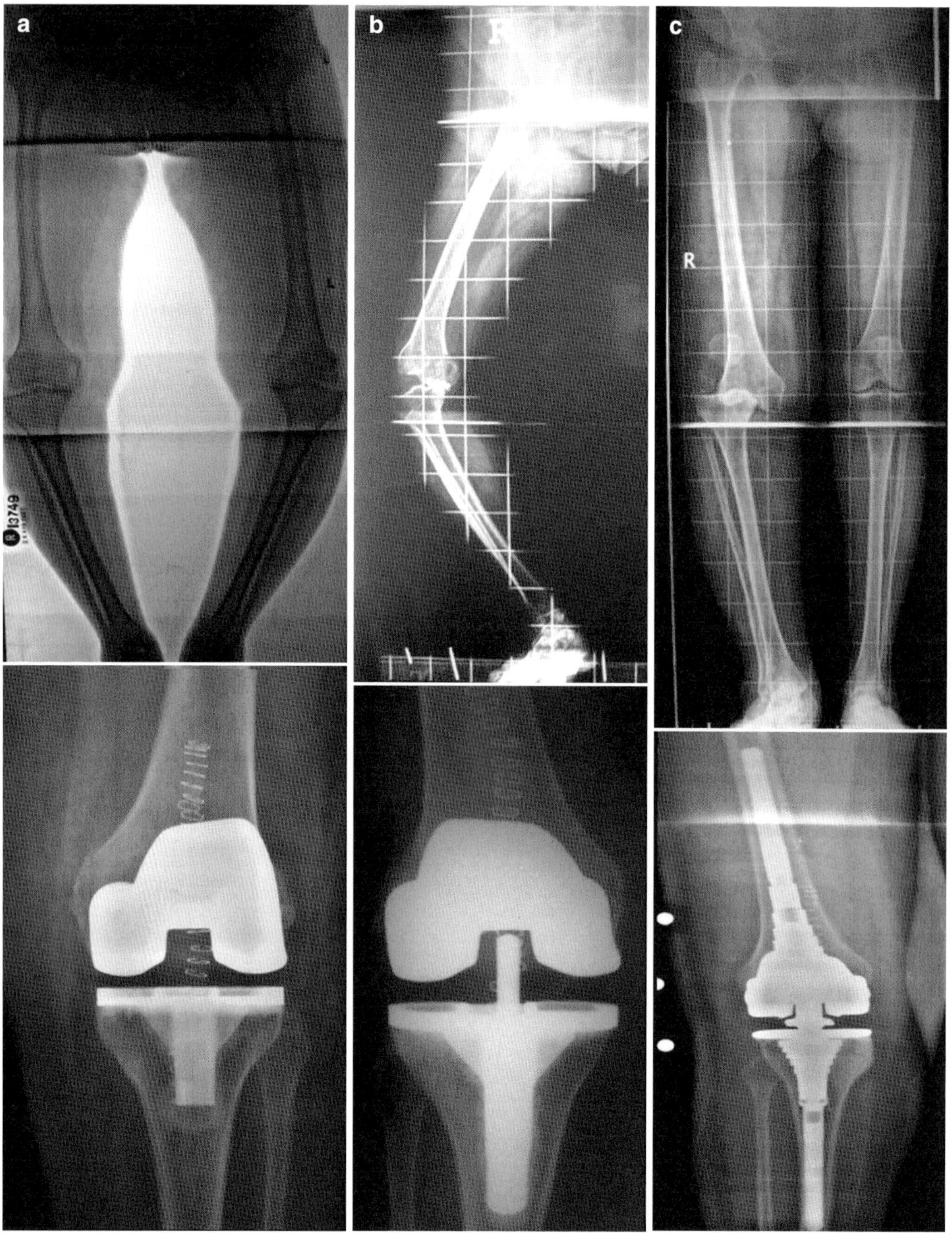

Fig. 1.12 Different types of implant. (**a**) Case 1 where despite severe varus deformity a standard cruciate-substituting design was adequate. (**b**) Case 2 where the presence of severe varus deformity and excessive lateral laxity warranted the use of a TC3 insert. (**c**) Case 3 showed gross instability and dislocation of the arthritic joint which required a hinge prosthesis

Computer Navigation

Although the authors follow a similar surgical technique workflow for both conventional and navigated TKA, computer-assisted TKA requires the use of additional instruments for registration, navigation and verification during the procedure. Different navigation systems for TKA use different types of technical workflow depending on the manufacturer and the version of software being used. The surgeon needs to be well versed with the instruments, hardware and computer software workflow of the system before using navigation for TKA. The authors use the image-free Ci navigation system (Brainlab, Munich, Germany) for all their TKAs where the surgeon can not only quantify the alignment of limb and component but also determine gaps throughout the entire range of motion. A well-trained technician who can operate the navigation system during surgery can be very helpful to ensure smooth operability of the system. Broadly, the components of this navigation system include:

(a) Infrared-emitting *camera unit*
(b) Computer *monitor unit* with the navigation software
(c) Instruments:
Reflective arrays which are attached to the femur and tibia and whose position is tracked during navigation.
Marker spheres which are attached to the arrays and which reflect back the infrared beams emitted by the camera.
Pointer with attached marker spheres is used to register various anatomic landmarks, lines and surfaces during the registration process.
Cutting block adaptor helps to verify position of cutting blocks and the bone cuts.
Schanz pins which help fix arrays to the femur and tibia.

The basic setup of the camera and monitor unit with respect to the surgeon and the limb being operated needs to be determined by the surgeon beforehand (Fig. 1.13). The camera unit needs to be placed in such a manner that both femoral and tibial arrays are in range and easily tracked throughout the entire procedure. The monitor unit needs to be in full view so that the surgeon can visualise and control the navigation process. The reflective arrays need to be fixed to the tibia and femur at a proper angle and distance in such a way that their tracking is not hindered during the surgical procedure. The

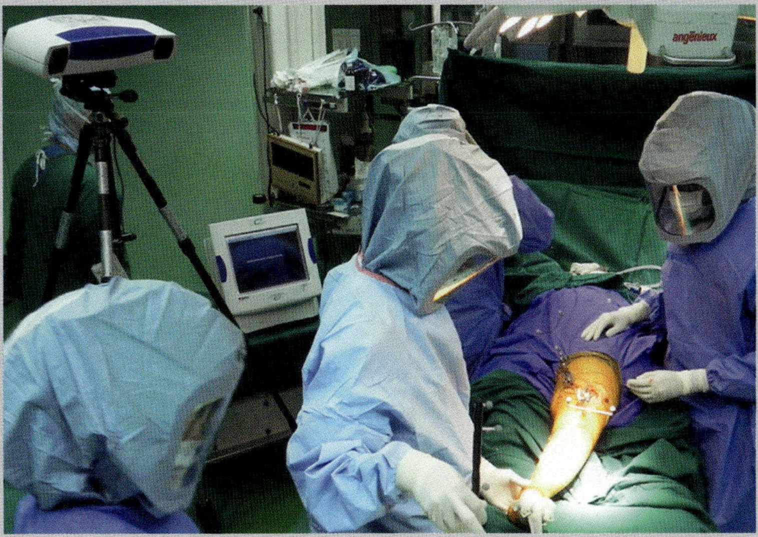

Fig. 1.13 Navigation system setup during total knee arthroplasty (TKA). Setup for a left side TKA where the arrays are fixed on the medial side of the femur and tibia and the camera and display unit are placed on the right side. Note the surgeon holding a pointer with marker spheres for registration

surgeon needs to ensure that the arrays are securely fastened to the Schanz pins and the marker spheres fully tightened to the arrays before the start of the procedure. Whenever an additional procedure maybe indicated such as a corrective or an epicondylar osteotomy or a long stem is likely to be used, pins for fixing the arrays should be placed away from the operative site (preferably closer to the diaphysis of the bone). The Schanz screws must be firmly fixed to the bone, and we use two screws each for the femoral and tibial arrays and these have a unicortical purchase. In poor-quality bone, bicortical fixation is preferred. At any stage if the arrays/Schanz screws loosen out, the navigation process has to be abandoned.

Glossary

Coronal component malalignment Components outside the acceptable ±3° range from a neutral alignment of 90° in the coronal and sagittal plane.

Coronal limb malalignment Postoperative HKA angle outside the acceptable ±3° range from a neutral alignment of 180°.

Femoral anatomic axis Mid-diaphyseal line of the femur passing proximally from the piriformis fossa just medial to the greater trochanter distally just medial to the intercondylar notch of the femur.

Femoral mechanical axis Line passing from the centre of the femoral head to the apex of the intercondylar notch on the femoral articular surface.

Femorotibial angle (FTA) Medial angle formed by the distal femoral anatomic axis and the proximal tibial anatomic axis.

Hip-knee-ankle (HKA) angle Medial angle formed by the mechanical axis of the femur and the tibia and denotes the coronal alignment of the limb.

Joint divergence angle (JDA) Angle formed by the proposed distal femoral cut and proximal tibial cut each drawn perpendicular to their respective mechanical axes. This generally equals the HKA angle.

Joint line This is the distance between the tip of the fibula and the tangent drawn to the distal end of the femoral condyles on lateral radiographs.

Mechanical axis of the limb Line passing from the centre of the femoral head and the centre of the ankle plafond.

Patellar height This is the distance between the distal tip of the patellar component and the tangent drawn to the distal part of the femoral component on lateral radiographs. Intraoperatively, this distance is assessed as the gap between the distal tip of the patellar component and the tibial polyethylene insert when the knee is put through an arc of flexion.

Tibial mechanical axis Line passing from the midpoint between the tibial spines to the centre of the talar dome.

Valgus correction angle (VCA) Angle formed by the mechanical and distal anatomic axes of the femur and denotes the amount of valgus angulation required for the distal femoral cut.

Appendix 1

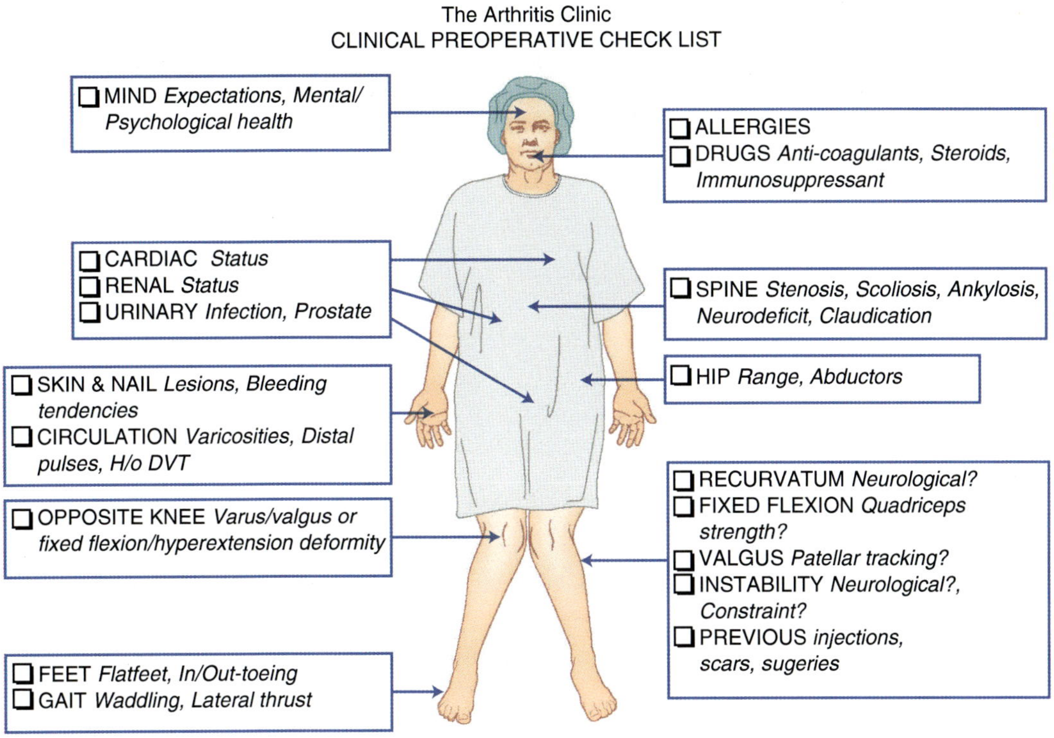
The Arthritis Clinic
CLINICAL PREOPERATIVE CHECK LIST
❑ MIND *Expectations, Mental/ Psychological health*
❑ ALLERGIES
❑ DRUGS *Anti-coagulants, Steroids, Immunosuppressant*
❑ CARDIAC *Status*
❑ RENAL *Status*
❑ URINARY *Infection, Prostate*
❑ SPINE *Stenosis, Scoliosis, Ankylosis, Neurodeficit, Claudication*
❑ SKIN & NAIL *Lesions, Bleeding tendencies*
❑ CIRCULATION *Varicosities, Distal pulses, H/o DVT*
❑ HIP *Range, Abductors*
❑ OPPOSITE KNEE *Varus/valgus or fixed flexion/hyperextension deformity*
❑ RECURVATUM *Neurological?*
❑ FIXED FLEXION *Quadriceps strength?*
❑ VALGUS *Patellar tracking?*
❑ INSTABILITY *Neurological?, Constraint?*
❑ PREVIOUS *injections, scars, sugeries*
❑ FEET *Flatfeet, In/Out-toeing*
❑ GAIT *Waddling, Lateral thrust*

Appendix 2

THE ARTHRITS CLINIC
RADIOGRAPHIC PREOPERATIVE CHECK LIST

- ❑ Hip-Knee-Ankle Angle
- ❑ Valgus Correction Angle
- ❑ Joint Divergeence Angle
- ❑ Femoral/Tibial Bowing, Tibia Vara, Extra-articular Deformity
- ❑ Osteophytes/Loose bodies
- ❑ Bone defect
- ❑ Extremes of implant size
- ❑ Implant in-situ, prior Osteotomy
- ❑ Patella position
- ❑ Condition of hip joints

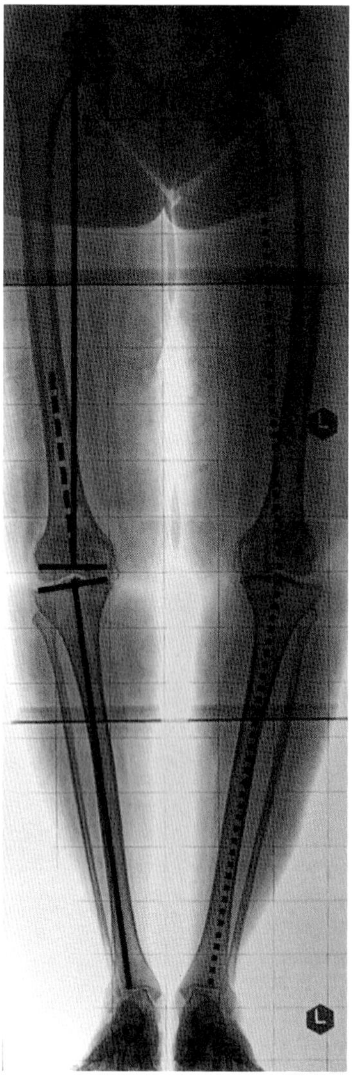

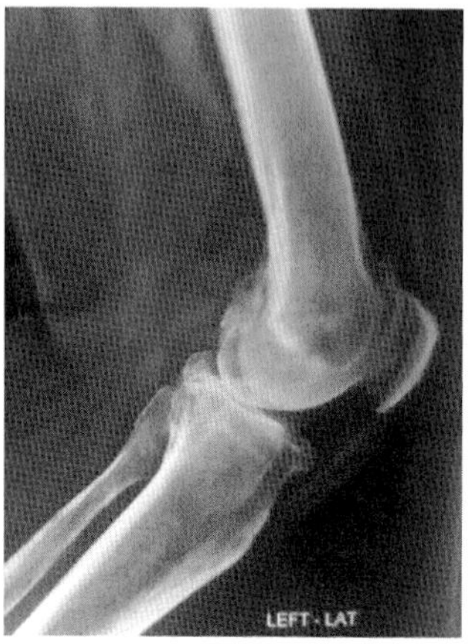

References

1. Singh JA. Epidemiology of knee and hip arthroplasty: a systematic review. Open Orthop J. 2011;5:80–5.
2. Ravi B, Croxford R, Reichmann WM, Losina E, Katz JN, Hawker GA. The changing demographics of total joint arthroplasty recipients in the United States and Ontario from 2001 to 2007. Best Pract Res Clin Rheumatol. 2012;26:637–47.
3. Meneghini RM, Russo GS, Lieberman JR. Modern perceptions and expectations regarding total knee arthroplasty. J Knee Surg. 2014;27:93–8.
4. Lingard EA, Riddle DL. Impact of psychological distress on pain and function following knee arthroplasty. J Bone Joint Surg Am. 2007;89:1161–9.
5. Brander VA, Stulberg SD, Adams AD, Harden RN, Bruehl S, Stanos SP, Houle T. Predicting total knee replacement pain: a prospective, observational study. Clin Orthop Relat Res. 2003;416:27–36.
6. Riediger W, Doering S, Krismer M. Depression and somatisation influence the outcome of total hip replacement. Int Orthop. 2010;34:13–8.
7. Shetty GM, Mullaji A, Bhayde S, Chandra Vadapalli R, Desai D. Simultaneous bilateral versus unilateral computer-assisted total knee arthroplasty: a prospective comparison of early postoperative pain and functional recovery. Knee. 2010;17:191–5.
8. Mullaji A, Shetty GM. Persistent hindfoot valgus causes lateral deviation of weightbearing axis after total knee arthroplasty. Clin Orthop Relat Res. 2011;469:1154–60.
9. Kim TK, Chang CB, Kang YG, Kim SJ, Seong SC. Causes and predictors of patient's dissatisfaction after uncomplicated total knee arthroplasty. J Arthroplasty. 2009;24:263–71.
10. Patel DV, Ferris BD, Aichroth PM. Radiological study of alignment after total knee replacement. Short radiographs or long radiographs? Int Orthop. 1991; 15:209–21.
11. McGrory JE, Trousdale RT, Pagnano MW, Nigbur M. Preoperative hip to ankle radiographs in total knee arthroplasty. Clin Orthop Relat Res. 2002;404:196–202.
12. Odenbring S, Berggren AM, Peil L. Roentgenographic assessment of the hip-knee-ankle axis in medial gonarthrosis. A study of reproducibility. Clin Orthop Relat Res. 1993;289:195–6.
13. Petersen TL, Engh GA. Radiographic assessment of knee alignment after total knee arthroplasty. J Arthroplasty. 1988;3:67–72.
14. Hsu RW, Himeno S, Coventry MB, Chao EY. Normal axial alignment of the lower extremity and load-bearing distribution at the knee. Clin Orthop Relat Res. 1990;255:215–27.
15. Rauh MA, Boyle J, Mihalko WM, Phillips MJ, Bayers-Thering M, Krackow KA. Reliability of measuring long-standing lower extremity radiographs. Orthopedics. 2007;30:299–303.
16. Mullaji AB, Marawar SV, Mittal V. A comparison of coronal plane axial femoral relationships in Asian patients with varus osteoarthritic knees and healthy knees. J Arthroplasty. 2009;24:861–7.
17. Mullaji A, Shetty GM. Computer-assisted total knee arthroplasty for arthritis with extra-articular deformity. J Arthroplasty. 2009;24:1164–9.
18. Mullaji AB, Shetty GM, Kanna R, Vadapalli RC. The influence of preoperative deformity on valgus correction angle: an analysis of 503 total knee arthroplasties. J Arthroplasty. 2013;28:20–7.
19. Mullaji AB, Shetty GM. Surgical technique: computer-assisted sliding medial condylar osteotomy to achieve gap balance in varus knees during TKA. Clin Orthop Relat Res. 2013;471:1484–91.
20. Mullaji A, Shetty G. Total knee arthroplasty for arthritic knees with tibiofibular stress fractures: classification and treatment guidelines. J Arthroplasty. 2010;25:295–301.
21. Mullaji AB, Lingaraju AP, Shetty GM. Alignment of computer-assisted total knee arthroplasty in patients with altered hip center. J Arthroplasty. 2011;26:1072–7.
22. Aslam N, Lo S, Nagarajah K, Pasapula C, Akmal M. Reliability of preoperative templating in total knee arthroplasty. Acta Orthop Belg. 2004;70:560–4.
23. Peek AC, Bloch B, Auld J. How useful is templating for total knee replacement component sizing? Knee. 2012;19:266–9.
24. Mullaji AB, Marawar SV, Simha M, Jindal G. Cruciate ligaments in arthritic knees: a histologic study with radiologic correlation. J Arthroplasty. 2008;23:567–72.
25. Mullaji AB, Marawar SV, Luthra M. Tibial articular cartilage wear in varus osteoarthritic knees: correlation with anterior cruciate ligament integrity and severity of deformity. J Arthroplasty. 2008;23: 128–35.
26. Hopley CD, Crossett LS, Chen AF. Long-term clinical outcomes and survivorship after total knee arthroplasty using a rotating platform kneeprosthesis: a meta-analysis. J Arthroplasty. 2013;28:68–77.
27. Aggarwal AK, Agrawal A. Mobile vs fixed-bearing total knee arthroplasty performed by a single surgeon: a 4- to 6.5-year randomized, prospective, controlled, double-blinded study. J Arthroplasty. 2013;28: 1712–6.
28. Shi X, Shen B, Yang J, Kang P, Zhou Z, Pei F. In vivo kinematics comparison of fixed- and mobile-bearing total knee arthroplasty during deep knee bending motion. Knee Surg Sports Traumatol Arthrosc. 2012 [Electronic publication ahead of print]
29. Gioe TJ, Maheshwari AV. The all-polyethylene tibial component in primary total knee arthroplasty. J Bone Joint Surg Am. 2010;92:478–87.
30. Han HS, Kang SB, Yoon KS. High incidence of loosening of the femoral component in legacy posterior stabilised-flex total knee replacement. J Bone Joint Surg Br. 2007;89:1457–61.
31. Zelle J, Janssen D, Van Eijden J, De Waal Malefijt M, Verdonschot N. Does high-flexion total knee arthroplasty promote early loosening of the femoral component? J Orthop Res. 2011;29:976–83.

2 Basic Technique of Total Knee Arthroplasty

Introduction

With rapid advancement in technology and materials in total knee arthroplasty (TKA), long-term survival and function of the total knee are increasingly more dependent on optimum surgical technique [1–3]. Adherence to basic surgical principles ensures a successful outcome. Surgical technique in TKA is akin to a game of chess where every move has predictable and logical consequences. Hence, every step of the surgical technique needs to be well thought of before execution. The aim of the authors, like most surgeons, is to ensure a well-aligned, well-balanced and well-fixed TKA. Ligament balancing is an integral part of TKA, and soft-tissue release should follow a functional and anatomic rationale to achieve correct alignment and ligament balance throughout the range of flexion and extension. Any deviation from this principle may lead to stiffness, imbalance or instability during TKA.

The two basic techniques commonly used in TKA are the measured resection technique and the gap-balancing technique. The authors have successfully used the gap-balancing technique in all their cases. This technique has proved reliable to achieve a well-aligned and well-balanced knee across various types and severity of knee deformity. The present chapter aims to outline the basic principles of TKA being followed by the authors. The chapter begins with a brief "disclaimer" listing the characteristic features of surgical technique being followed by the authors.

"Disclaimer"

- Only posterior cruciate-substituting (CS) TKAs have been used by the authors. The rationale of using only CS knees is based on the finding that the posterior cruciate ligament may undergo marked structural and functional deterioration in arthritic knees especially in severe grades of arthritis [4–7] and that the functional outcome and kinematics may be more predictable with a CS knee [8–10].
- Tibial preparation is performed as the first step in the majority of the knees.
- The gap-balancing technique has been used in all knees. Ligament balancing and gap balancing are done with balancing in extension first followed by femoral sizing and creating a flexion gap equal to the extension gap.
- Ligament balancing is predictable and can be ensured throughout the full knee range of motion in most knees. The authors mainly check ligament balance in full extension and at 90° flexion (and can also now quantify it throughout knee range of motion using navigation). However, balancing around deep knee flexion is still an area of controversy and is unclear [11].
- Only cemented components have been used in all knees, and all knees undergo patellar resurfacing.
- Standard approach with medial parapatellar arthrotomy has been used in all knees.
- Computer navigation described here is not only utilised to ensure accurate limb and component alignment but also to quantify ligament

A.B. Mullaji, G.M. Shetty, *Deformity Correction in Total Knee Arthroplasty*,
DOI 10.1007/978-1-4939-0566-9_2, © Springer Science+Business Media New York 2014

balancing and the amount of bone resection and soft-tissue release performed. Hence, navigation has been used by the authors more as a tool for verification where the computer navigation system provides real-time feedback of various surgical steps.

Ligament Balancing: The *"Kaizen"* Approach

Kaizen, Japanese for "improvement", or "change for the better", refers to philosophy or practices that focus upon continuous improvement of processes and techniques [12]. In simple language, this concept implies performing *several small, continuous steps of improvement to achieve significant results* [12]. The principles of ligament balancing we use during TKA are very similar to the Kaizen concept. Optimum limb alignment and soft-tissue balancing are achieved during TKA by executing several small, interrelated steps involving bone cuts and soft-tissue release and varying the size and position of the femoral component.

Basically, soft-tissue balancing in TKA involves achieving "equality and equipoise" (i.e. equal width and equal tension) between the medial and the lateral compartments within the extension or flexion gap and between the extension and flexion gaps. Hence, the two aims are to achieve a rectangular extension and flexion gap and a flexion gap equal in width to the extension gap. Soft-tissue releases to achieve balance in TKA involve deciding what to release, when to release and how much to release for a given knee deformity. It is crucial to keep in mind that intra-articular soft-tissue release and bone cuts are intended to deal with intra-articular deformities. Attempts to tackle an associated extra-articular deformity of the femur or tibia using this technique may involve significant release of important soft-tissue stabilizers of the knee joint like the collaterals which may subsequently result in imbalance. Hence, cases with a concomitant extra-articular deformity may require an additional procedure like corrective or epicondylar osteotomy [13].

How to Assess Soft-Tissue Tension?

Numerous devices have been described to assess soft-tissue tension during TKA. We use a tensioner made up of a single fixed tibial plate which sits on the tibial cut surface and two separate moveable plates for the medial and the lateral femoral condyles (Fig. 2.1a). These two femoral plates can be moved independently using a screw mechanism to increase or decrease the tension medially and laterally. In full extension, the aim while assessing ligament tension is to achieve a limb alignment as close to neutral as possible and equal tension both medially and laterally as assessed by the surgeon (Fig. 2.1b). The final stability is checked in full extension using spacer blocks where a valgus and a varus stress are applied to determine the degree of laxity (Fig. 2.1c). This step is again repeated in 90° flexion using the tensioning device and also using a spacer block with the AP cutting block in place (Fig. 2.1d, e). The aim is not only to ensure that there is optimum stability in full extension and 90° flexion but also to confirm that any opening on stressing is equal on both sides and which also springs back equally.

What to Release?

Based on the type of knee deformity and the degree of initial soft-tissue imbalance, the site and the structures to be released vary from knee to knee. A thorough knowledge of what structures can be released during TKA for any given deformity is essential. For a varus knee, no release on the lateral side should be performed, and for a valgus knee the opposite is true. Similarly, for a knee with flexion deformity, posterior release is necessary, whereas

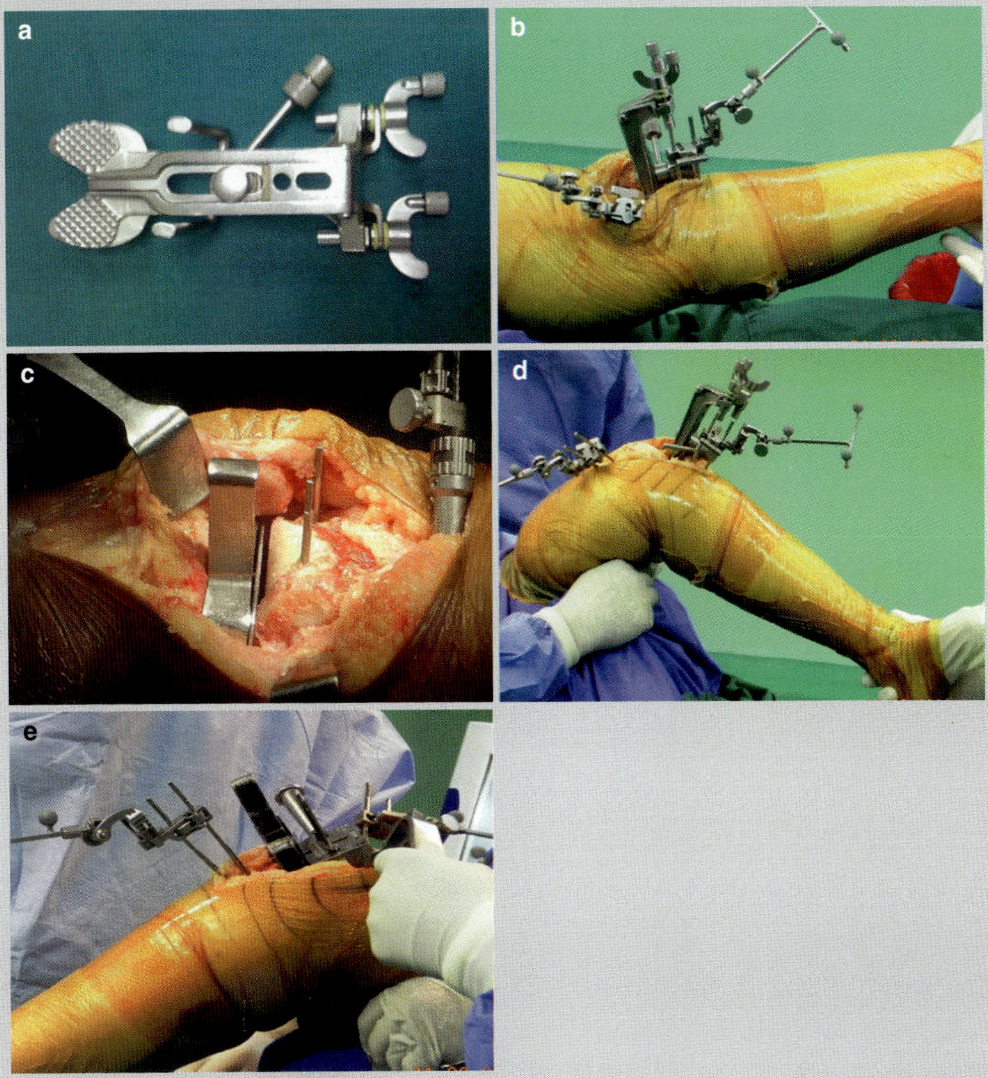

Fig. 2.1 Various steps for assessing soft-tissue tension during TKA. (**a**) Soft-tissue tensioner used by the authors during TKA. It is made up of a single fixed tibial plate which sits on the tibial cut surface and two separate moveable plates for the medial and the lateral femoral condyles. (**b**) Assessment of medial and lateral soft-tissue tension using the tensioner with the limb held in neutral alignment and the knee held in full extension. (**c**) Assessment of medial and lateral soft-tissue tension using a spacer block with the knee held in full extension. (**d**) Assessment of medial and lateral soft-tissue tension using the tensioner with the knee held in 90° flexion. Note that the thigh is supported by an assistant to nullify the effect of the weight of the limb during the assessment. (**e**) Assessment of medial and lateral soft-tissue tension using a spacer block with the knee held in 90° flexion. This is done before the posterior cut is performed with the femoral AP block pinned in place

in a hyperextending knee it should be strictly avoided. We completely avoid performing any sort of release of the collaterals and avoid completely releasing the pes anserinus or dividing the popliteus tendon. Most deformities and imbalance can be corrected releasing capsular structures and adhesions rather than the collaterals and supplementing these releases with osteotomies. It must be pointed out that the collateral ligaments themselves do not undergo contracture/shortening.

When and How Much to Release?

We follow a graduated, controlled and stepwise approach to soft-tissue release during TKA. Removal of osteophytes as the initial step considerably improves deformity and decreases the quantum of soft-tissue release required. A preliminary soft-tissue release is performed as part of exposure and following osteophyte excision. Rigid deformities may not be fully corrected with a preliminary release. Similarly, although soft-tissue release may achieve full correction of deformity, it may fail to achieve medio-lateral balance. Such cases with residual deformity or medio-lateral imbalance will require further, extended releases supplemented by a reduction osteotomy [14].

Equalising Medial and Lateral Gap in Extension

With the knee in full extension, the tibial and the distal femoral resection are made perpendicular to their respective mechanical axes (Fig. 2.2a). The aim is to create a rectangular extension gap equal on both medial and lateral side. However, despite accurate bone cuts, the extension gap may be unequal or quadrilateral owing to medio-lateral soft-tissue imbalance as determined by spacer blocks (Fig. 2.2b). This disparity needs to be rectified using appropriate soft-tissue releases to restore limb alignment and medio-lateral balance (Fig. 2.2c). The extent of medio-lateral soft-tissue disparity in extension after the bone cuts can be predicted using the joint divergence angle on preoperative full-length radiographs (see Chap. 1).

Equalising Medial and Lateral Gap in 90° Flexion

With the knee in 90° flexion, the tibial and posterior femoral cuts should generally be parallel to the epicondylar axis and perpendicular to the anteroposterior axis of the femur (Fig. 2.3a). We mark the level of the tentative posterior femoral cut after assessing flexion gap balance using the tensioner (Fig. 2.3b, c). However, it is very important to achieve good medio-lateral balance in flexion before determining the level and performing the posterior femoral cut. In varus knees, if the posterior femur is cut in the presence of excessive medial tightness, then the femoral component may get placed in excessive external rotation and vice versa (Fig. 2.3d–e). Similar to when the knee is in full extension, the aim at 90° knee flexion is to create a rectangular flexion gap equal on both medial and lateral side. Hence, the determinants of flexion gap include distal femoral and tibial cuts, medio-lateral soft-tissue tension in 90° flexion, femoral component size and position and the tibial insert thickness.

Equalising Flexion Gap to the Extension Gap

Based on our technique of creating the extension gap first, the way to flexion-extension gap balancing involves creating a flexion gap matching in dimension to the previously created extension gap. The key to achieving this is the size and position of the femoral component. Using the method previously described, the flexion gap is assessed using

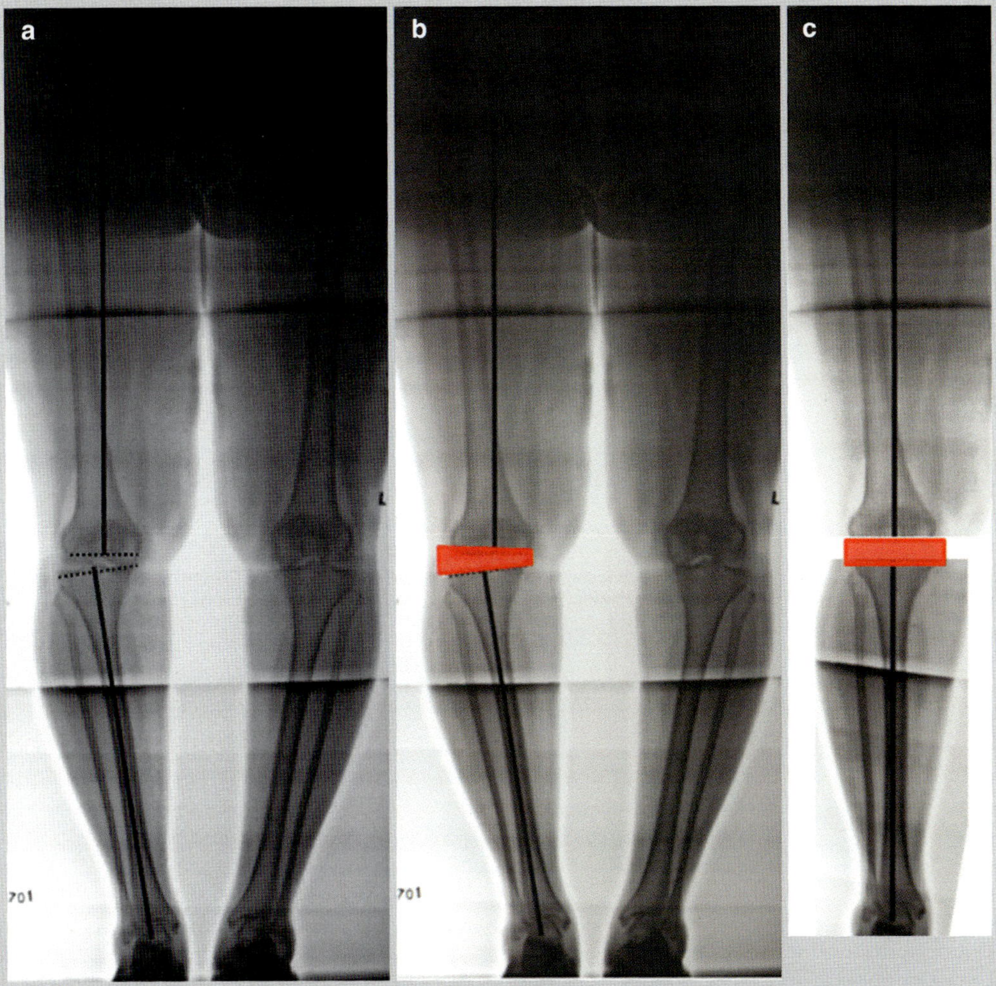

Fig. 2.2 Equalising medial and lateral gaps in full extension. (**a**) The tibial and the distal femoral resections (*dotted lines*) are made perpendicular to their respective mechanical axes (*solid lines*). (**b**) Despite accurate cuts, the resultant extension gap may be quadrilateral instead of rectangular due to medio-lateral soft-tissue imbalance as determined by a spacer block. (**c**) This requires appropriate soft-tissue releases to restore limb alignment and medio-lateral balance and a rectangular extension gap

a spacer block with the AP cutting block of the estimated femoral component size pinned in place. This must have no slots posteriorly. Using a stylus or "angel wing", we ensure that there is no notching. If the flexion gap is tighter for the corresponding spacer block used previously in the assessment of extension gap, the femoral component needs to be undersized or moved anteriorly in order to equalise the flexion-extension gaps. Slight flexion or posterior shift of the femoral component may also be helpful to tackle a flexion gap that exceeds the extension gap. However, the surgeon needs to be cautious in not overdoing this and causing either anterior notching or post impingement against the box in extension. The AP block is placed accurately before performing the anterior and posterior femoral cuts by using "combined referencing" where multiple references are used to ascertain the position of the AP cutting block and subsequently the femoral component (Fig. 2.4).

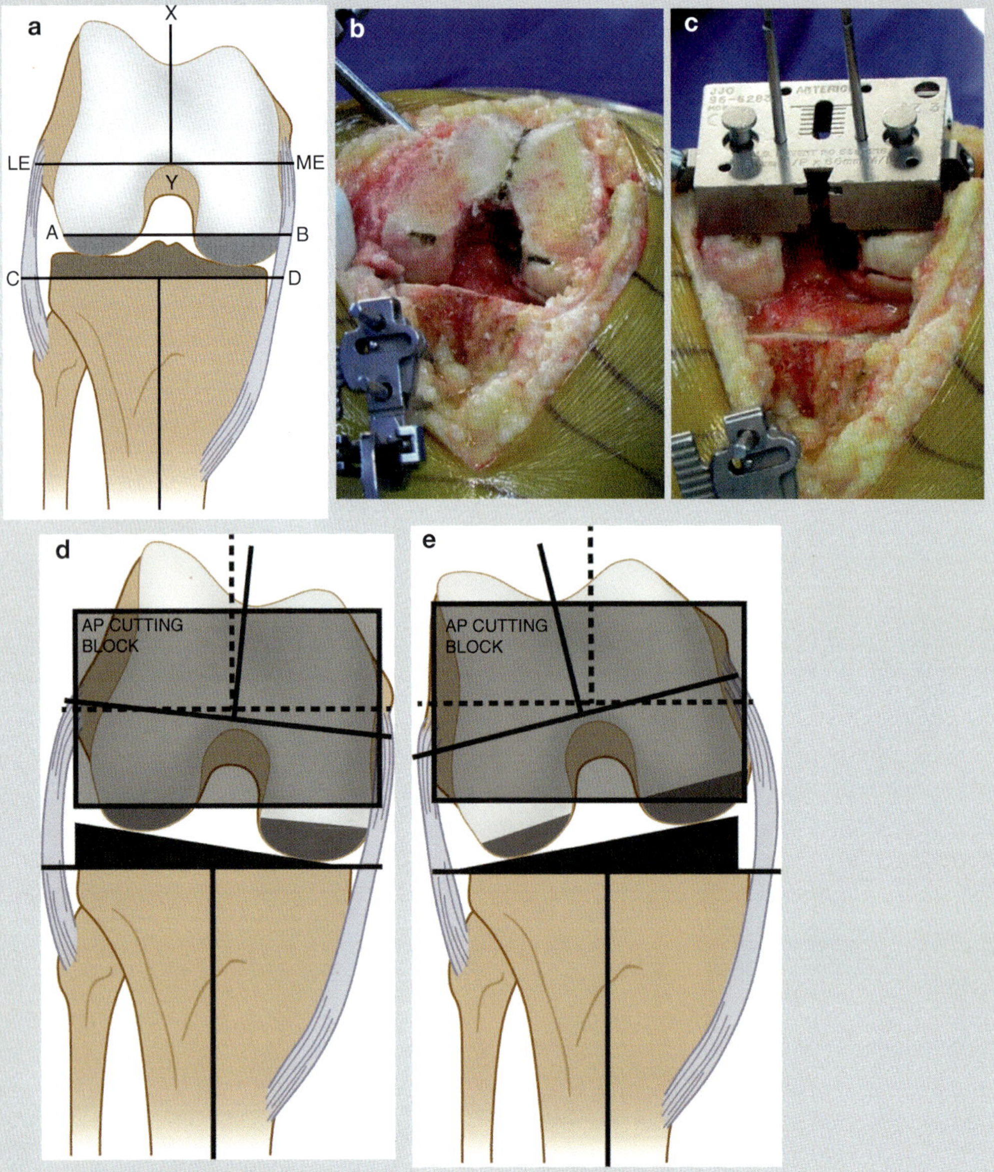

Fig. 2.3 Equalising medial and lateral gaps in 90° flexion. (**a**) Relation of various distal femoral rotational axes to the posterior femoral (line AB) and tibial (line CD) cuts with the knee in 90° flexion. The tibial and posterior femur cuts should generally be parallel to the epicondylar axis (line LE–ME) and perpendicular to the anteroposterior (AP) axis of the femur (line XY). (**b**) The tentative posterior femoral cut marked after assessing flexion gap balance using the tensioner and its relation to the AP axis. (**c**) The AP cutting block pinned in position and its relation to the previously marked distal cut. Note that the cutting block has been positioned based on "combined referencing". (**d**) If the AP cutting block is placed and the posterior femur is cut in the presence of excessive medial tightness, then the femoral component may get placed in excessive external rotation. (**e**) Similarly, if the AP cutting block is placed and the posterior femur is cut in the presence of excessive lateral tightness, then the femoral component may get placed in excessive internal rotation

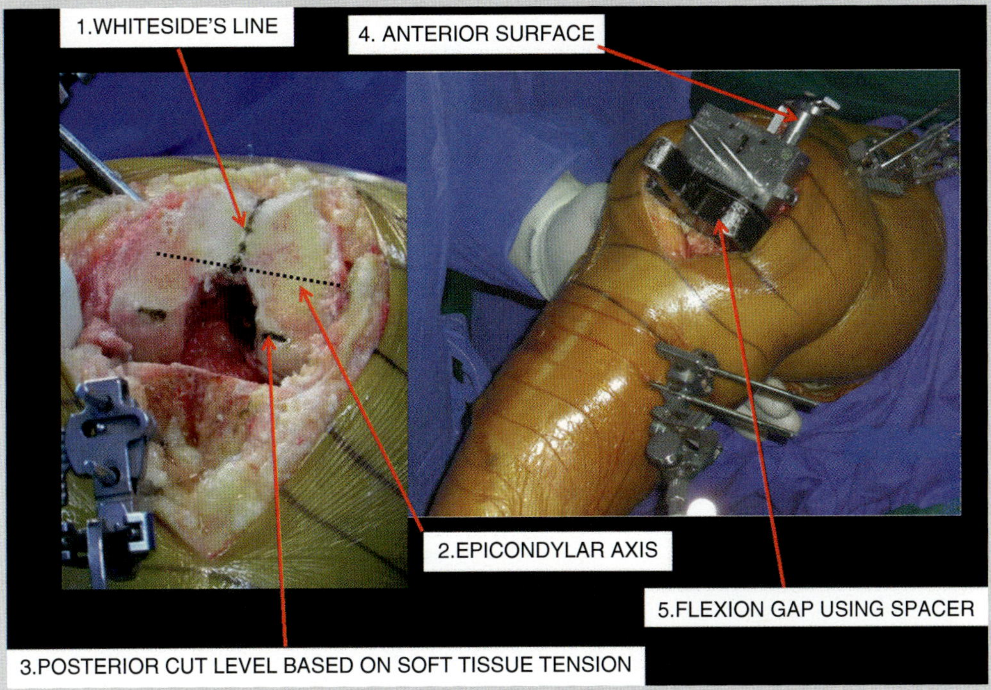

Fig. 2.4 The concept of "combined referencing" and its five components in order to accurately place the AP cutting block

Surgical Approach and Exposure

The authors use the classical anterior skin incision with the medial parapatellar arthrotomy to approach the knee. This approach has served us well in almost all of our TKA cases. Rare exceptions where an alternative approach was used include knees with severe valgus arthritis and patellar maltracking which required a lateral parapatellar arthrotomy and stiff arthritic knees where a tibial tubercle osteotomy was performed to improve exposure.

We use a pneumatic tourniquet in all our cases which is inflated before the incision is taken. The pressure set is typically 100 mmHg over the systolic pressure of the patient in thin or nonobese patients or 150 mmHg over and above if the patient is obese. Rarely, if the patient is morbidly obese and the thigh size is too big for the largest cuff, tourniquet is applied but inflated after all the bone cuts have been performed and just before cementing.

The tibial cut is always performed first in all our cases. Using seven simple steps during exposure will help in easily dislocating the knee and bringing the tibia forwards without having to perform excessive, unnecessary soft-tissue release or having to apply a Hohmann's retractor on the posterior aspect of the tibia. This approach allows for laterally displacing the extensor apparatus (quadriceps tendon and patella) easily without having to evert the patella and adequately exposing the tibial articular surface to perform the tibial cut (Fig. 2.5). Like any surgical procedure, approaching the knee to perform TKA is facilitated by using the right surgical instruments. After the medial parapatellar arthrotomy, the following seven steps are performed to adequately expose the knee for TKA:

1. *Patella* – Division of the patellofemoral ligament, excision of the infrapatellar fat pad and removal of patellar osteophytes and peripatellar synovium to facilitate lateral displacement of the extensor apparatus and patella for resurfacing.

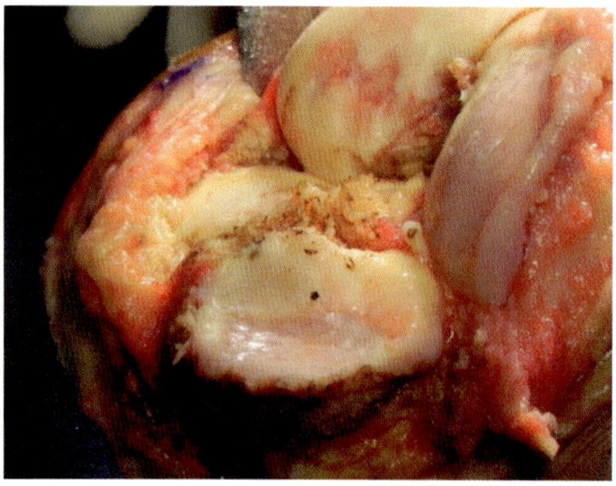

Fig. 2.5 Complete anterior dislocation of the tibia following excision of cruciates and menisci. The laterally displaced extensor apparatus (quadriceps tendon and patella) is held in place with an angled Hohmann's retractor without having to evert the patella and adequately exposing the tibial articular surface to perform the tibial cut

2. *Anterior surface of femur* – Elevation of the synovium, fat and soft tissue from over the anterior surface of distal femur not only for registering the surface for CAS but by adequate visualisation notching can be avoided.
3. *Cruciates* – Complete excision of both cruciates is essential prior to balancing.
4. *Anterior osteophytes* – Removal of osteophytes around the distal end of the femur and the medial or lateral aspect of the proximal tibia. Excision of the osteophyte usually present in the medial corner of the medial femoral condyle just beneath the femoral attachment of the MCL is important in varus knees to reduce tenting of the MCL (Fig. 2.6a). Osteophytes are often seen posteromedially deep in the intercondylar notch and should be excised as well (Fig. 2.6b).
5. *Knee dislocation* – The knee is now flexed maximally and the tibia gently externally rotated by an assistant while the surgeon simultaneously releases the deep MCL and capsule along the medial and posteromedial edge of the tibial articular surface using diathermy. This safely dislocates the knee and brings the tibia fully forwards. An angled Hohmann's retractor then applied to the posterolateral aspect of the tibia adjacent to the laterally displaced patella helps to completely expose the tibial articular surface (Fig. 2.5).
6. *Menisci* – Excision of both menisci with cauterisation of the lateral genicular vessels.
7. *Posterior osteophytes* – Excision of posteromedial tibial osteophytes with a broad flat osteotome (Fig. 2.6c) and removal of posterior femoral osteophytes using a curved osteotome (Fig. 2.6d). Removal of the medial meniscus beforehand improves access to the posterior surface of the femoral condyle for removal of these osteophytes.

After completing these seven basic exposure steps, the knee is now extended and checked for amount of correction achieved with these preliminary soft-tissue releases by applying a valgus stress for a varus knee (and a varus stress for a valgus knee) and the amount of soft-tissue laxity present on the opposite side by applying a varus stress for a varus knee (and a valgus stress for a valgus knee).

Tibial Resection

The tibial cut affects both the extension and the flexion gaps. How much minimum thickness of tibia needs to be resected with reference to the less involved side is governed by the type and severity of knee deformity and the knee prosthesis design. The standard tibial cut involves resecting an amount equal to the combined thinnest insert and tray thickness available with an implant system. However, this needs to be varied depending on the type and severity of deformity. More severe the coronal plane deformity (varus or valgus), less should be the amount of tibial resection. Similarly, less bone needs to be resected in knees with severe ligamentous instability or in a hyperextending knee. More than 8 mm of tibia can occasionally be resected in knees with a severe fixed flexion deformity or in knees with a large defect where resecting an additional few mm may provide a uniform flat surface.

The coronal plane of tibial resection is based on using either the mechanical axis of the tibia or the medullary axis of the tibia. The position of

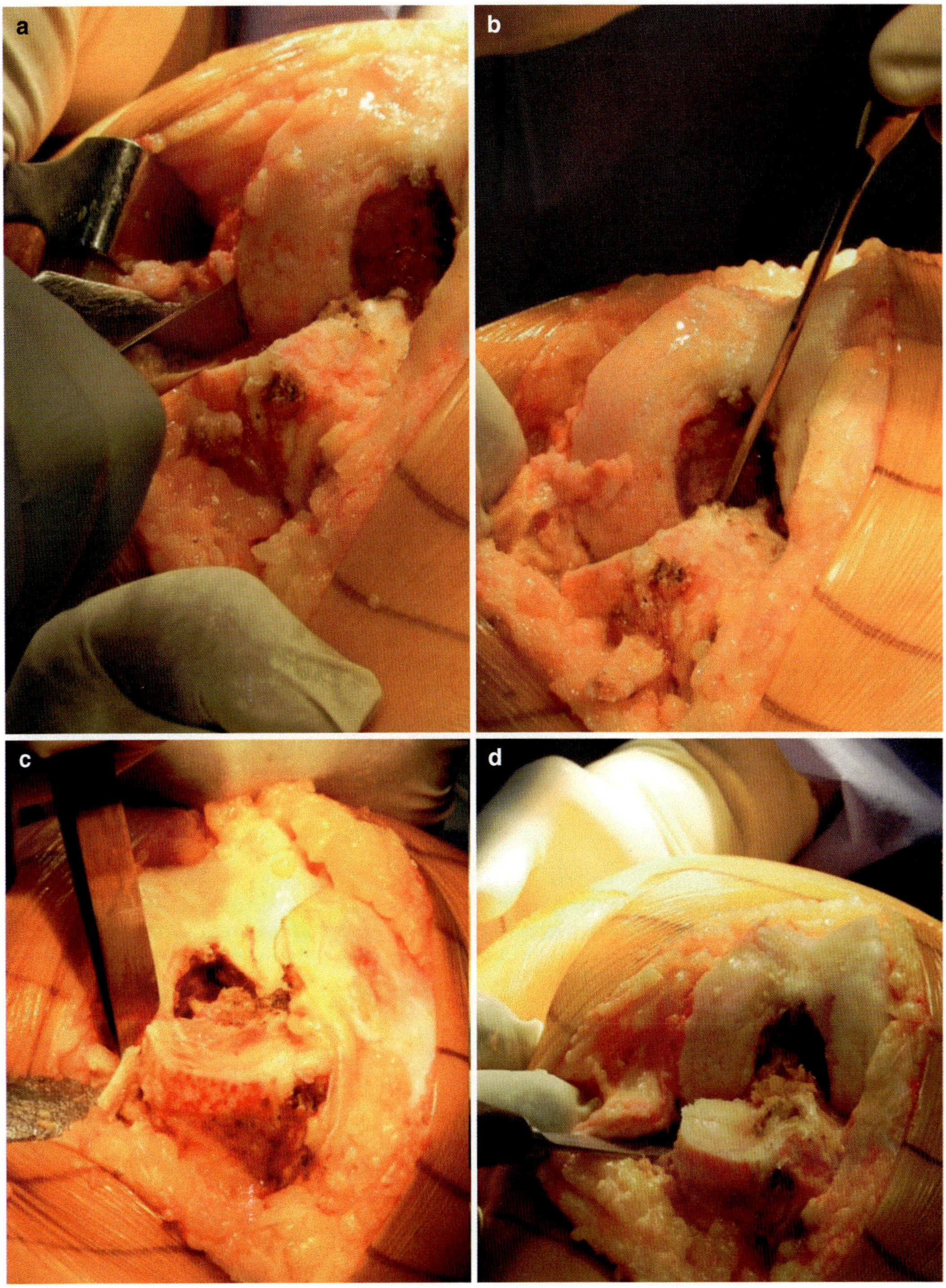

Fig. 2.6 Removal of osteophytes as part of the exposure for TKA. (**a**) Excision of osteophyte usually present in the medial corner of the medial femoral condyle just beneath the femoral attachment of the MCL with a flat narrow osteotome. (**b**) Excision of osteophytes posteromedially deep in the intercondylar notch with a flat narrow osteotome. (**c**) Excision of posteromedial tibial osteophytes with a flat broad osteotome. (**d**) Excision of posterior femoral osteophytes using a curved osteotome. Note that the tibia has been displaced anteriorly as much as possible to allow better access for the osteotome posteriorly

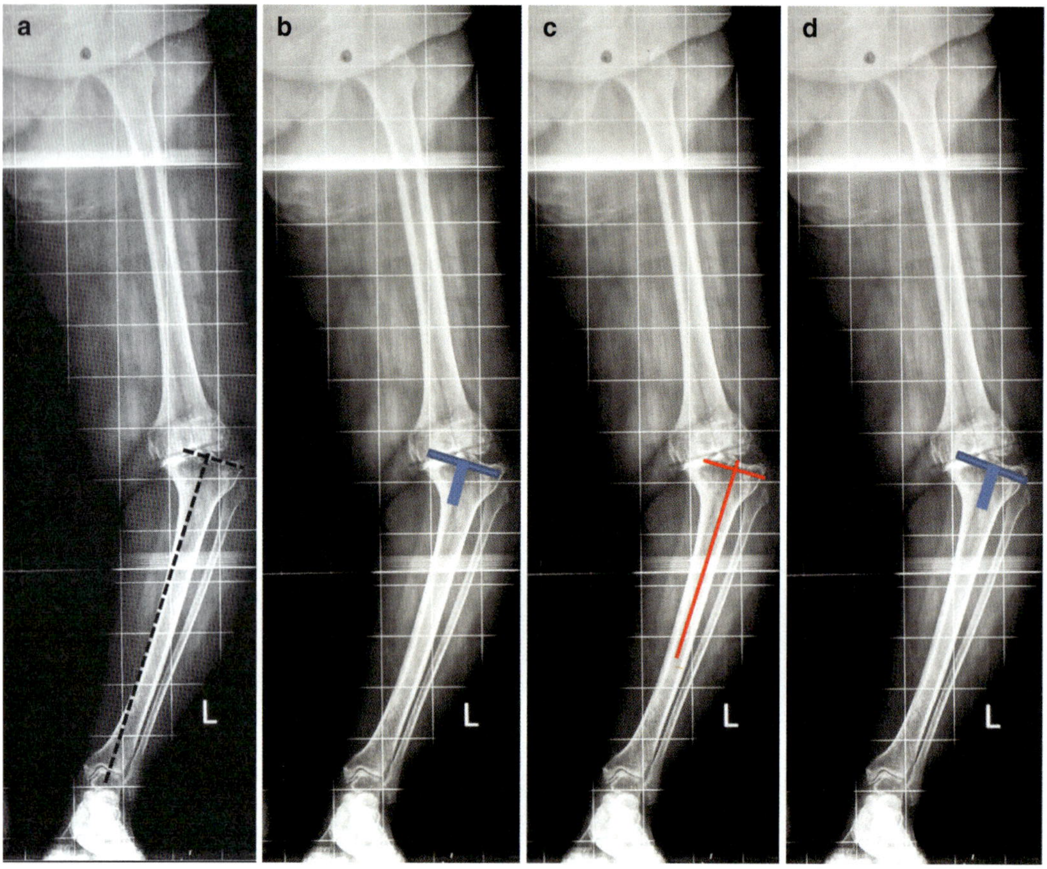

Fig. 2.7 Reference for tibial cut in the coronal plane. (**a**) Position of the tibial mechanical axis in a curved tibia. (**b**) Position of the tibial tray when the mechanical axis of the tibia is used to decide the coronal plane of the tibial cut in the presence of tibial bowing or tibial vara. Note that the entry point and subsequently the tibial tray and stem may be placed too medially. (**c**) Using the medullary axis of the middle third of the tibial shaft as reference to decide the coronal plane of the tibial cut in the presence of tibial bowing or tibial vara results in shift of the entry point laterally. (**d**) This facilitates lateralising the tibial component which helps in decreasing the area of medial bone defect, performing a reduction osteotomy for deformity correction and ligament balancing and placing the tibial stem at the centre of the proximal medullary canal of the tibia

tibial tray in the coronal plane and the amount of tibial resection may vary depending on which axis is used. The coronal plane of tibial resection has been classically recommended to be perpendicular to the mechanical axis of the tibia or the proximal tibial medullary axis. Although this may be appropriate in a straight tibia, the same may not hold true for tibiae which show coronal plane bowing (Fig. 2.7). When the mechanical axis of the tibia is used to decide the coronal plane of the tibial cut in the presence of tibial bowing or tibial vara, the entry point and subsequently the tibial tray and stem may be placed too medially (Fig. 2.7a-b). Similarly when the proximal medullary axis of the tibia is used in a deformed tibia, the tibial component may be placed too medially. A third way of deciding the coronal plane of the tibial cut is based on the medullary axis of the middle third of the tibial shaft (Fig. 2.7c). Although using this axis in tibia with bowing or varus deformity shifts the entry point laterally, this facilitates lateralising the tibial component which helps in decreasing the area of medial bone defect, performing a reduction osteotomy for deformity correction and ligament balancing and placing the tibial stem at the centre of the proximal medullary canal of the tibia (Fig. 2.7c-d).

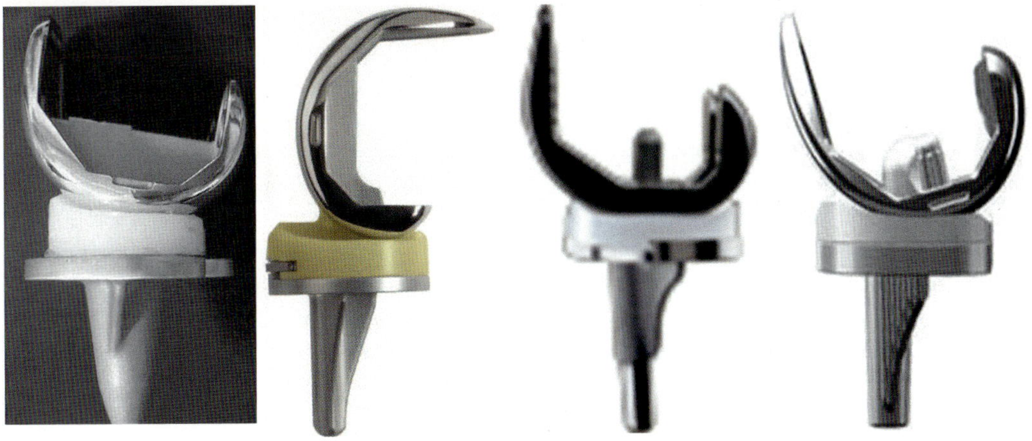

Fig. 2.8 Variations in the tibial slope based on the design of the insert and tibial tray

Slope of the tibial cut is governed by the implant being used and the manufacturer's recommendation for that implant. Certain designs have a built-in slope in the polyethylene insert, whereas others have a slope built in the cutting block (Fig. 2.8). The tibia should be cut at neutral with respect to the sagittal plane if the implant polyethylene already has an inbuilt slope. Adding a slope to the tibial cut in this situation will increase the flexion gap and also limit terminal knee extension. Tibial resection affects both the extension and flexion gap. Hence, proper execution of the tibial cut in both coronal and sagittal plane is crucial to avoid further errors in gap balancing. Using the medullary axis of the middle third of the tibial shaft, especially in bowed tibiae, will not only minimise tibial cutting error but also component placement errors in the coronal plane.

Balancing in Extension and Distal Femoral Resection

The distal femoral cut affects only the extension gap. After the tibial cut, a soft-tissue tensioning device is used to tension the medial and lateral soft tissues so as to achieve an equal medial and lateral gap while checking the alignment of the limb in full extension (Fig. 2.1b). It is important to remove all osteophytes especially from the posterior aspect of femoral condyle before this step as their presence may lead to underestimation of the extension gap. If either the medio-lateral gaps or the limb alignment in full extension is suboptimal, then additional soft-tissue release needs to be performed to achieve a balanced extension gap and satisfactory limb alignment.

The distal femoral cut is made perpendicular to the mechanical axis of the femur. The thickness of distal femoral resection needs to be conservative in cases with severe bone loss, severe lateral or medial laxity in varus or valgus, recurvatum deformity and in knees with gross instability. More than usual amount of distal femur may have to be occasionally resected in knees with fixed flexion deformity to achieve correction. Conventionally, the cut is performed using intramedullary guides which are commonly set at an angle of 5–7° valgus. However, choosing this fixed range for the distal femoral valgus cut is fraught with risks especially in knees with severe deformities. A recent prospective study [15] done by the authors has shown wide variations in this angle among patients with the distal femoral valgus correction angle (VCA) varying from 2° to 11° and almost 45 % of limbs having a VCA outside the conventional 5–7° range [15]. This is commonly due to bowing of the femoral shaft in the coronal plane which is frequently encountered in Asian patients undergoing TKA. Evaluation of femoral bowing in our patients undergoing TKA revealed that one in five varus limbs had significant femoral bowing in the coronal plane [16]. Using an intramedullary guide (straight rod) in a bowed femur (curved canal) will lead to displacement of the cutting jig and an inaccurate cut vis-à-vis the mechanical axis of the femur. Hence, to avoid malalignment of femoral component in the coronal plane, the distal femoral cut should be tailored in each limb based on VCA determined on preoperative full-length hip-to-ankle radiographs.

After the tibial and distal femoral cuts, limb alignment and medio-lateral extension gap balance can be verified using a spacer block (Fig. 2.1c). Again varus and valgus stressing is performed to assess imbalance. Any soft-tissue imbalance and limb malalignment at this stage can be addressed with a further release.

Balancing in Flexion, Femoral Sizing and Rotation

After achieving a well-balanced extension gap, the flexion gap is assessed using a soft-tissue tensioner. The aim is to achieve a flexion gap equal to the previously created extension gap. Medio-lateral soft-tissue tension is assessed at 90° flexion with an assistant supporting the weight of the limb at the proximal thigh (Fig. 2.1d). Ideally the medial and the lateral gaps should have equal tension. However, arthritic knees in general, based on the authors' experience, tend to be more lax laterally. Hence, 2 mm of disparity between the medial and lateral gaps (lateral more lax than the medial side in varus knees) may be accepted and does not seem to affect the overall function of the knee. This rectangular gap achieved after soft-tissue tensioning is marked on the distal femoral cut surface to denote the posterior femoral cut (Fig. 2.3b). In varus knees, the presence of excessive medial tightness may encourage the femoral component to get placed in excessive external rotation and vice versa.

The AP cutting block equivalent to the femoral component size estimated is now selected and placed in the AP axis. The surgeon references the anterior cortex of the distal femur to avoid notching and the previously made mark on the posterior aspect of the distal femoral cut surface based on soft-tissue tension. For rotation, the AP cutting block is generally placed parallel to the epicondylar axis and perpendicular to Whiteside's line. After pinning the AP cutting block to the distal femur, the flexion gap balance is assessed using a spacer block (Fig. 2.1e). If the flexion gap seems too tight compared to the extension gap, the femur needs to be downsized or vice versa. Hence, the authors use the concept of "combined referencing" to determine the position, size and rotation of the femoral component (Fig. 2.4). Preparation of the distal femur is then completed using a notch cutting block of appropriate size to perform the notch and chamfer cuts.

Tibial Sizing and Rotation

After the femoral chamfer and notch cuts, limb alignment, extension and flexion gap balance are assessed using trial components. In varus knees showing excessive medial tightness and/or excessive lateral laxity, additional soft-tissue release with or without a reduction osteotomy and downsizing of the tibial component may be needed. In such a situation, a thicker insert will have to be used to achieve soft-tissue stability.

Tibial component rotation is determined by putting the knee through an arc of flexion and extension, and the optimum position of the tray is marked using cautery on the anterior aspect of the tibia. Tibial tray size is governed by its compatibility with the femoral component size (some systems require both to be matched, others allow one and two sizes up or down) and the need for a reduction osteotomy which consequently calls for downsizing of the tibia. The tibial tray is placed along the lateral cortex of the tibial surface. Uncapped bone medially may be removed with an osteotome to prevent tenting of the medial soft-tissue sleeve. Tibial torsion may be seen with severe deformity. Tibial torsion calls for greater caution in accurately rotating the tibial component so as not to result in in-toeing [17].

Patella

The authors resurface the patella in all cases of TKA. A rare exception includes a very thin native patella where leaving behind at least 12 mm thickness of patellar bone is not feasible. The aim is to leave behind at least 12–14 mm of patellar bone with the component placed slightly more medially and superiorly. Usually more thickness of bone is removed medially than laterally (as the patella is asymmetric in thickness) so as to end up with a symmetrically thick remnant. A thorough excision of peripatellar synovium is performed at the outset during exposure, and peripatellar cauterisation is performed before patellar implantation to prevent postoperative patellar crepitus or clunk. The authors use an onlay-type, oval dome, 3-pegged, all-polyethylene, cemented patellar component in all cases. After implantation, excessive patellar bone around the component is removed using a large bone rongeur or bone cutter to obtain an even slope around the patella so as to prevent crepitus or impingement.

Cementing

The authors use cemented components in all TKAs. A thorough preparation of femoral, tibial and patellar cancellous bone surfaces is essential to ensure good penetration of bone cement and fixation of the components. The authors use normal saline sprayed with a 50-cc syringe along with an ETO-sterilised toothbrush to clean and prepare the cancellous bone surface [18]. This has proved to be an effective and inexpensive alternative in our setup where using pulse lavage adds to the cost of the procedure. Besides, using pulse lavage in patients with poor bone quality (which is often the case in our patients) may result in inadvertent surface removal of fragile bony trabeculae. However, pulse lavage may have to be used in certain cases where the tourniquet has not been used and the field is excessively bloody. The bone surfaces need to be inspected for any cysts which need to be curetted out and any loose cancellous bone from the canal needs to be removed. Most small to medium well-contained cysts or small to medium uncontained cysts can be tackled by a bone cement fill. However, large cysts need to be grafted using cancellous bone pieces obtained from the femoral cuts. A large peripheral defect should be first refashioned using a saw to prepare a step-cut defect in which one can ensure good fit of the solid bone graft which should be then fixed using Kirschner wires [19]. This construct should then be supplemented with a long stem to ensure additional stability of the tibial component.

Closure

We deflate the tourniquet after the cement has hardened. While the cement is setting, excessive cement around the components is curetted out, and the periarticular soft-tissue sleeve is infiltrated with an analgesic "cocktail" [20]. Once the cement is set, the tourniquet is deflated, and the knee is put through a range of flexion and extension to check patellar tracking. Any sign of lateral maltracking or patellar component lift-off is dealt with by a lateral retinacular release. The authors perform this with an inside-out technique. The knee is then dislocated to remove any cementophytes around the posterior aspect of the knee. After a thorough haemostasis with special care to cauterise the superior lateral genicular vessels which may get transected during the lateral release, the incision is closed in layers over a negative suction drain placed within the knee joint. After closure of the capsule, the knee is again put through a range of flexion and extension to check patellar tracking, maximum flexion obtained on table, watertight closure of the capsule and the patency of the drain tube.

Technique of Computer-Assisted TKR

The basic surgical technique followed by the authors is the same as described above when computer navigation is used. Navigation acts as a verification tool during bone cuts, soft-tissue release and implant positioning to achieve accurate and consistent results. However, it is important to note that when computer navigation is being used, the surgeon needs to be aware about its limitations and may have to override some of its recommendations whenever required. It may be unwise to use computer navigation on an "auto-pilot mode" with the surgeon's experience and clinical judgement taking a back seat. Although it does involve a learning curve and may add to surgical time initially, in the authors' experience the surgical time during computer-assisted TKA quickly becomes equivalent to conventional TKA technique with experience. This section gives a brief overview of the basic setup of computer navigation and its use during TKA. The authors have used the image-free Ci navigation system with its software (Brainlab, Munich, Germany) for all their cases. The computer navigation system consists of a camera unit, a computer screen and the arrays. The Ci navigation system is based on infrared technology where infrared light emitted by the camera unit is reflected back by tibial and femoral reflective arrays and is detected by two cameras. The use of computer navigation system involves the following basic steps:

Fixation of Arrays: The tibial and femoral arrays, each with three reflective spheres, are fixed to the bone using two 4-mm Schanz pins placed unicortically. The position of the pins is usually confined to the proximal third of the tibia and the distal third of the femur (Fig. 2.9). The arrays may be fixed within the surgical wound or outside of it using small stab incisions. When placed within the surgical wound, care should be taken so that the pins do not impede the cutting blocks or the components. For the tibial pins, the authors fix the first pin one thumb below the tibial articular surface with both the pins directed away from the position of the tibial stem. For the femur, the distal-most pin is placed midway between the articular cartilage margin and the medial epicondyle.

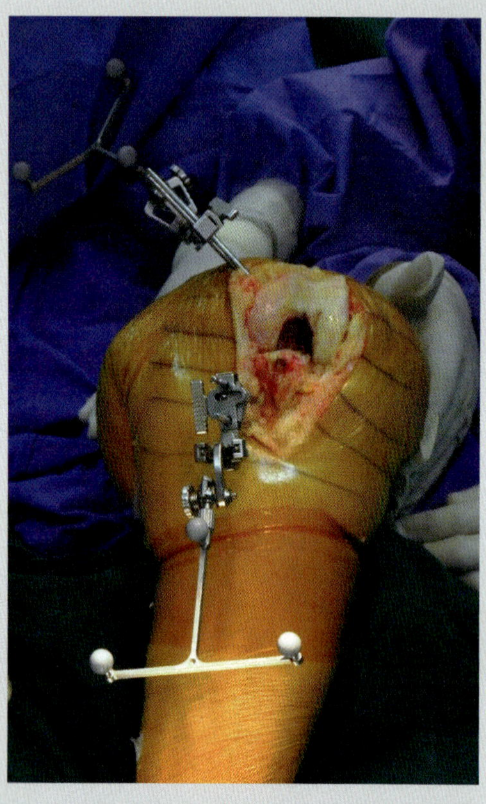

Fig. 2.9 The position of the array pins confined to the proximal third of the tibia and the distal third of the femur within the surgical incision

Registration: Registration is done in the standard fashion as described for the navigation system. Registration starts by kinematic identification of the centre of the femoral head, mapping of the lower femur, upper tibia and bony landmarks of the ankle. The centre of the femoral head is computed by pivoting the femur and moving the entire limb in a circular motion while the pelvis is steadied. It is accepted if the accuracy

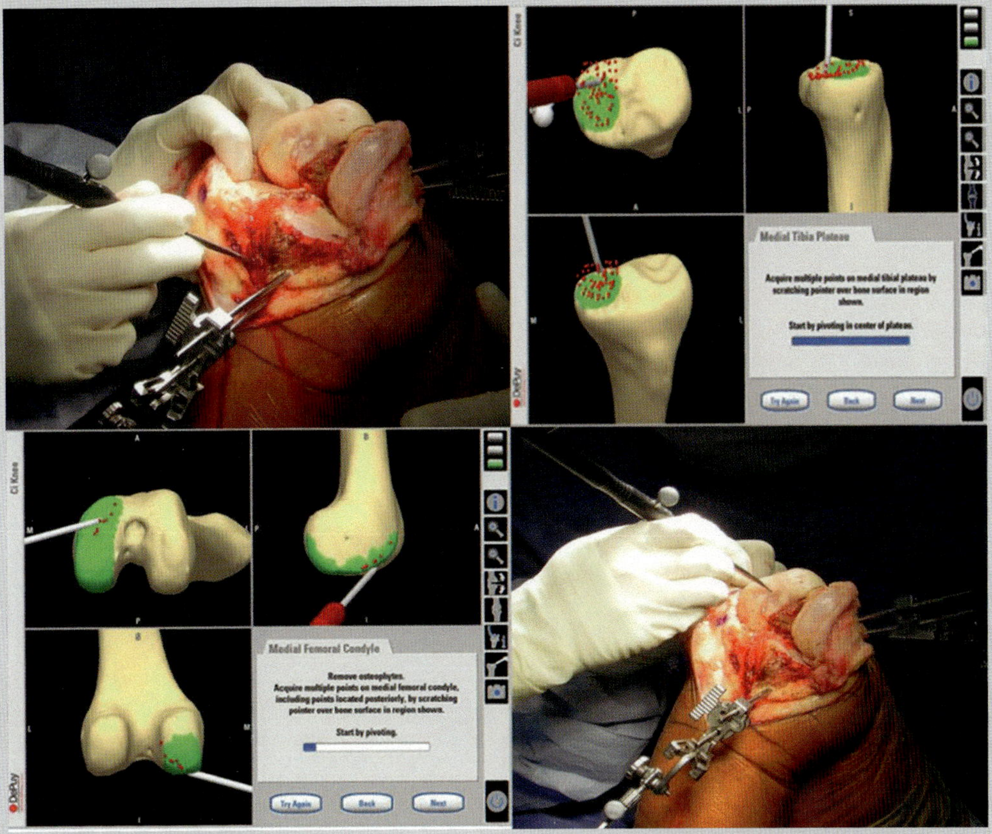

Fig 2.10 Registration of surfaces on the distal femur and upper tibia

is within 3 mm. The computer calculates the centre of the femoral head as the apex of a cone described in space by the arrays as the leg is pivoted. This is followed by registration of bony landmarks, lines and surfaces on the distal femur and upper tibia (Fig. 2.10). The initial mechanical axis of the lower limb is then determined by the computer using the centre of the femoral head, centre of the knee and the centre of the ankle.

Navigating Cutting Blocks: Conventional cutting blocks for the tibial, distal femoral and anteroposterior femoral cuts can be navigated in position (Fig. 2.11a) to match the default recommendations of the computer in order to obtain the desired cuts. The positions of these cutting blocks are verified using the flat verification arrays. The surgeon can choose to alter the thickness and orientation of the cuts if desired.

Verification of Bone Cuts: After initial registration, different steps of TKA can be verified using computer navigation. The amount and plane of tibial, distal femoral cut and anterior femoral cut are verified (Fig. 2.11b) and can be compared to the desired settings.

Gap Balancing in Extension and Flexion: In extension, navigation allows quantification of medial and lateral gaps and the limb alignment for a given spacer. It also allows visualising the degree of medio-lateral laxity present for a given spacer. In flexion, medio-lateral gap balance can be assessed

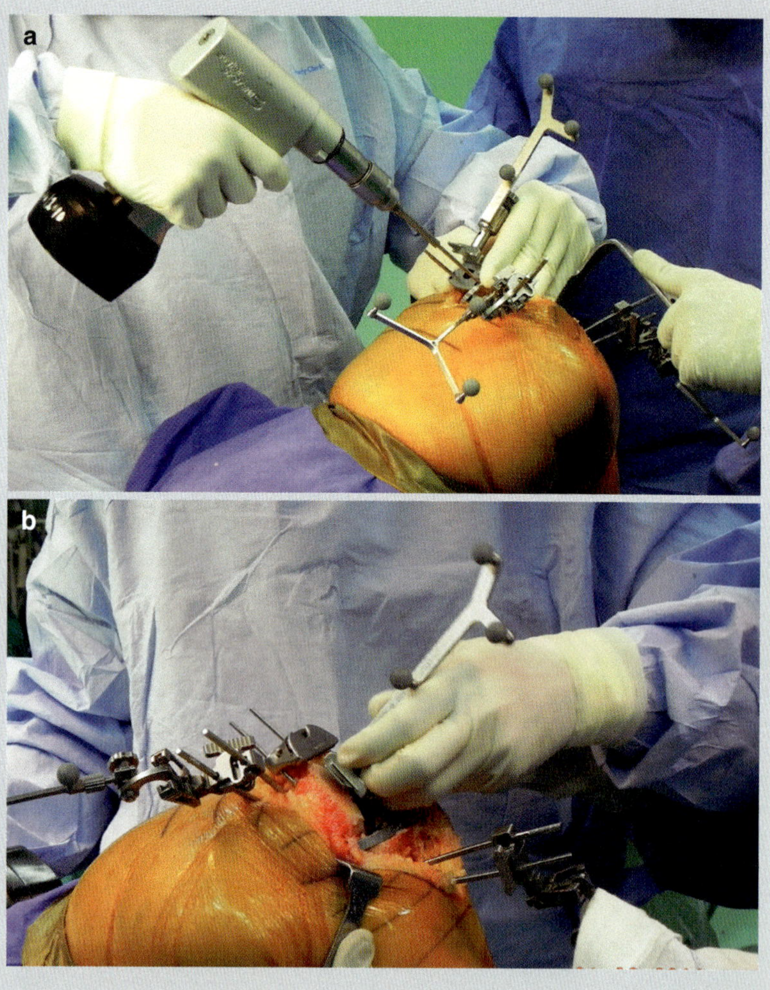

Fig. 2.11 Verification of cutting block position and bony cut accuracy with navigation using a flat pointer. (**a**) The distal femoral cutting block is pinned in position while simultaneously verifying its position with navigation. (**b**) The distal femoral cut is verified for accuracy with navigation

with respect to the position of distal femoral bony landmarks such as the transepicondylar line, Whiteside's line and the posterior condylar axis. The optimised version of the Ci navigation software allows the surgeon to simulate the effect of change in rotation, flexion or extension, upsizing or downsizing of the femoral component on the flexion gap vis-à-vis the extension gap (Fig. 2.12) without actually performing the cuts.

Final Alignment: The final alignment of the limb and gaps can be confirmed with trial components and again after implantation of the prosthesis especially when the cement is setting. Holding the limb in the appropriate position while the cement is setting is crucial to avoid malalignment of tibial and femoral components due to an uneven cement mantle or incomplete seating of the components. Navigation allows for real-time continuous visualisation of the limb position in both the coronal and sagittal plane while the cement is curing.

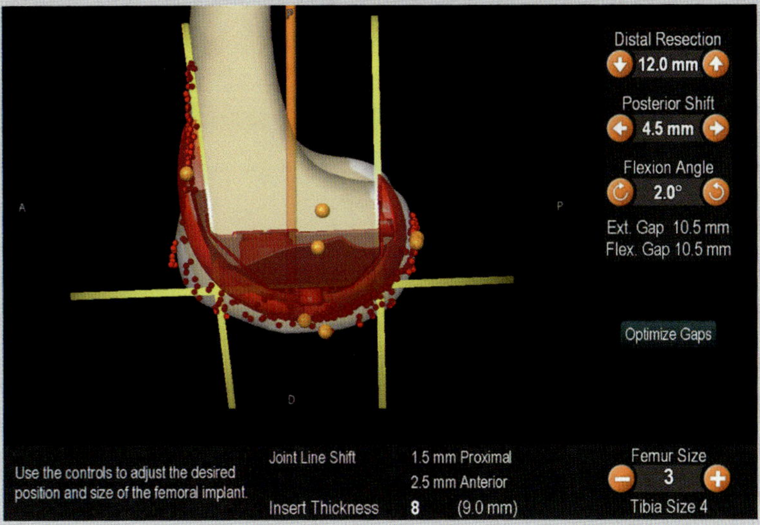

Fig. 2.12 Optimised version of the Ci navigation software allows the surgeon to simulate the effect of change in rotation, flexion or extension, upsizing or downsizing of the femoral component on the flexion gap vis-à-vis the extension gap before performing any cuts on the femur

Appendix Surgical Technique Workflow Chart for TKA

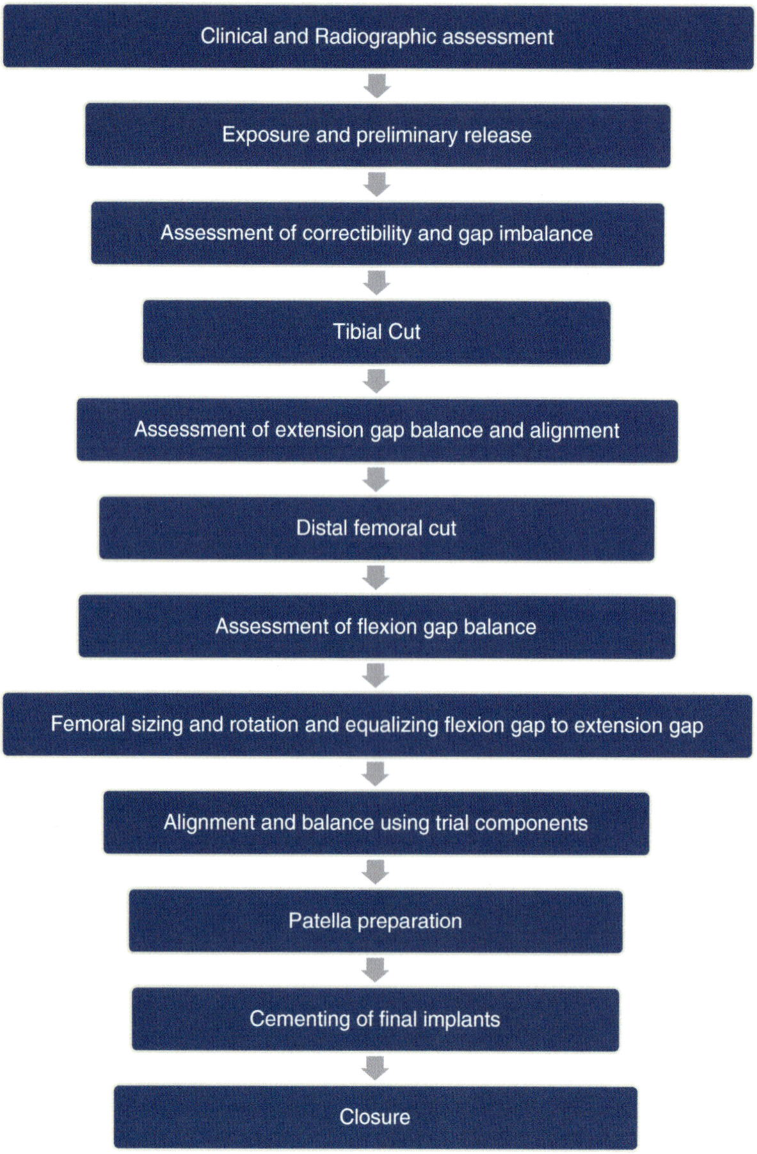

References

1. Namba RS, Inacio MC, Paxton EW, Ake CF, Wang C, Gross TP, Marinac-Dabic D, Sedrakyan A. Risk of revision for fixed versus mobile-bearing primary total knee replacements. J Bone Joint Surg Am. 2012;94:1929–35.
2. Cheng CH, Cheng YT, Chen JS. A learning curve of total knee arthroplasty (TKA) based on surgical volume analysis. Arch Gerontol Geriatr. 2011;53:e5–9.
3. Dalury DF, Pomeroy DL, Gorab RS, Adams MJ. Why are total knee arthroplasties being revised? J Arthroplasty. 2013;28(8 Suppl):120–1.
4. Mullaji AB, Marawar SV, Simha M, Jindal G. Cruciate ligaments in arthritic knees: a histologic study with radiologic correlation. J Arthroplasty. 2008;23:567–72.
5. Albert A, Forthomme JP, Vandenhooft A, Van Eeckhout P, Feoli F. Are lesions of the posterior cruciate ligament predictable before knee arthroplasty? A histological study of 434 ligaments in osteoarthritic knees. Acta Orthop Belg. 2008;74:652–8.
6. Stubbs G, Dahlstrom J, Papantoniou P, Cherian M. Correlation between macroscopic changes of arthrosis and the posterior cruciate ligament histology in the osteoarthritic knee. ANZ J Surg. 2005;75:1036–40.
7. Mullaji AB, Marawar SV, Luthra M. Tibial articular cartilage wear in varus osteoarthritic knees: correlation with anterior cruciate ligament integrity and severity of deformity. J Arthroplasty. 2008;23:128–35.
8. Seon JK, Park JK, Shin YJ, Seo HY, Lee KB, Song EK. Comparisons of kinematics and range of motion in high-flexion total knee arthroplasty: cruciate retaining vs. substituting designs. Knee Surg Sports Traumatol Arthrosc. 2011;19:2016–22.
9. Luo SX, Zhao JM, Su W, Li XF, Dong GF. Posterior cruciate substituting versus posterior cruciate retaining total knee arthroplasty prostheses: a meta-analysis. Knee. 2012;19:246–52.
10. Harato K, Bourne RB, Victor J, Snyder M, Hart J, Ries MD. Midterm comparison of posterior cruciate-retaining versus -substituting total knee arthroplasty using the Genesis II prosthesis. A multicenter prospective randomized clinical trial. Knee. 2008;15:217–21.
11. Yoon JR, Jeong HI, Oh KJ, Yang JH. In vivo gap analysis in various knee flexion angles during navigation-assisted total knee arthroplasty. J Arthroplasty. 2013;28(10):1796–800.
12. Graban M, Swartz JE. Kaizen and continuous improvement. In: Graban M, Swartz JE, editors. Healthcare Kaizen: engaging front-line staff in sustainable continuous improvements. New York: Productivity Press; 2012. p. 3–27.
13. Mullaji A, Shetty GM. Computer-assisted total knee arthroplasty for arthritis with extra-articular deformity. J Arthroplasty. 2009;24:1164–9.
14. Mullaji AB, Shetty GM. Correction of varus deformity during TKA with reduction osteotomy. Clin Orthop Relat Res. 2014;472(1):126–32.
15. Mullaji AB, Shetty GM, Kanna R, Vadapalli RC. The influence of preoperative deformity on valgus correction angle: an analysis of 503 total knee arthroplasties. J Arthroplasty. 2013;28:20–7.
16. Mullaji AB, Marawar SV, Mittal V. A comparison of coronal plane axial femoral relationships in Asian patients with varus osteoarthritic knees and healthy knees. J Arthroplasty. 2009;24:861–7.
17. Mullaji AB, Sharma AK, Marawar SV, Kohli AF. Tibial torsion in non-arthritic Indian adults: a computer tomography study of 100 limbs. Indian J Orthop. 2008;42:309–13.
18. Shetty GM, Mullaji A. The humble toothbrush – a simple and inexpensive tool for bone surface preparation in cemented total knee arthroplasty. J Maharashtra Orthop Assoc. 2011;6:1–4.
19. Mullaji A, Marawar S, Sharma A. Correcting varus deformity. J Arthroplasty. 2007;22(4 Suppl 1):15–9.
20. Mullaji A, Kanna R, Shetty GM, Chavda V, Singh DP. Efficacy of periarticular injection of bupivacaine, fentanyl, and methylprednisolone in total knee arthroplasty: a prospective, randomized trial. J Arthroplasty. 2010;25:851–7.

Part II

Coronal Plane Deformities

Varus Deformity

3

Introduction

Varus deformity, the most commonly encountered deformity in patients undergoing total knee arthroplasty (TKA), is associated with a limb alignment (hip-knee-ankle angle) of less than 180° and varying degrees of contracture of medial soft-tissue structures, laxity of the lateral soft-tissue structures, flexion deformity and medial bone erosion at the knee joint. Medial osteophytes cause tethering and functional shortening of the medial soft-tissue structures in a varus deformity; posterior osteophytes exert the same effect on the posterior capsule leading to flexion contracture and obstruction to deep flexion. There may also be associated lengthening and attenuation of the lateral soft-tissue structures especially in severe varus deformities [1].

Hence, the challenges in performing TKA in a varus arthritic knee include restoration of limb alignment, balancing the medial and lateral soft-tissue tension, equalising flexion and extension gaps and restoring medial bone loss. Severe varus deformities may be associated with malrotation of the distal femur and tibia which makes conventional bony landmarks less reliable to determine rotational alignment of the femoral and tibial components [2–4]. Furthermore, severe varus deformities may also be associated with extra-articular deformities such as excessive coronal bowing of the femoral shaft and proximal tibia vara which makes TKA technically challenging [5]. The current chapter describes the principles of dealing with a varus deformity, both mild to moderate and severe deformities, during TKA.

Pathoanatomy

Stability and function of the knee joint involve a dynamic interplay of various soft-tissue structures around the knee joint. A sound knowledge of these structures, both under normal and diseased conditions, is crucial to achieve optimum alignment, balance and kinematics after TKA for the arthritic knee. The issue of stability and balancing of soft tissues around the knee joint during TKA is compounded by the fact that ligaments and muscles around the knee joint are dynamic structures which behave differently in knee extension and flexion.

A sequential release of soft-tissue structures has been recommended to achieve equal medial and lateral gaps during TKA [1, 6–9]. It is hence important to know the soft-tissue structures around the medial aspect of the knee joint and the effect of release of these structures on gaps and alignment.

Traditionally, medial soft-tissue structures of the knee joint have been described in three layers [10–12]. The first and most superficial layer consists of the deep crural fascia of the knee joint including the retinacula and the pes anserinus (sartorius, gracilis and semitendinosus) attachment on the anteromedial aspect of the

A.B. Mullaji, G.M. Shetty, *Deformity Correction in Total Knee Arthroplasty*,
DOI 10.1007/978-1-4939-0566-9_3, © Springer Science+Business Media New York 2014

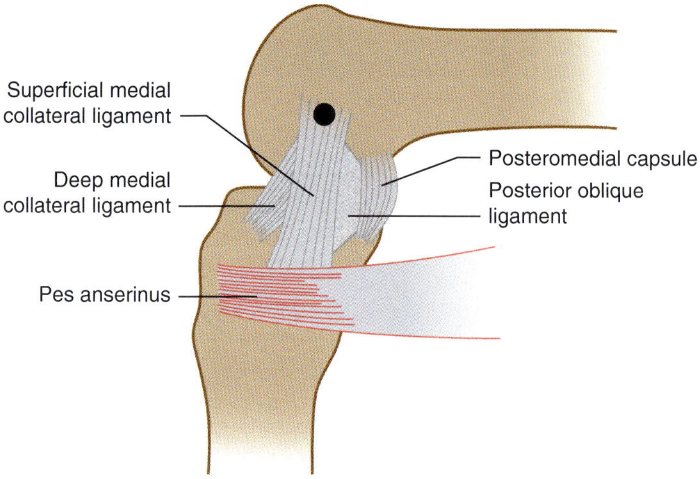

Fig. 3.1 Medial soft-tissue structures of the knee joint

proximal tibia distally. The second layer consists of the superficial part of the medial collateral ligament (MCL) which also gives rise to the posterior oblique ligament (POL) posteromedially (Fig. 3.1). The third and the deepest layer consists of the deep part of MCL, the deep capsular layer and the insertion of the semimembranosus tendon at the posteromedial corner of the tibia just below the joint line. We performed a cadaveric study to quantify the effect of sequential posteromedial release on flexion and extension gaps using an image-free computer navigation system [13]. Our study demonstrated that sequential soft-tissue releases led to an incremental and differential effect on flexion and extension gaps [13]. Hence, judicious and titrated use of this posteromedial soft-tissue releases sequence and following an algorithmic approach will help in correcting deformity and restoring limb alignment and balance during TKA. Although several authors have described different sequence of soft-tissue release for varus deformities [1, 6–9], we follow our technique of sequential soft-tissue release as described here for a cruciate-substituting TKA (Fig. 3.2).

As described in Chap. 1 , a lot of information can be derived about the pathologic soft-tissue and bony changes which have occurred in an arthritic knee based on preoperative radiographic features and examination of the knee under anaesthesia during TKA. Depending on the clinicoradiographic features presented by each varus arthritic knee, the surgeon will have to individualise the amount of bone resection, soft-tissue release and component size and position for each TKA in order to achieve optimum limb alignment and gap balance. Based on our experience of nearly 10,000 TKAs over the last 20 years, the authors have identified several clinical and radiographic features in varus arthritic knees which form the basis of their surgical technique.

The three principal clinical features of varus deformity on clinical examination (under anaesthesia) which need to be noted are (1) correctibility of the deformity (rigid, partially correctible, fully correctible and unstable) with knee in maximum extension, (2) associated sagittal plane deformity (fixed flexion or hyperextension) and (3) extent of lateral side soft-tissue laxity (mild, moderate or severe) (Fig. 3.3). The degree of correctibility of deformity will decide the amount of soft-tissue release required medially in order to achieve correction and balance. Similarly, amount of soft-tissue laxity on the lateral side of the knee in a varus deformity decides the extent of medial soft-tissue release required in order to equalise the medial and lateral soft-tissue gaps. Any associated sagittal plane deformity will require titrating the amount of tibial and distal femoral bony resection and posterior soft-tissue release to achieve deformity correction and flexion-extension gap balance.

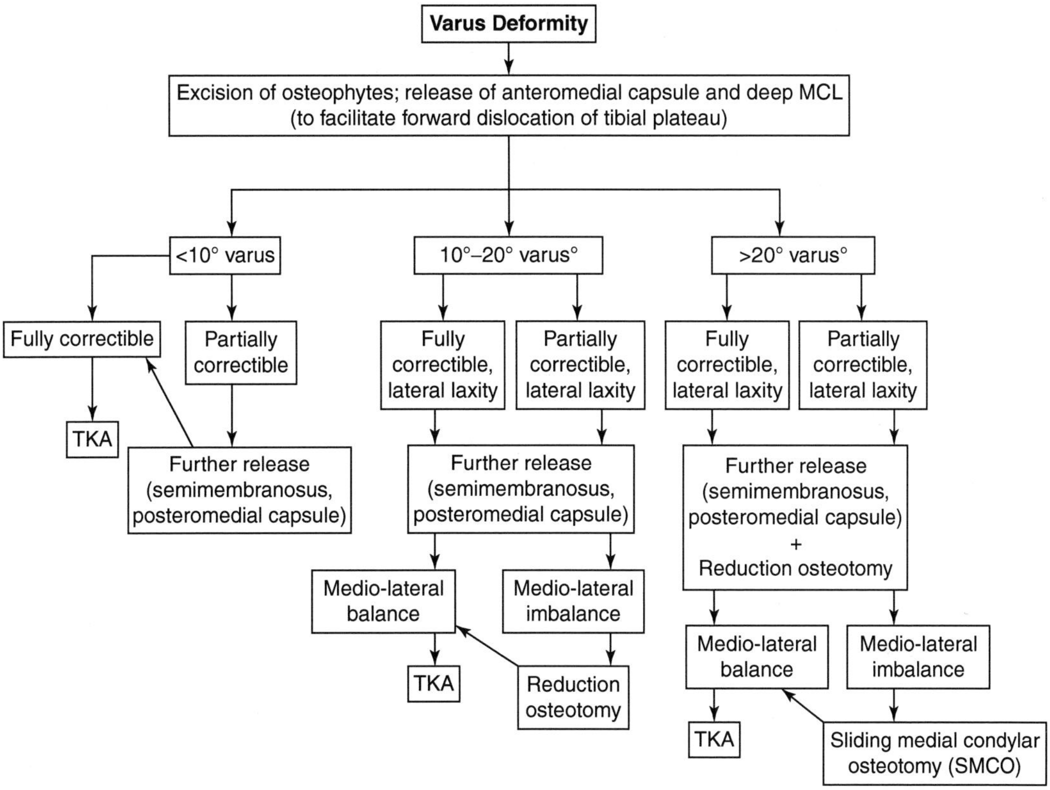

Fig. 3.2 Algorithmic approach to achieve limb alignment and soft-tissue balance in varus deformity during TKA

Preoperative radiographic features will usually provide hints as to what manoeuvres need to be carried out to correct the deformity and achieve optimum soft-tissue balance and can also help predict the difficulty a surgeon may face in achieving these goals. The five radiographic features of varus arthritic knees which need attention are (1) degree of deformity (as measured on full-length hip-to-ankle radiographs), (2) amount of lateral laxity (based on joint divergence angle and lateral translation of tibia), (3) presence of extra-articular deformity (coronal femoral bowing based on valgus correction angle, tibia vara based on tibial plateau angle), (4) medial bone loss (mild, moderate, severe) and (5) presence of osteophytes (minimal, moderate, abundant) (Fig. 3.4).

Several of the above features may be present or absent primarily based on the severity of arthritic involvement and the degree of knee deformity. Rigidity, associated sagittal plane deformities, excessive lateral laxity, abundant osteophytes and severe medial bone loss are more commonly seen in knees with severe longstanding varus deformities (especially ≥20°) than in knees with mild to moderate varus deformities [4]. In some knees, where the degree of arthritic involvement and the amount of intra-articular deformity is less severe, the above features may be absent. However, in these knees the degree of deformity may be confounded by the presence of an extra-articular deformity (commonly excessive coronal bowing of the femur) which adds to the overall severity of limb deformity and makes the case more challenging to treat (Fig. 3.5). Furthermore, increase in varus deformity may also cause variation in the distal valgus correction angle (VCA) and rotational profile of the distal femur and the tibia which needs to be accounted for while positioning the femoral and tibial components [2–4, 14–19].

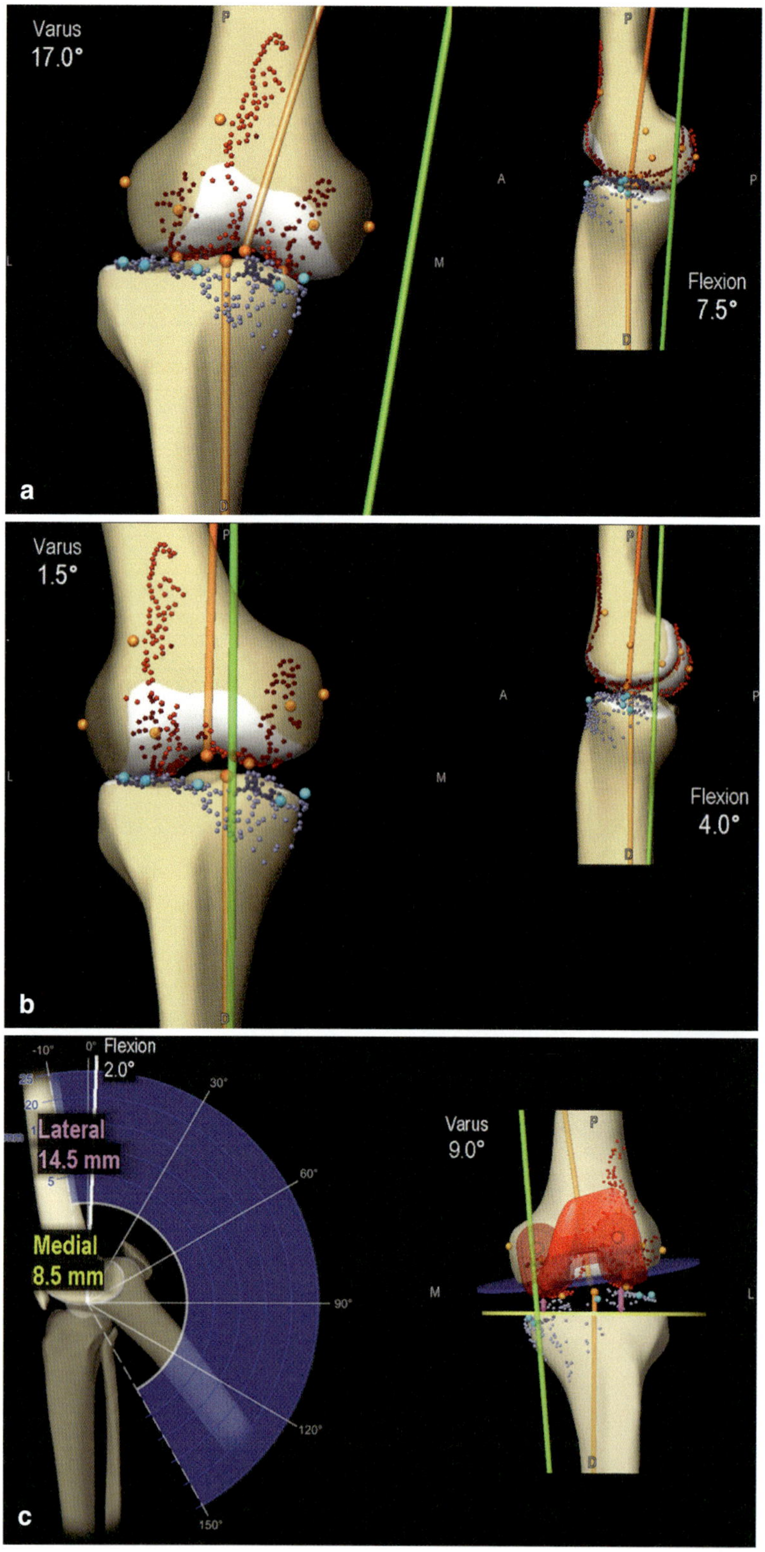

Fig. 3.3 The three principal clinical features of varus arthritic deformity which needs to be noted during TKA (shown here using computer navigation screen shot images). (**a**) Maximum varus deformity (using a varus stress at the knee joint in maximum extension) and maximum knee deformity in the sagittal plane (flexion). (**b**) Maximum correctibility of varus deformity (using a valgus stress at the knee joint in maximum extension). (**c**) Maximum lateral soft-tissue laxity (using a varus stress at the knee joint in maximum extension)

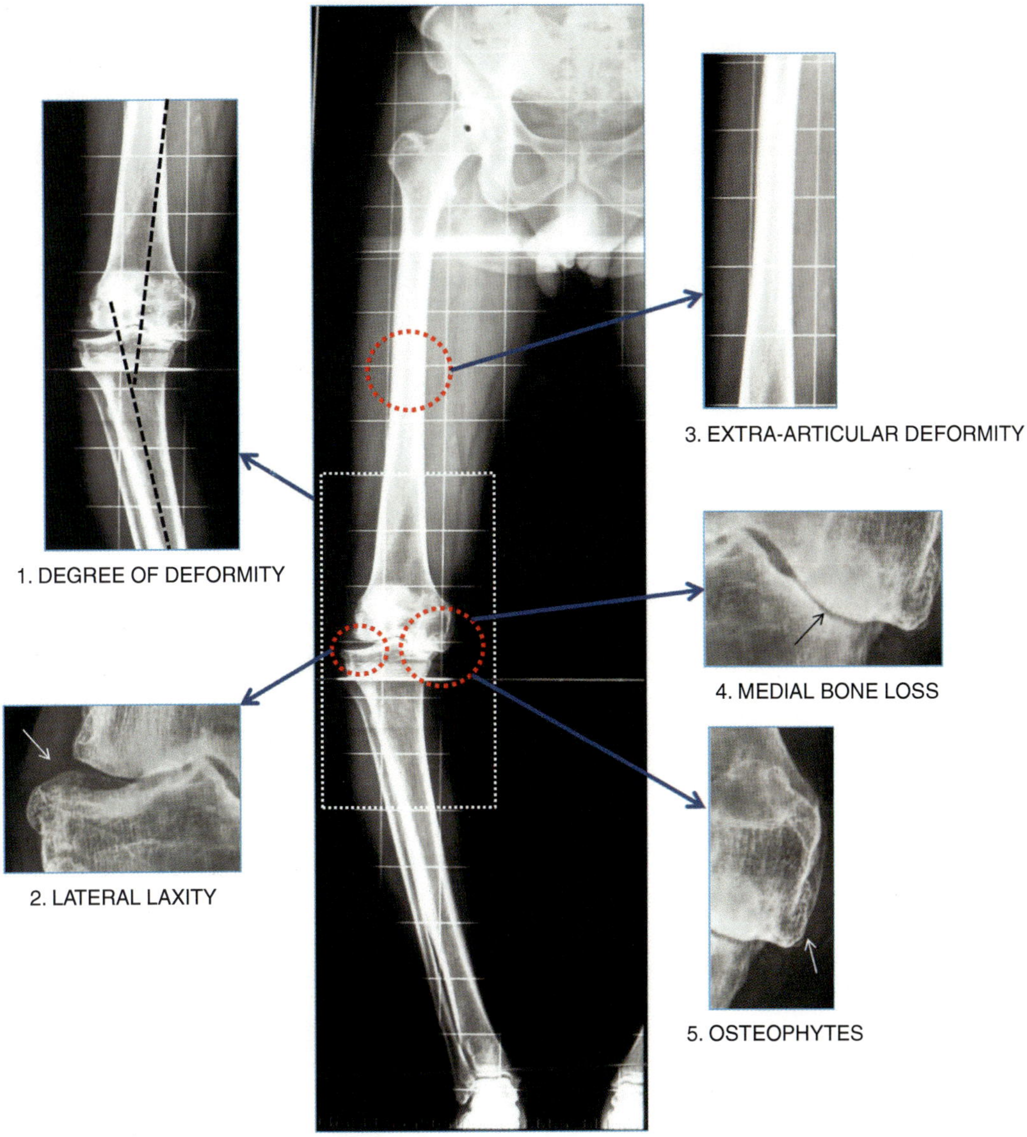

Fig. 3.4 The five principal radiographic features of varus arthritic deformity which needs to be noted on preoperative full-length hip-to-ankle radiographs

Based on radiographic analysis of 1,500 computer-assisted TKAs [5], the authors have described features of an "*at-risk*" *knee* which can be identified on preoperative standing, full-length hip-to-ankle radiographs (Fig. 3.6). The presence of these preoperative radiographic features put the knee at greater risk for malalignment after TKA [5]. Hence, the surgeon should identify such "at-risk" knees, and every measure must be undertaken to ensure optimum limb and component alignment and soft-tissue balance during TKA.

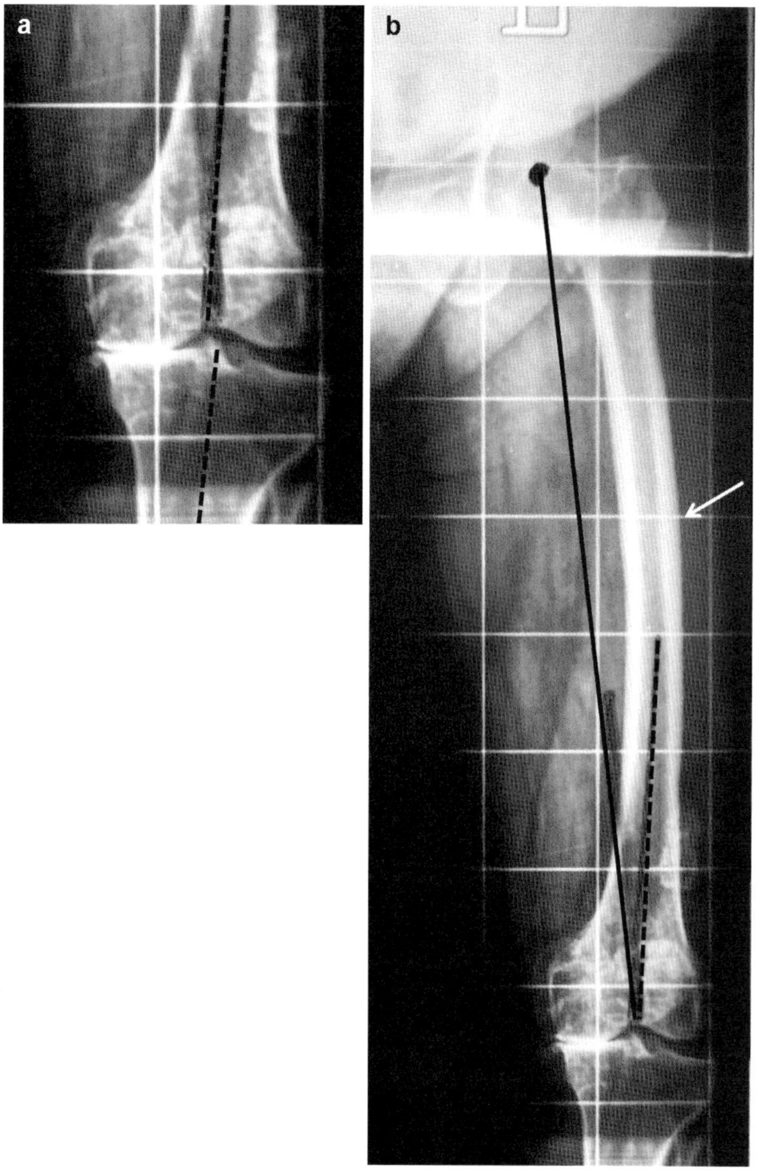

Fig. 3.5 Extra-articular deformity confounding the severity of deformity in an arthritic knee. (**a**) Preoperative standing knee radiograph showing mild changes in terms of deformity, bone loss, osteophytes and lateral laxity. Dotted line shows femoro-tibial angle. (**b**) Preoperative standing, full-length hip-to-ankle radiograph of the same patient (**a**) showing significant coronal bowing of the femoral shaft (*arrow*) because of which the distal femoral valgus correction angle (*VCA*) in this patient is almost 10.5°. *Dotted line* is the anatomic axis of the distal femur and the black line shows the femoral mechanical axis; the angle formed by the two lines is the VCA

Surgical Technique

The surgical technique followed by the authors for varus TKA is based on the presence of any combination of the three clinical and five radiographic features present in the arthritic knee. The basic technique followed is one of gap balancing where bone resection and soft-tissue release are tailored to each individual knee based on the presence or absence of the above clinico-radiologic features. The varus arthritic knee is treated with progressive release of medial soft-tissue structures to achieve full correction of deformity and to achieve "equipoise" with the

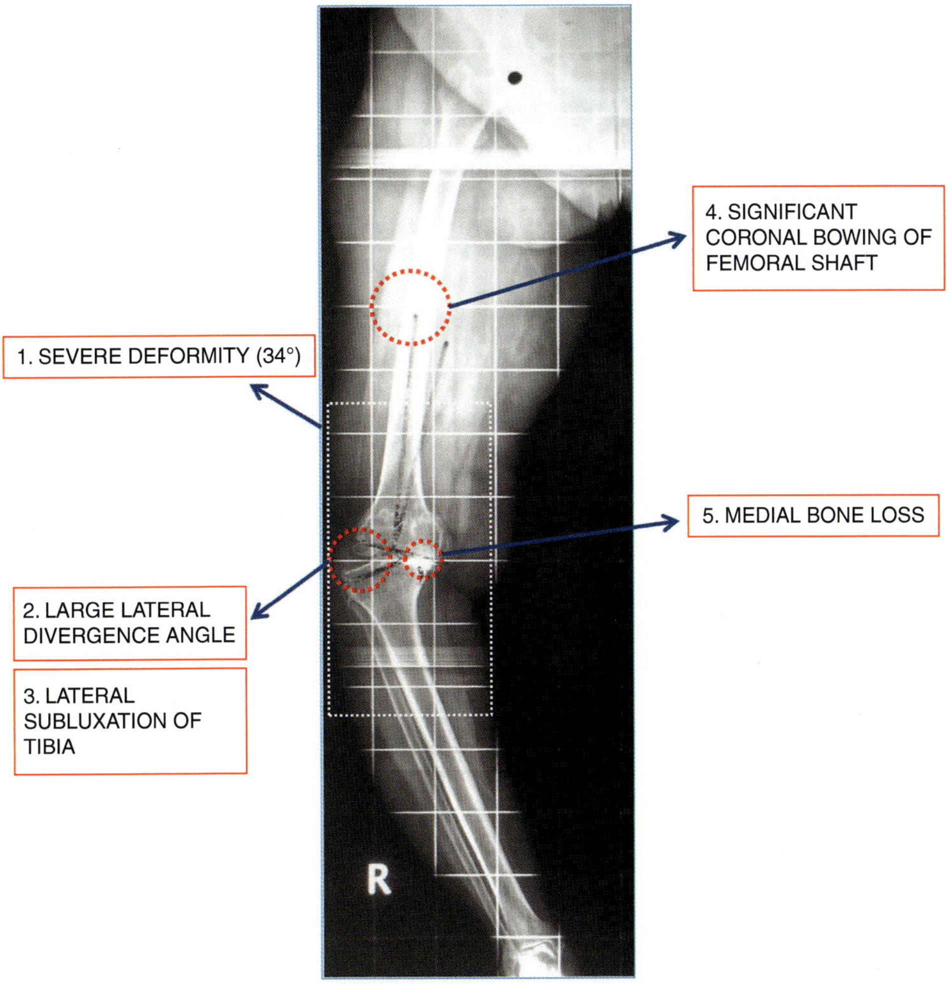

Fig. 3.6 The "at-risk" knee showing five features on preoperative full-length hip-to-ankle radiographs which may increase the risk of malalignment in this patient

lateral soft-tissue structures. However, this release of medial soft-tissue structures needs to be controlled and measured to avoid overcorrection or instability.

The first step to achieve these goals is to remove all osteophytes around the knee joint which will not only free the tethered soft-tissue structures but also helps avoid unnecessary soft-tissue release. Following this principal step, the surgeon can accurately assess in full extension how much residual deformity and soft-tissue tightness persists and which may require a formal soft-tissue release. Based on whether the deformity is fully correctible, partially correctible, rigid or unstable, further soft-tissue release may be required in order to correct the deformity. Most partially correctible deformities get fully corrected with removal of osteophytes and the preliminary soft-tissue release (deep MCL and semimembranosus) performed for exposure of the joint and anterior dislocation of tibia. However, the medial release required may be extensive (posteromedial capsular attachment to proximal tibia and segmental excision of the posteromedial capsule) in cases with rigid deformities or knees with severe medio-lateral soft-tissue imbalance and may also require performing a reduction osteotomy of the tibia (see Chap. 11 for technique) with or without undersizing the tibial component [20]. In contrast, soft-tissue releases should be restricted and controlled in knees which are unstable in coronal and or sagittal planes.

The next step after achieving deformity correction is to assess how lax the lateral soft-tissue structure vis-à-vis the medial structures. This is best done by giving a varus stress with a spacer block placed in the extension gap to determine how much the LCL is elongated. Although a varus deformity may appear to be fully corrected with medial soft-tissue release as evidenced by correct alignment being achieved with a spacer block in extension with a valgus stress being applied, medio-lateral soft-tissue balance may still prove to be elusive due to excessive lateral soft-tissue laxity. Similarly, in the presence of an extra-articular deformity, achieving optimum deformity correction and soft-tissue balance may not be possible despite extensive medial release. Both these scenarios warrant performing either a sliding medial condylar osteotomy or a corrective osteotomy of the extra-articular deformity (see Chap. 11 for technique) [21, 22].

Knee Deformity <10°

Typically, knees with mild deformities (<10° varus or HKA angle >170–180°) have minimal or no osteophytes, medial bone loss or extra-articular deformities and no associated sagittal plane deformities. Such knees are easily correctible with a preliminary medial soft-tissue release and standard bone cuts. However, these deformities may be sometimes associated with mild to moderate lateral laxity or an associated sagittal plane deformity. Excessive lateral laxity maybe dealt with by proportionately extending the amount of medial soft-tissue release. An associated fixed flexion deformity may get corrected by a thorough posterior clearance (osteophyte excision and capsular release) and as a last resort resecting additional distal femoral bone. However, when an associated hyperextension deformity is present, conservative tibial and distal femoral bone resection should be performed and posterior soft-tissue release avoided. Rarely, some of these knees may have an associated "reverse" bowing of the femoral shaft (Fig. 3.7) when analysed on preoperative full-length hip-to-ankle radiograph. This puts the knee at greater risk for overcorrecting the limb axis into valgus alignment. In such cases, the surgeon should strictly avoid over-release on the medial side and reduce the valgus correction angle (VCA) for the distal femoral cut.

Knee Deformity 10–20°

Such varus deformities are commonly associated with mild to moderate degree of lateral laxity, medial bone loss, sagittal plane deformity or extra-articular deformity. The amount of osteophytes present may vary from mild to moderate. Again, although most of these deformities can be easily tackled using the standard procedure, an associated extra-articular deformity either in the femur (excessive coronal bowing) or the tibia (proximal tibia vara) may make deformity correction and soft-tissue balancing a challenge. The presence of such extra-articular deformity will require more than the usual medial soft-tissue release to achieve limb realignment and gap balance. Rarely, when even extensive soft-tissue release fails to achieve the surgical goals (due to excessive lateral laxity with or without excessive medial tightness), a sliding medial condylar osteotomy (SMCO) may be required. The need for SMCO in such cases can usually be predicted on preoperative radiographs by the presence of an extra-articular deformity confounding the lesser degree of intra-articular knee deformity, often in combination with the presence of excessive lateral laxity of the knee joint (lateral divergence angle), lateral translation of the tibia and lack of osteophyte, excision of which would otherwise contribute to deformity correction without the need for excessive medial release.

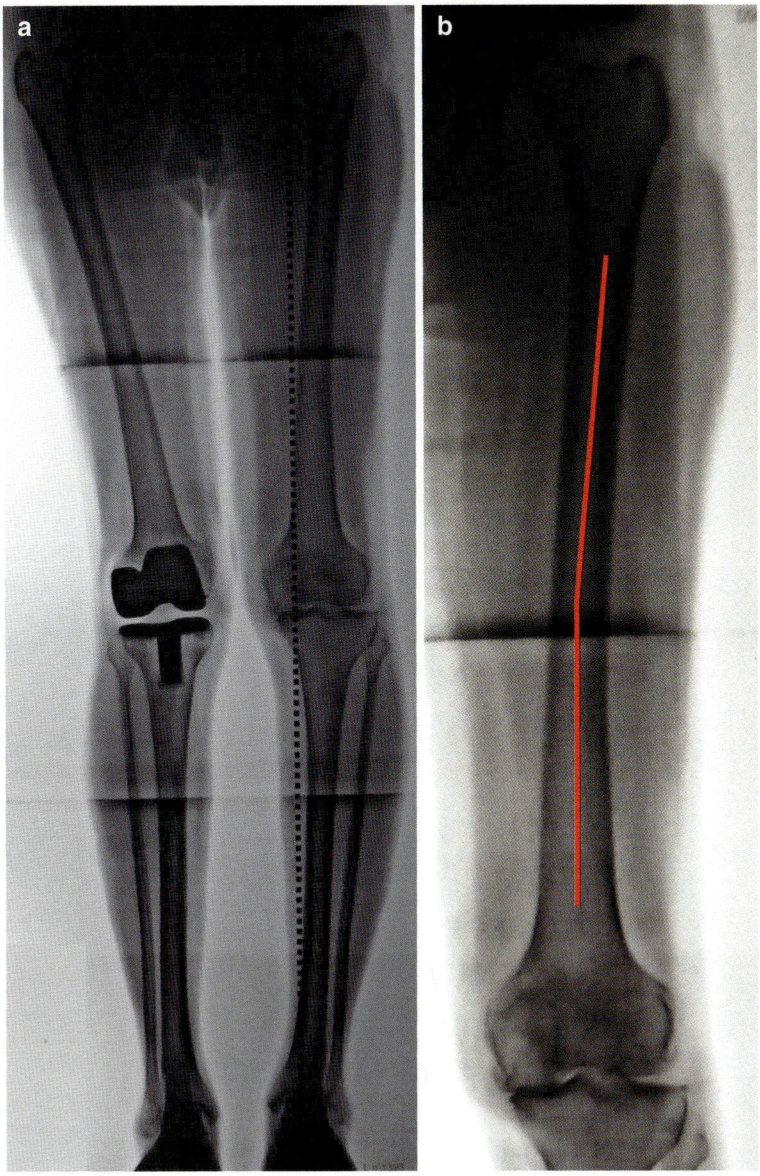

Fig. 3.7 Reverse bowing of the femoral shaft in the coronal plane. (**a**) Preoperative standing, full-length hip-to-ankle radiograph showing mild varus deformity of the left knee. Failure to recognize reverse bowing has led to valgus malalignment of the right knee. *Dotted black line* shows mechanical axis of lower limb. (**b**) An enlarged view of the femoral shaft shows reverse bowing in the coronal plane. *Red line* shows reverse bowing angle of the femoral shaft

Knee Deformity >20°

Severe varus deformities pose several challenges during TKA including severe extra-articular deformity, severe lateral laxity, medial bone loss and associated moderate to severe sagittal plane deformities. The degree of soft-tissue release is governed by the amount of soft-tissue tightness assessed using a tensioning device. An extensive, graded, stepwise soft-tissue release (subperiosteal elevation of the deep medial collateral ligament (MCL), posteromedial capsule and semimembranosus) is performed as per the technique previously described by the authors (Fig. 3.2). Excision of osteophytes along the posteromedial tibia and medial femoral condyle is initially performed. Tibial resection is restricted at approximately 6–7 mm of bone with respect to the lateral tibial condyle when the deformity is associated with excessive lateral laxity or an associated hyperextension deformity [23]. In the presence of a medial tibial bone defect, this cut

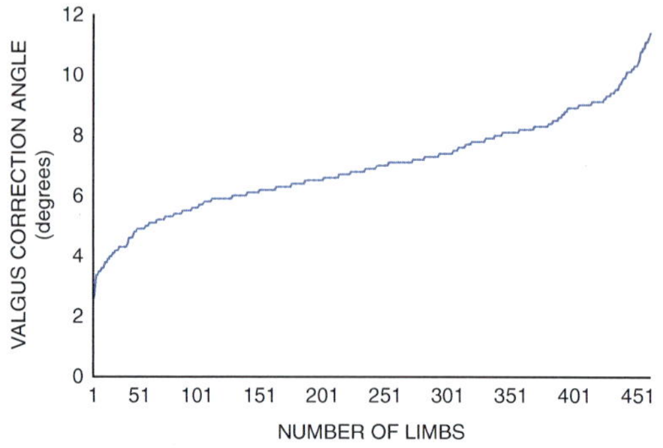

Fig. 3.8 Graph showing distribution of the valgus correction angle (*VCA*) in our series of 459 varus limbs. The VCA in 47 % of varus limbs was >7°

usually passes some distance above it and not through its base. An additional 1–2 mm is resected if it reduces the size of the bone defect. By lowering the tibial surface with this additional resection, a smaller tibial component could be used, which in turns helps in increasing the amount of reduction osteotomy which can be performed for deformity correction and/or medio-lateral soft-tissue balancing [20].

The distal femur is cut at a valgus correction angle (VCA) determined on preoperative long hip-to-ankle radiographs for each individual limb since this may show wide variation among individuals (Fig. 3.8). The thickness of the distal cut is determined by the extent of medial femoral condylar bone defect and the severity of the flexion contracture. The thickness must be reduced if the medial condyle shows significant bone loss or in the presence of an associated hyperextension deformity or severe instability. Additional bone may have to be resected from the distal femur in the presence of a significant flexion deformity which has not improved with removal of posterior osteophytes and release of posterior capsular adhesions. In the presence of excessive coronal bowing of the femur, a short intramedullary guide rod should be used to avoid malposition of the distal cutting block with respect to the mechanical axis of the femur, or computer navigation should be used to accurately align the cutting block and to bypass the extra-articular deformity in the femur.

The medio-lateral gap balance in knee extension is assessed with a spacer block, and any discrepancy is address with additional soft-tissue release and reduction osteotomy. Usually the flexion gap may be larger than the extension gap (due to extensive soft-tissue release), and the femoral component may have to be upsized, flexed 2–5° and translated posteriorly to achieve balance. If the flexion gap is still larger than the extension gap, additional resection of distal femur is needed to accommodate a thicker spacer.

Despite associated femoral and tibial extra-articular deformities and excessive lateral laxity, the above technique of bone resection and soft-tissue release results in well-aligned and balanced knees in majority of limbs with severe varus deformity undergoing TKA. However, in a few cases of rigid deformities, medial tightness may persist even after extensive medial soft-tissue release, and a sliding medial condylar osteotomy (SMCO) may be required. This involves distalising and fixing the medial femoral condylar fragment using cancellous screws after the implant has been cemented (see Chap. 11 for technique). Rarely, in cases with persistent and severe lateral side soft-tissue laxity and severe instability, a constrained implant may have to be used.

Medial tibial bone defects may be significant even after the tibial cut has been performed. Bone defects are dealt with based on their size and position (Fig. 3.9). Usually, uncontained medial tibial bone defects less than 10 mm deep are filled with bone cement, whereas defects ≥10 mm are filled with autologous bone graft (typically using bone from the notch cut). The bone defect should be first gently fashioned into a step-cut defect using a saw and then the bone block shaped to match the defect. The graft is usually punched into position or fixed into place using 2-mm K-wires or cancellous screw if the size of the graft is large (Fig. 3.9). These should be directed parallel to the tibial surface to avoid the peg or stem of the tibial component. A tibial stem extender is usually used in cases with large medial bone defects of >10 mm (Fig. 3.9). Rarely, significant medial femoral bone defects may require the use of metal augments supplemented with a femoral stem (Fig. 3.10).

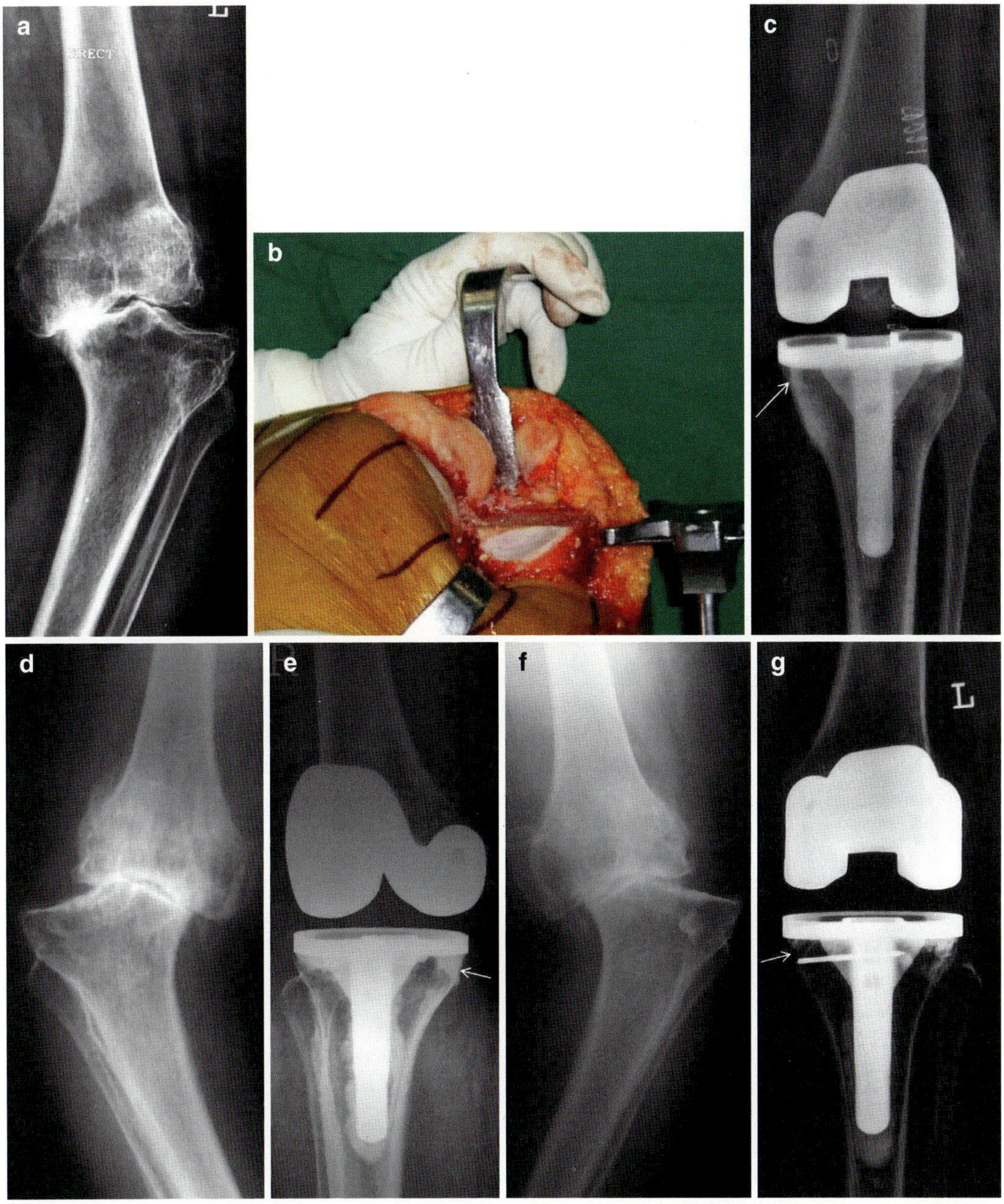

Fig. 3.9 Medial tibial bone defect in varus arthritic knees undergoing TKA. (**a**) Preoperative anteroposterior standing knee radiograph showing significant medial tibial bone defect. (**b**) Intraoperative photograph of the same patient (**a**) showing the medial tibial bone defect. Note that the tibial cut passes much above the deepest point of the bone defect. (**c**) Postoperative anteroposterior standing knee radiograph of the same patient (**a**) where the tibial bone defect was treated with autograft punched in position without fixation (*arrow*) and supported with a long stem tibial implant. (**d**) Preoperative anteroposterior standing knee radiograph showing significant medial tibial bone defect. (**e**) Postoperative anteroposterior standing knee radiograph of the same patient (**d**) where the tibial bone defect was not large enough to warrant grafting and hence was filled with bone cement (*arrow*) and supported with a long stem tibial implant. (**f**) Preoperative anteroposterior standing knee radiograph showing significant medial tibial bone defect. (**g**) Postoperative anteroposterior standing knee radiograph of the same patient (**f**) where the tibial bone defect was large enough to require bone grafting and fixation with wires (*arrow*) and supported with a long stem tibial implant. (**h**) Preoperative anteroposterior standing knee radiograph showing significant medial tibial bone defect and subluxation of the knee joint. (**i**) Postoperative anteroposterior standing knee radiograph of the same patient (**h**) where a constrained design was used and the tibial bone defect was treated with bone grafting and screw fixation

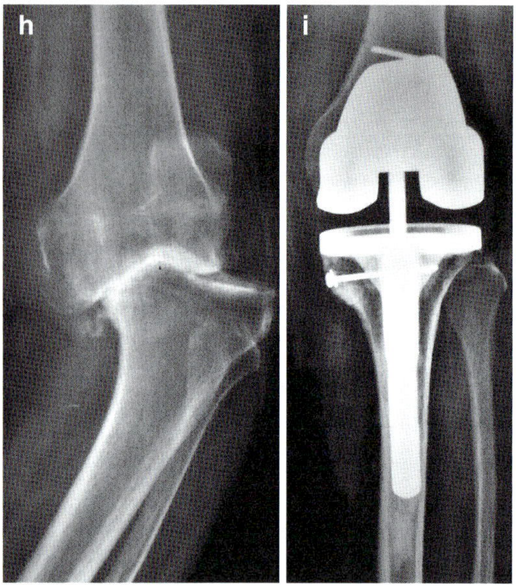

Fig. 3.9 (continued)

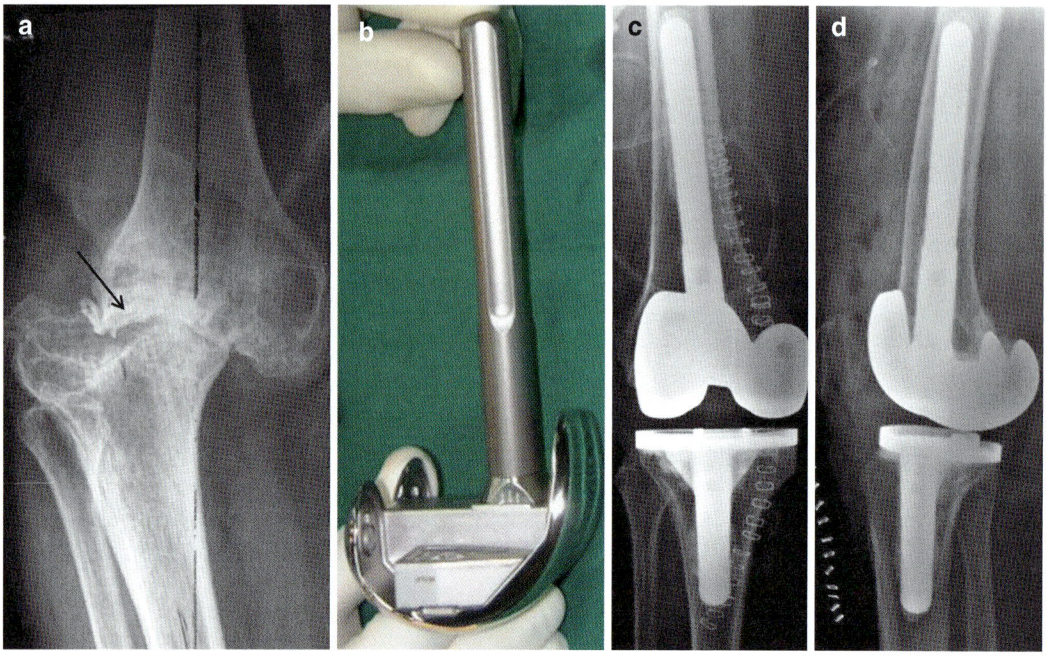

Fig. 3.10 Lateral femoral condyle bone defect in a varus arthritic knees undergoing TKA. (**a**) Preoperative anteroposterior standing knee radiograph showing substantial lateral femoral and tibial bone defect. *Arrow* shows substantial lateral femoral bone loss. (**b**) A distal femoral metal augment along with a femoral stem was used in the same patient (**a**) to treat the bone defect. (**c**) Postoperative anteroposterior standing knee radiograph of the same patient (**a**). (**d**) Postoperative lateral knee radiograph of the same patient (**a**)

Computer-Assisted Technique

The basic surgical technique for computer-assisted TKA in varus knees is similar to the one previously described for conventional TKA. Navigation allows for precise, quantitative and graduated medial soft-tissue release (as described above) to achieve rectangular balanced gaps and a fully restored mechanical axis. The navigation system with its software offers several advantages during TKA especially in severe varus arthritic knees. It bypasses extra-articular deformities such as excessive coronal bowing of the femur or malunited fractures or hardware from a previous surgery and avoids the difficulty in using intramedullary guide rods. Furthermore, in limbs where an additional reduction osteotomy or sliding medial condylar osteotomy may be required, navigation allows for precise, controlled, quantitative lengthening of the tight medial soft-tissue structures and proper restoration of soft-tissue balance and knee alignment [20, 21]. Similarly in rare cases where a corrective osteotomy for an extra-articular deformity in the femur or tibia is required, navigation allows for precise correction of the deformity and accurate realignment of the limb [22].

References

1. Mihalko WM, Saleh KJ, Krackow KA, Whiteside LA. Soft-tissue balancing during total knee arthroplasty in the varus knee. J Am Acad Orthop Surg. 2009;17:766–74.
2. Matsuda S, Miura H, Nagamine R, Urabe K, Mawatari T, Iwamoto Y. A comparison of rotational landmarks in the distal femur and the tibial shaft. Clin Orthop Relat Res. 2003;414:183–8.
3. Matsui Y, Kadoya Y, Uehara K, Kobayashi A, Takaoka K. Rotational deformity in varus osteoarthritis of the knee: analysis with computed tomography. Clin Orthop Relat Res. 2005;433:147–51.
4. Nagamine R, Miyanishi K, Miura H, Urabe K, Matsuda S, Iwamoto Y. Medial torsion of the tibia in Japanese patients with osteoarthritis of the knee. Clin Orthop Relat Res. 2003;408:218–24.
5. Mullaji AB, Shetty GM, Lingaraju AP, Bhayde S. Which factors increase risk of malalignment of the hip-knee-ankle axis in TKA? Clin Orthop Relat Res. 2013;471:134–41.
6. Whiteside LA. Soft tissue balancing: the knee. J Arthroplasty. 2002;17(4 Suppl 1):23–7.
7. Verdonk PC, Pernin J, Pinaroli A, Ait Si Selmi T, Neyret P. Soft tissue balancing in varus total knee arthroplasty: an algorithmic approach. Knee Surg Sports Traumatol Arthrosc. 2009;17:660–6.
8. Mullaji A, Marawar S, Sharma A. Correcting varus deformity. J Arthroplasty. 2007;22(4 Suppl 1):15–9.
9. Mullaji AB, Padmanabhan V, Jindal G. Total knee arthroplasty for profound varus deformity: technique and radiological results in 173 knees with varus of more than 20 degrees. J Arthroplasty. 2005;20:550–61.
10. LaPrade RF, Engebretsen AH, Ly TV, Johansen S, Wentorf FA, Engebretsen L. The anatomy of the medial part of the knee. J Bone Joint Surg Am. 2007;89:2000–10.
11. Warren LF, Marshall JL. The supporting structures and layers on the medial side of the knee: an anatomical analysis. J Bone Joint Surg Am. 1979;61:56–62.
12. De Maeseneer M, Van Roy F, Lenchik L, Barbaix E, De Ridder F, Osteaux M. Three layers of the medial capsular and supporting structures of the knee: MR imaging-anatomic correlation. Radiographics. 2000;20:83–9.
13. Mullaji A, Sharma A, Marawar S, Kanna R. Quantification of effect of sequential posteromedial release on flexion and extension gaps: a computer-assisted study in cadaveric knees. J Arthroplasty. 2009;24:795–805.
14. Mullaji AB, Sharma AK, Marawar SV, Kohli AF. Tibial torsion in non-arthritic Indian adults: a computer tomography study of 100 limbs. Indian J Orthop. 2008;42:309–13.
15. Siston RA, Patel JJ, Goodman SB, Delp SL, Giori NJ. The variability of femoral rotational alignment in total knee arthroplasty. J Bone Joint Surg Am. 2005;87:2276–80.
16. Mullaji AB, Sharma AK, Marawar SV, Kohli AF, Singh DP. Distal femoral rotational axes in Indian knees. J Orthop Surg (Hong Kong). 2009;17:166–9.
17. Sahin N, Atıcı T, Öztürk A, Özkaya G, Özkan Y, Avcu B. Accuracy of anatomical references used for rotational alignment of tibial component in total knee arthroplasty. Knee Surg Sports Traumatol Arthrosc. 2012;20:565–70.
18. Sun T, Lu H, Hong N, Wu J, Feng C. Bony landmarks and rotational alignment in total knee arthroplasty for Chinese osteoarthritic knees with varus or valgus deformities. J Arthroplasty. 2009;24:427–31.
19. Mullaji AB, Shetty GM, Kanna R, Vadapalli RC. The influence of preoperative deformity on valgus correction angle: an analysis of 503 total knee arthroplasties. J Arthroplasty. 2013;28:20–7.

20. Mullaji AB, Shetty GM. Correction of varus deformity during TKA with reduction osteotomy. Clin Orthop Relat Res. 2014;472:126–32.
21. Mullaji AB, Shetty GM. Surgical technique: computer-assisted sliding medial condylar osteotomy to achieve gap balance in varus knees during TKA. Clin Orthop Relat Res. 2013;471:1484–91.
22. Mullaji A, Shetty GM. Computer-assisted total knee arthroplasty for arthritis with extra-articular deformity. J Arthroplasty. 2009;24:1164–9.
23. Mullaji A, Lingaraju AP, Shetty GM. Computer-assisted total knee replacement in patients with arthritis and a recurvatum deformity. J Bone Joint Surg Br. 2012;94:642–7.

Valgus Deformity

4

Introduction

A valgus arthritic knee, compared to a varus knee, offers its own challenges during total knee arthroplasty (TKA). A valgus knee is less commonly encountered in arthritic knees undergoing TKA and involves a distinctly different set of pathoanatomic structural changes when compared to a varus knee. The incidence of valgus arthritic knees in patients undergoing TKA is less than 10 % in the senior surgeon's series [1, 2]. Restoration of optimal limb alignment and gap balance after TKA in valgus knees can be a formidable challenge because of several reasons. First, a surgeon may be less familiar with the surgical technique and soft-tissue releases involved and there is a paucity of soft-tissue structures available for release on the lateral side compared to the medial side. Second, there is a higher risk of common peroneal nerve palsy due to its proximity to lateral soft-tissue structures and stretching that may occur in correcting long-standing valgus deformity especially if associated with flexion deformity. Finally, osseous defects in the posterolateral aspect of the femur and tibia; hypoplastic lateral femoral condyle, an associated external rotation deformity of the distal femur or proximal tibia, and patellar maltracking may also be commonly encountered in valgus arthritic knees. Hence, a valgus knee is a different ball game when compared to varus arthritic knees, and this chapter aims to outline the management of the same with TKA.

Pathoanatomy

Valgus arthritic deformities commonly present with tightness of lateral soft-tissue structures which may be associated with varying degrees of laxity of the medial structures. Contracture of the iliotibial (IT) band, popliteus tendon, posterolateral capsule and popliteofibular ligament may be encountered in these knees (Fig. 4.1). We do not believe that the lateral collateral ligament (LCL) undergoes contracture and shortening. The surgeon should be aware which soft-tissue structures are taut in different positions of knee flexion and extension so that a calibrated, stepwise approach is followed during release and imbalance or instability avoided. Essentially, the LCL and popliteus tendon are taut in both flexion and extension, the IT band and posterolateral capsule are taut only in extension, and the popliteofibular ligament is taut only in flexion [3].

In addition, there may be asymmetric wear or hypoplasia of the posterior condyles with excessive wear of the posterolateral condyle of the femur and/or tibia (Fig. 4.2a, b) [4]. This is important to note intraoperatively as using the posterior femoral condyles as a reference to place the AP cutting block may cause excessive resection from the posterior femoral condyle laterally, thereby resulting in excessive internal rotation of the femoral component and patellar maltracking. Using the AP axis (as described by Arima and Whiteside [5]) as an alternative to achieving proper femoral component rotation is also fraught

A.B. Mullaji, G.M. Shetty, *Deformity Correction in Total Knee Arthroplasty*,
DOI 10.1007/978-1-4939-0566-9_4, © Springer Science+Business Media New York 2014

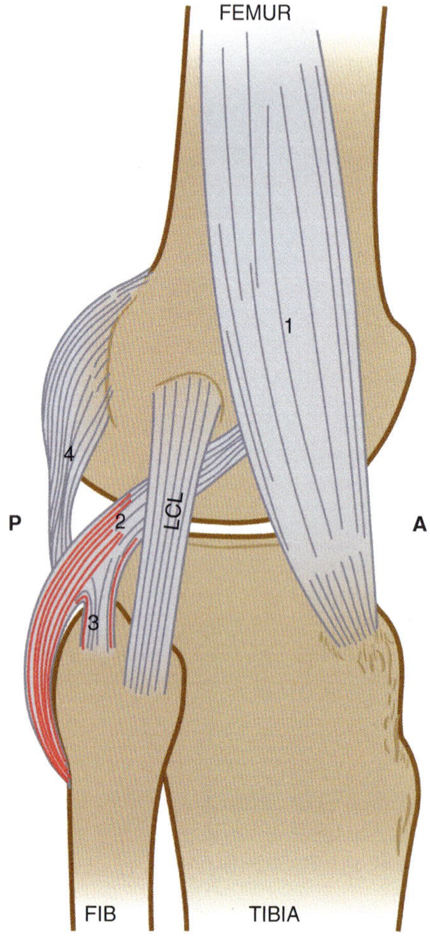

Fig. 4.1 Soft-tissue structures on the lateral and posterolateral aspect of the knee joint which may require release during TKA in a valgus arthritic knee. *1* Iliotibial band, *2* popliteus tendon, *3* popliteofibular ligament, *4* posterolateral capsule. *A* anterior, *P* posterior, *LCL* lateral collateral ligament

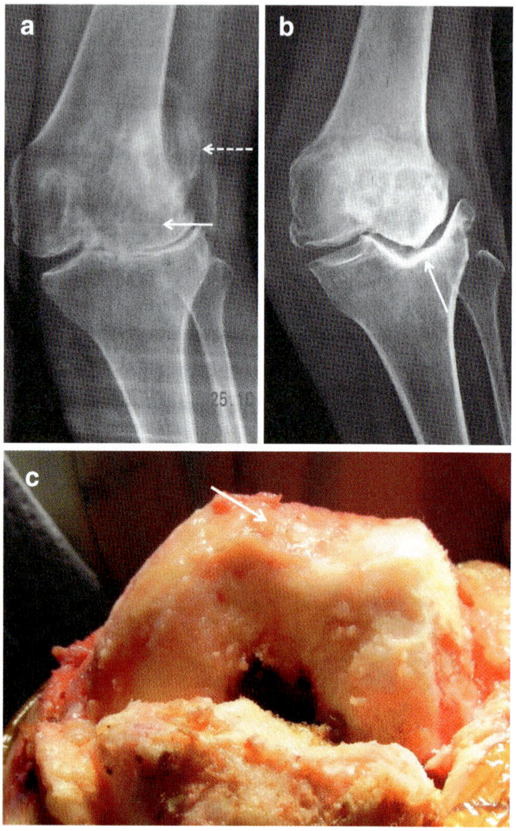

Fig. 4.2 Common pathoanatomic findings in a valgus arthritic knee. (**a**) Hypoplasia and distortion of the lateral femoral condyle (*solid arrow*) with associated patellar maltracking (*dashed arrow*) as seen on an anteroposterior standing knee radiograph. (**b**) Significant bone loss from the lateral tibial condyle (*arrow*) as seen on an anteroposterior standing knee radiograph. Note the large osteophyte on the lateral margin of the tibial plateau which must be excised before any soft-tissue release. (**c**) Intraoperative finding showing significant erosion and distortion of the femoral trochlear groove (*arrow*) due to severe patellofemoral arthritis and significant patellar maltracking. Using the anteroposterior axis as reference to determine femoral rotation in this case is risky

with risk especially if the patella is maltracking and leads to more lateral wear of the trochlear groove (Fig. 4.2c). Hence, the transepicondylar axis (TEA) is preferred by the authors in severe valgus deformities as a landmark for determining femoral rotation. Patellar maltracking, commonly seen in severe valgus deformities (Fig. 4.2a), is usually the consequence of an excessive Q angle due to valgus malalignment, excessive external tibial torsion and excessive tightness of the lateral retinaculum [6]. Valgus knees may also be associated with external rotation deformity of the proximal tibia due to a tight iliotibial tract [6]. Lastly, the valgus arthritic knee just like the varus knee may also be associated with a sagittal plane deformity such as flexion or hyperextension deformity or an extra-articular deformity which may further complicate the surgical technique. Most patients with a valgus deformity at the knee have associated hindfoot valgus (flatfeet) (Fig. 4.3) and even distortion of the midfoot [7, 8]. The authors have reported that despite restoring the hip-knee-ankle (HKA) axis in such patients, the ground mechanical axis may still pass lateral to the centre of the knee joint, and this may need to be factored in while deciding what should be the final knee alignment during TKA [7].

Valgus knees form a spectrum of deformities with important differences which impact surgical technique. All valgus knees are not alike! Ranawat et al. [9] had classified valgus arthritic knees into three major variants based on the degree of deformity, status of medial collateral ligament (MCL) and the amount of lateral release required – variant 1 showing minimal valgus deformity and medial soft-tissue stretching; variant 2 showing substantial deformity (>10°), bone loss and medial stretching; and variant 3 showing severe deformity and osseous deficiency with an incompetent medial soft-tissue sleeve. The authors have modified this classification to include six types of valgus knees based on (1) severity and correctibility of valgus deformity, (2) associated flexion, hyperextension or extra-articular deformity and (3) status of the medial collateral ligament (MCL) (Table. 4.1, Figs. 4.4, 4.5, 4.6, 4.7, 4.8 and 4.9).

The majority of valgus knees are correctible under anaesthesia with a varus stress. These are typically knees where the valgus deformity present in extension disappears on flexing the knee (type 1) (Fig. 4.4). Type 2 knees are those in which

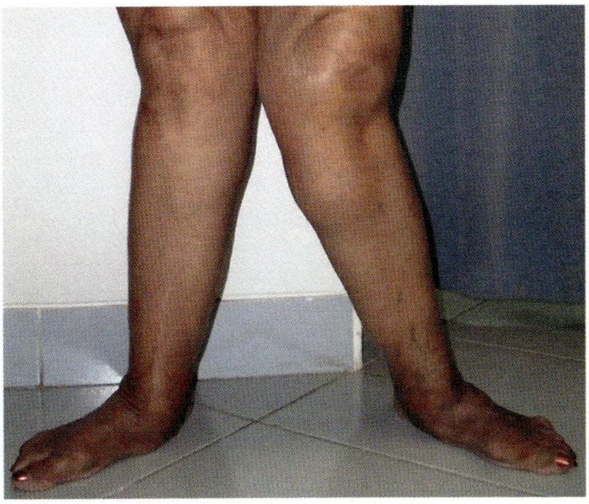

Fig. 4.3 Bilateral valgus knees associated with significant hindfoot valgus

Table 4.1 Classification of valgus knees

Type 1:	Correctible valgus, no associated deformity, MCL intact
Type 2:	Rigid valgus, no associated deformity, MCL intact
Type 3:	Valgus with hyperextension deformity, MCL intact
Type 4:	Valgus with flexion deformity, MCL intact
Type 5:	Severe valgus with incompetent MCL
Type 6:	Valgus with extra-articular deformity

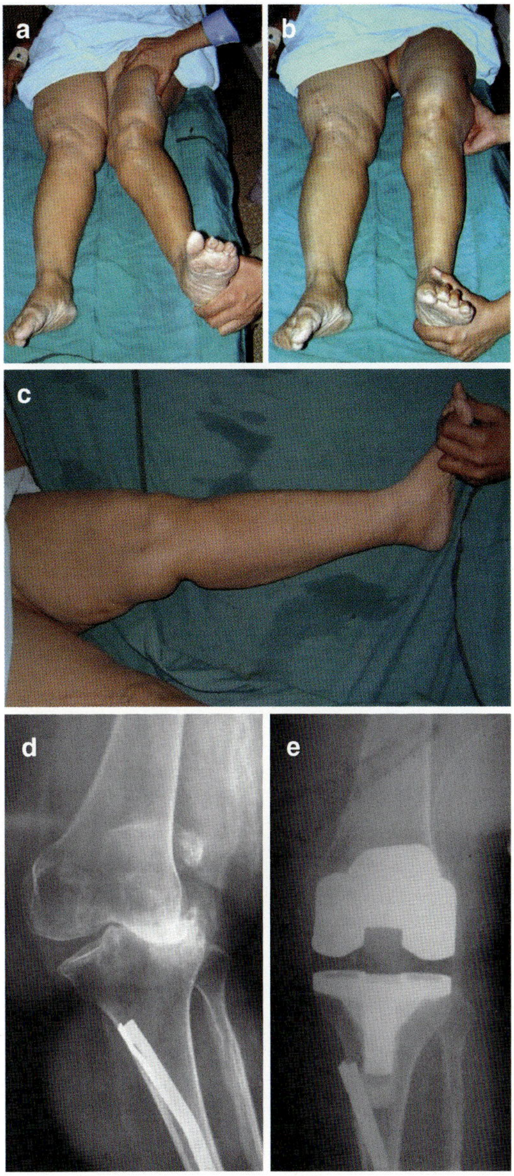

Fig. 4.4 Type 1 valgus deformity. (**a**) Clinical photograph showing maximum valgus deformity with a valgus stress applied with patient under anaesthesia. (**b**) Clinical photograph showing complete correctibility of valgus deformity with a varus stress applied with patient under anaesthesia. (**c**) Clinical photograph showing no associated flexion or hyperextension deformity with patient under anaesthesia. (**d**) Preoperative standing anteroposterior knee radiograph showing the valgus deformity. (**e**) Postoperative standing anteroposterior knee radiograph showing restoration of knee alignment with a cruciate-substituting design

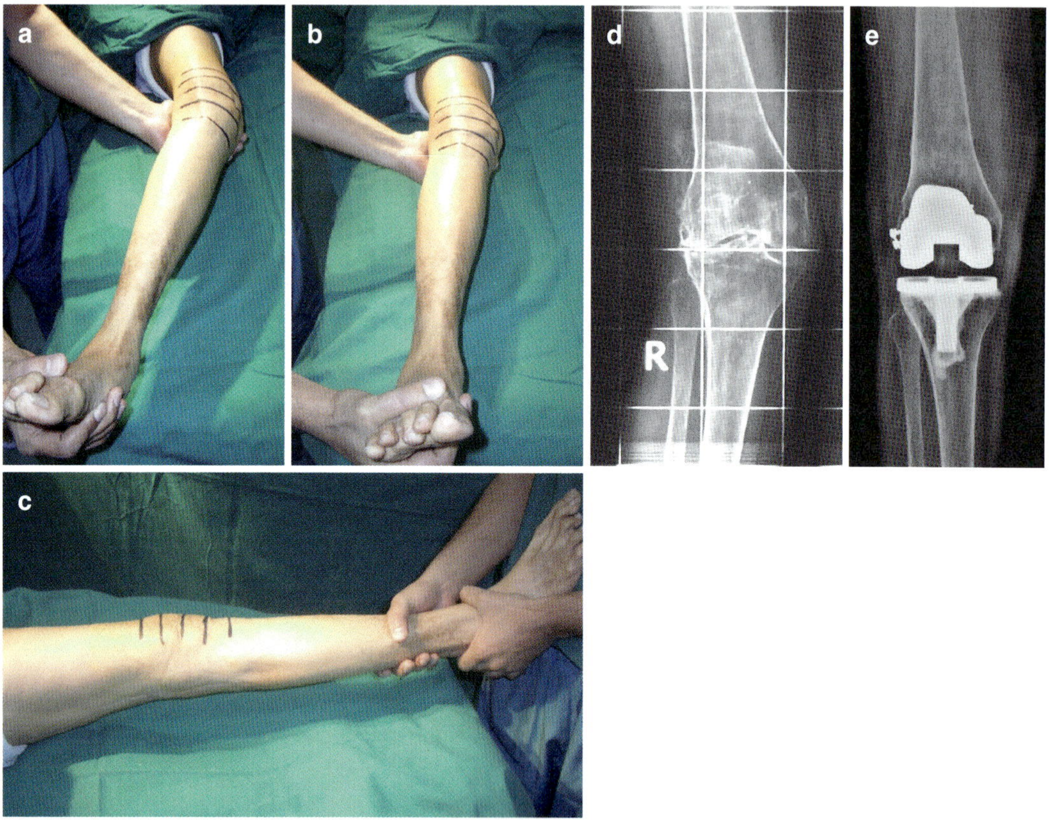

Fig. 4.5 Type 2 valgus deformity. (**a**) Clinical photograph showing maximum valgus deformity with a valgus stress applied with patient under anaesthesia. (**b**) Clinical photograph showing partial correctibility of valgus deformity with a varus stress applied with patient under anaesthesia. (**c**) Clinical photograph showing no associated flexion or hyperextension deformity with patient under anaesthesia. (**d**) Preoperative standing anteroposterior knee radiograph showing the valgus deformity. (**e**) Postoperative standing anteroposterior knee radiograph showing restoration of knee alignment with a cruciate-substituting design. A lateral epicondylar osteotomy (*LEO*) was required in this case due to the rigid nature of the deformity

the valgus deformity is rigid in both extension and flexion and are most likely to be associated with a hypoplastic lateral femoral condyle (Fig. 4.5). In type 3 knees, the deformity is usually correctible (Fig. 4.6), while in type 4 there may be a trapezoidal flexion gap due to contracture of posterolateral structures (Fig. 4.7). Any long-standing valgus deformity which is severe may develop attenuation of the MCL (type 5) (Fig. 4.8).

Surgical Technique

The authors follow an algorithmic approach to deal with a valgus knee during TKA principally based on their classification (Fig. 4.10). Although the classical medial parapatellar approach is effective in the majority of valgus knees for TKA, a lateral parapatellar approach is indicated in cases where severe valgus deformity is associated with patellar maltracking. This approach provides greater access to lateral soft-tissue structures in severe valgus since a medial approach and lateral displacement of the quadriceps complex here will externally rotate the tibia, pushing the contracted posterolateral corner of the tibia away from the operative field. Besides, a lateral release is a part of this approach which will help in restoring normal patellar tracking. Advocates of this approach have also cited better preservation of blood supply to the extensor mechanism with a lateral arthrotomy as

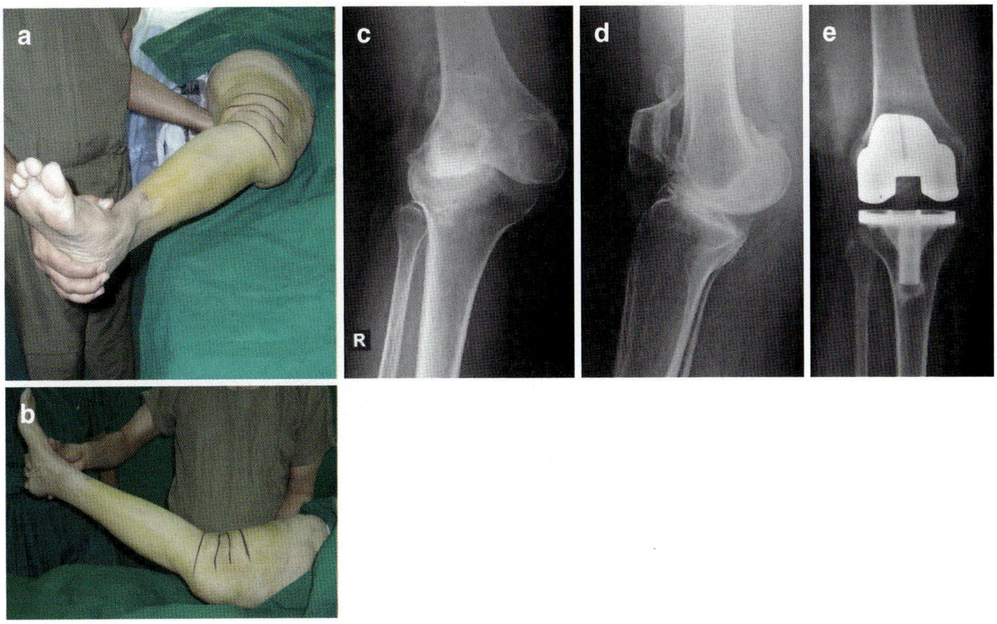

Fig. 4.6 Type 3 valgus deformity. (**a**) Clinical photograph showing maximum valgus deformity with a valgus stress applied with patient under anaesthesia. (**b**) Clinical photograph showing associated hyperextension deformity with patient under anaesthesia. (**c**) Preoperative standing anteroposterior knee radiograph showing the valgus deformity. (**d**) Preoperative lateral knee radiograph showing hyperextension at the knee joint. (**e**) Postoperative standing anteroposterior knee radiograph showing restoration of knee alignment with a cruciate-substituting design

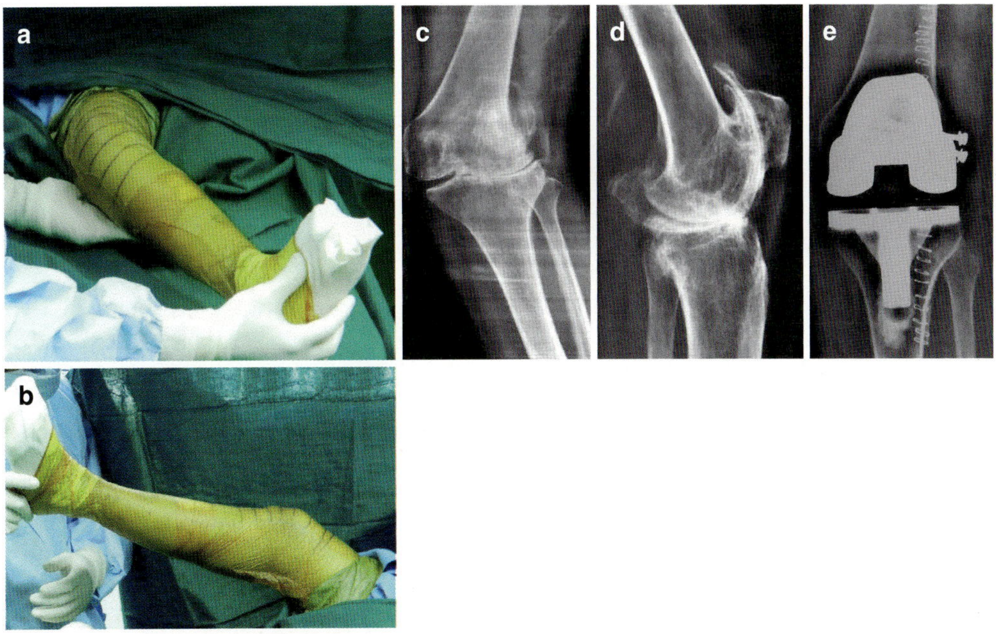

Fig. 4.7 Type 4 valgus deformity. (**a**) Clinical photograph showing maximum valgus deformity with a valgus stress applied with patient under anaesthesia. (**b**) Clinical photograph showing associated fixed flexion deformity with patient under anaesthesia. (**c**) Preoperative standing anteroposterior knee radiograph showing the valgus deformity. (**d**) Preoperative lateral knee radiograph showing large posterior femoral osteophyte. (**e**) Postoperative standing anteroposterior knee radiograph showing restoration of knee alignment with a cruciate-substituting design. A lateral epicondylar osteotomy (*LEO*) was required in this case to achieve correction of valgus and flexion deformity and achieve medio-lateral soft-tissue balance

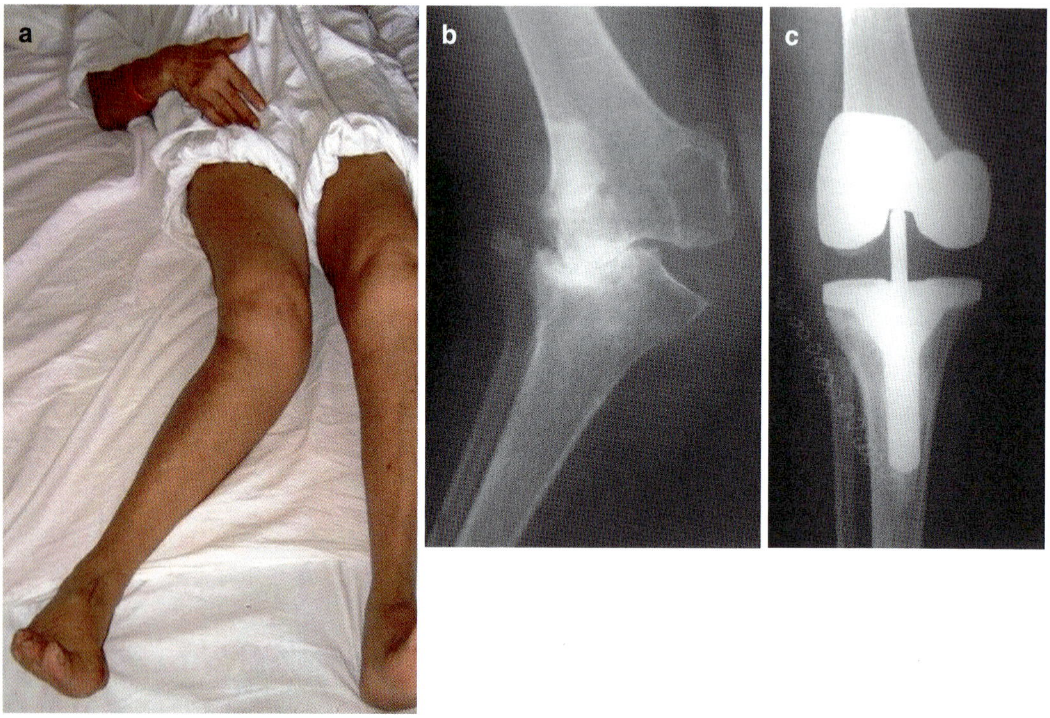

Fig. 4.8 Type 5 valgus deformity. (**a**) Clinical photograph showing severe valgus deformity of the knee. (**b**) Preoperative standing anteroposterior knee radiograph showing severe valgus deformity with a large medial joint space opening indicating an extremely lax or incompetent medial collateral ligament (MCL). (**c**) Postoperative standing anteroposterior knee radiograph showing restoration of knee alignment with a constrained design. Note the subperiosteal excision of fibular head to reduce risk of peroneal nerve palsy

compared to a medial arthrotomy combined with extensive lateral retinacular release for patellar maltracking [10, 11]. However, an inherent risk of this approach is the difficulty of achieving closure because of post-release deficiency of the flimsy soft-tissues inferior to the patella laterally. This may require achieving closure using a fat pad flap harvested from the infrapatellar fat pad [10]. Another disadvantage is the difficulty in accessing the medial aspect of the knee which may sometimes necessitate the need for a tibial tubercle osteotomy which carries the risk of patellar tendon failure and non-union.

The knee should be dislocated after excision of the cruciates with minimal or no release on the medial side. Any release here will only add to the excessive laxity of medial soft-tissue structures and will make medio-lateral soft-tissue balancing more difficult subsequently. Prior to any lateral soft-tissue release, all osteophytes from the lateral and posterolateral aspect of tibia and femur should be removed (Fig. 4.2a, b). Although removal of lateral tibial or femoral osteophytes has minimal effect on the LCL, this helps in reducing the tethering of posterolateral capsule. In severe valgus deformities, a subperiosteal excision of the fibular head, made easier through a lateral arthrotomy, helps in significantly reducing the tenting of LCL and also reduces the risk of stretching of the common peroneal nerve after the deformity has been fully corrected (Fig. 4.11). After excision of the PCL, an initial release of the IT band with the knee in full knee extension helps in reducing lateral tightness. The IT band is typically released from the Gerdy's tubercle but can also be lengthened using multiple small incisions at the level of the knee joint with the knee placed in full extension with a varus stress to feel the taut IT band. Lateral tightness in full extension can be further reduced by releasing the posterolateral capsule. The authors perform this as close to the tibia as

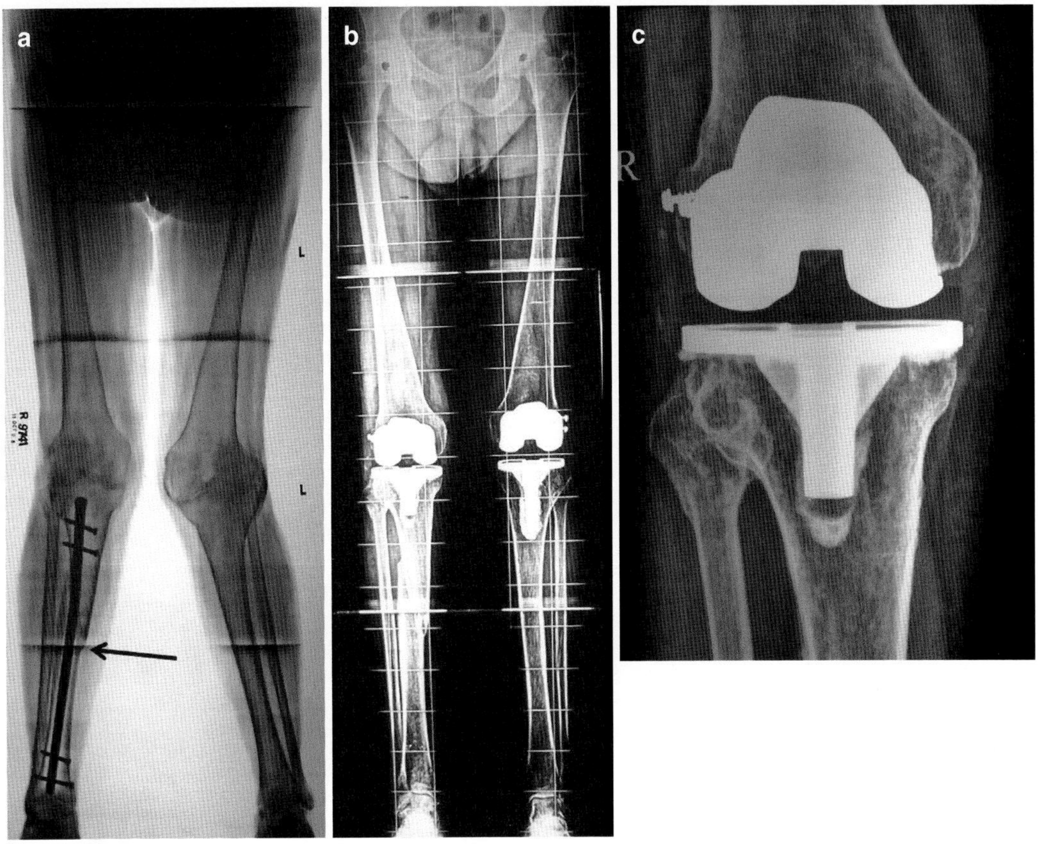

Fig. 4.9 Type 6 valgus deformity. (**a**) Preoperative standing hip-to-ankle radiograph showing valgus deformity with an associated extra-articular deformity at the mid-shaft of the right tibia (*arrow*) due to malunited fracture with an intramedullary nail in situ. (**b**) Postoperative standing hip-to-ankle radiograph showing complete restoration of the hip-knee-ankle axis. The intramedullary nail had to be removed before starting the total knee arthroplasty (TKA) procedure in order to accommodate the stem of the tibial tray. (**c**) Postoperative standing knee radiograph showing restoration of the knee alignment with a cruciate-substituting design. A lateral epicondylar osteotomy (LEO) was performed in this case to achieve deformity correction and medio-lateral soft-tissue balance

possible using electrocautery. Another method is by using multiple stab incisions with the knee placed in full extension. However, this technique is fraught with risk of damaging the common peroneal nerve [12] which maybe between 7 and 9 mm from the posterolateral capsule in full extension [13].

The tibial and distal femoral cuts are typically decided based on the degree and complexity of deformity with the medial side as reference. Minimal amount of bone needs to be resected in both severe valgus deformities and in knees with associated instability or hyperextension. The valgus correction angle (VCA) for distal femoral resection in valgus knees may be much lesser than for varus knees and is typically set at 3°. However, in an analysis of 503 limbs undergoing TKA by the authors, the mean VCA in 44 valgus limbs was found to be 5.9° ± 1.9° (range, 3.5–10°) [1]. Although the mean VCA in valgus limbs was significantly lesser when compared to mean VCA in varus limbs, 70 % of valgus limbs had a VCA of >5° (Fig. 4.12). Hence, owing to wide variation, VCA for distal femoral cut needs to be individualised for each case based on preoperative full-length hip-to-ankle radiographs.

Lateral tightness in flexion is reduced by freeing the popliteus tendon from surrounding fibrous tissue and releasing the popliteofibular

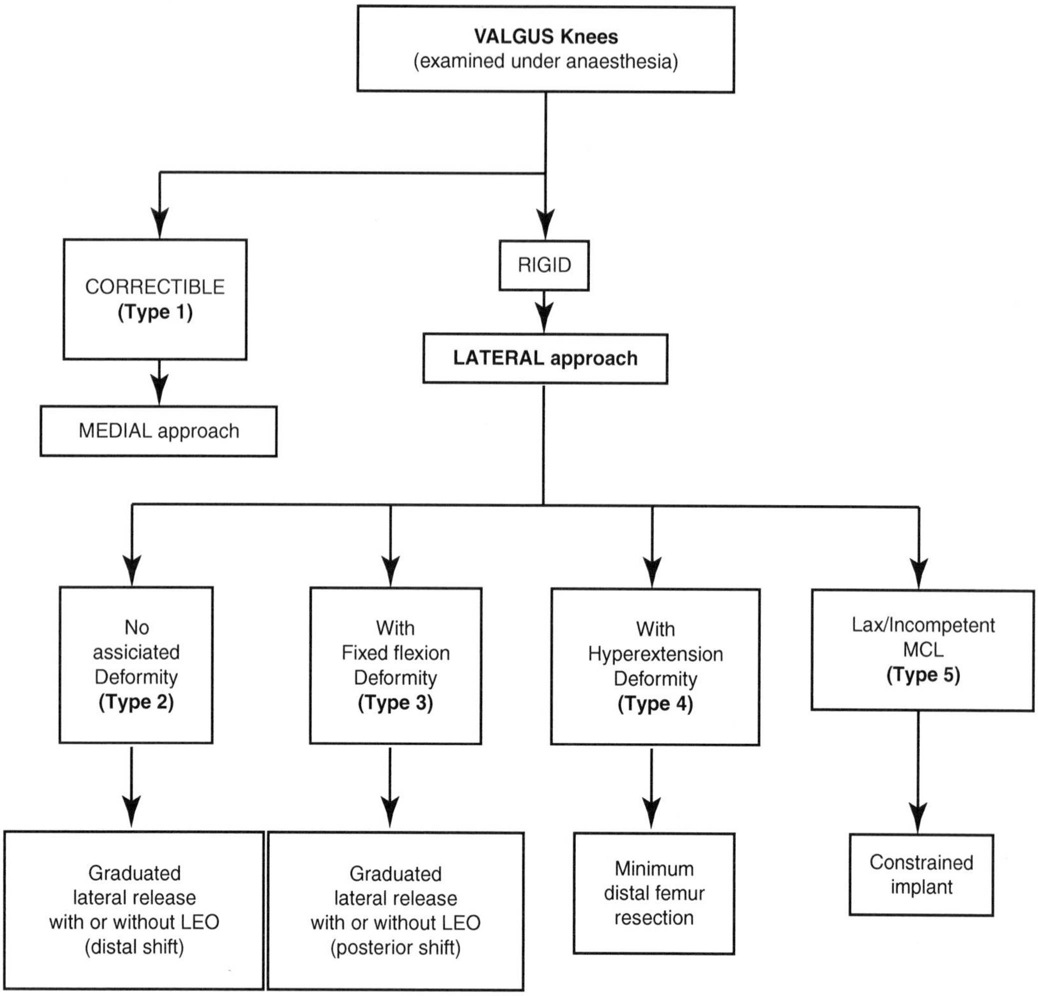

Fig. 4.10 Algorithm (based on the type of deformity) used by the authors to treat valgus deformity during TKA. *LEO* lateral epicondylar osteotomy

ligament. The popliteofibular ligament is a thin structure which runs from the inferior margin of the popliteus ligament to the head of the fibula. This structure is released by running the tip of the electrocautery below the inferior border of the popliteus tendon along the posterolateral corner of the knee joint (Fig. 4.13). If the posterior femur is resected in the presence of excessive lateral tightness, then the femoral component may get placed in excessive internal rotation. Hence, lateral tightness in flexion needs to be addressed and soft-tissue balance achieved before performing the posterior cuts.

The AP cutting guide is placed perpendicular to the transepicondylar axis (TEA). The size and position of the femoral component may have to be altered based on the extension gap previously achieved. The final alignment and balance are then checked using trial components. In full extension, a medial or lateral opening of >2 mm is considered abnormally lax. Similarly, in 90° flexion, a medial opening of >2 mm and a lateral opening of >4 mm are considered abnormally lax.

Patellar tracking is then checked throughout the knee range of motion with the trial components in place. Both abnormal tracking and lateral tilt of the patella are dealt with by serial, graduated release of the lateral retinaculum till the tracking is normal and there is no tilt. Very rarely, persistent maltracking of

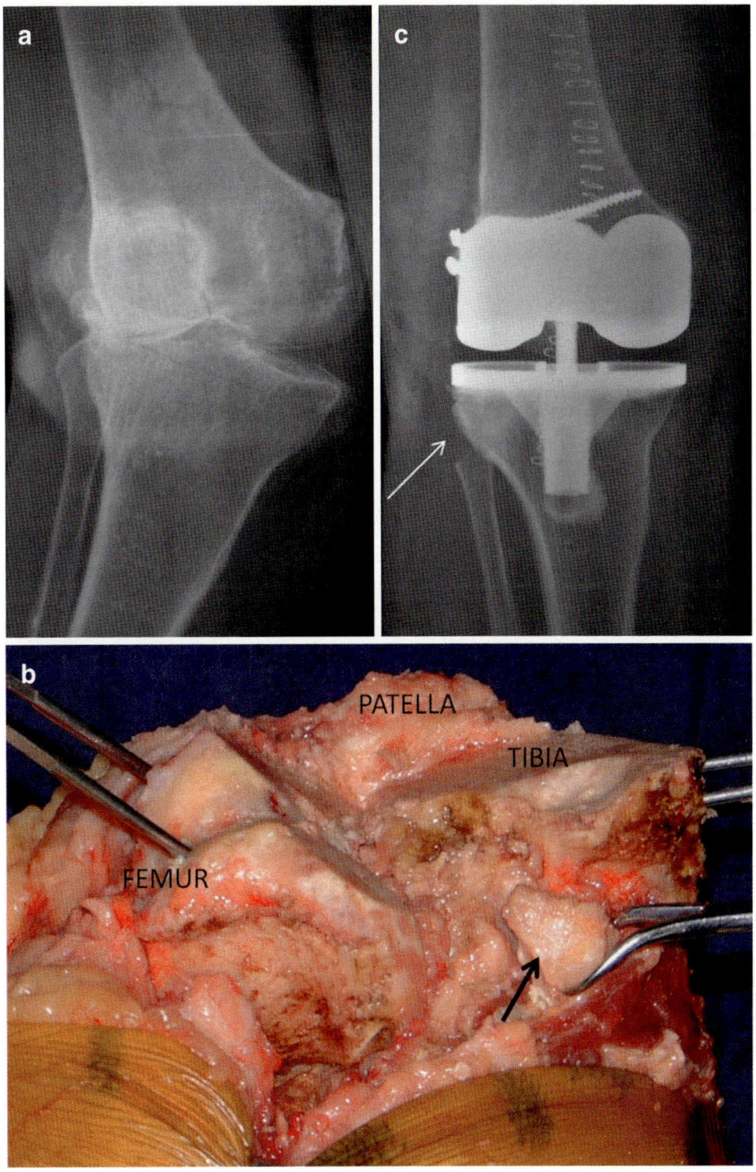

Fig. 4.11 Subperiosteal excision of the fibular head. (**a**) Preoperative standing knee radiograph showing severe valgus deformity. The fibular head adds to the tenting of the lateral collateral ligament (LCL). (**b**) Intraoperative photograph showing the exposed fibular head (*arrow*) which needs to be excised. A lateral approach was used in this case. (**c**) Postoperative standing anteroposterior knee radiograph showing restoration of knee alignment with a cruciate-substituting design. A lateral epicondylar osteotomy (LEO) along with subperiosteal excision of the fibular head (*arrow*) was required in order to restore alignment and balance in this rigid valgus deformity

the patella despite extensive lateral retinacular release may require plication and double breasting of the medial retinaculum during closure of the arthrotomy.

Severe Valgus Deformities (Type 5 and 6)

Profound valgus deformities of ≥15° present with their own challenges during TKA. Similar to profound varus knees, these can be associated with excessive laxity medially or excessive tightness laterally, severe bone loss on the lateral side and an associated extra-articular or sagittal plane deformity. Excessive valgus deformity may warrant the use of a lateral approach to facilitate easy access and release of lateral soft-tissue structures (Fig. 4.14). Excessive femoral bowing in the coronal plane commonly seen in severe varus deformities may also be present in severe valgus arthritic knees. However, in valgus knees the bowing may be in the reverse direction (i.e. excessive curvature of the femoral shaft medially) which may result in a low valgus correction angle (VCA) [1]. This

Fig. 4.12 Graph showing distribution of the valgus correction angle (VCA) in our series of 44 valgus limbs. The VCA in 70 % of valgus limbs was >5°

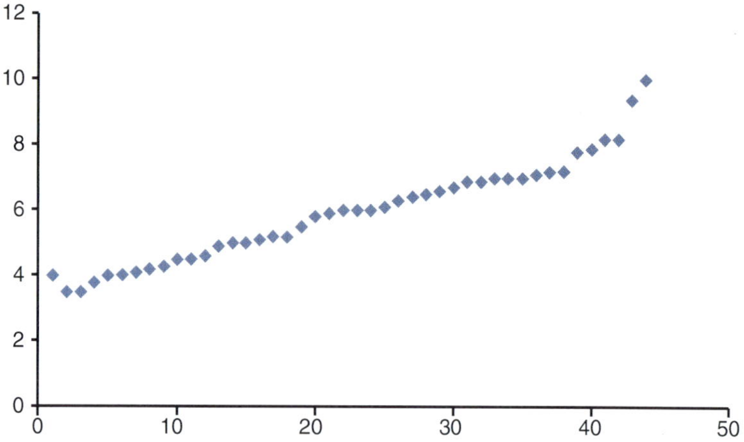

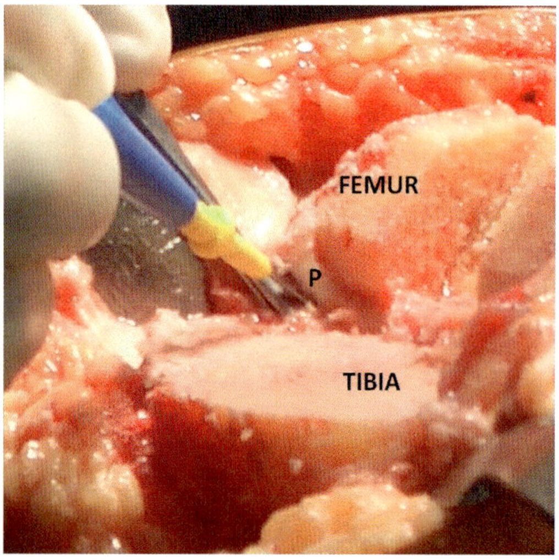

Fig. 4.13 Intraoperative photograph showing technique of releasing the popliteofibular ligament using cautery just below the popliteus tendon (*P*) close to the tibial cut surface

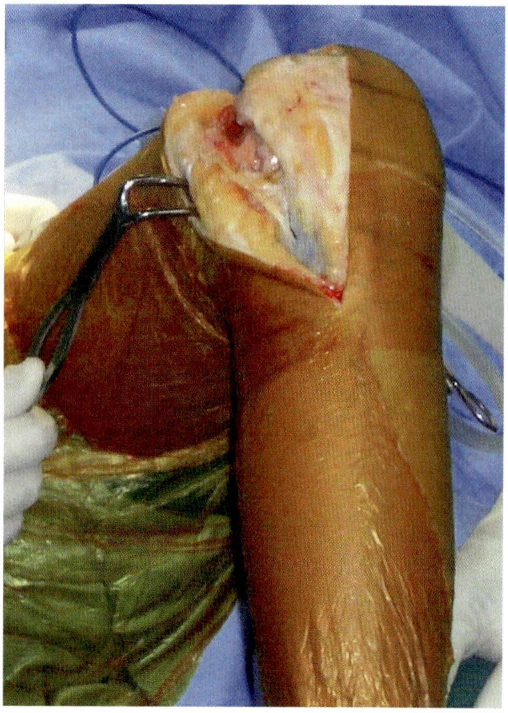

Fig. 4.14 Lateral approach to the knee used in rigid severe valgus deformities

needs to be determined on preoperative full-length radiographs and the calculated VCA used intraoperatively to execute the distal femoral cut. Similar to varus knees, in knees with severe valgus deformity, the amount of resection of the proximal tibia and distal femur needs to be kept at a minimum especially when associated with severe ligament laxity or an associated recurvatum deformity.

Very rarely, when substantial soft-tissue release laterally fails to correct deformity or achieve medial-lateral soft-tissue balance, a sliding lateral epicondylar osteotomy (LEO) may be indicated (Fig. 4.15) [14]. This should be ideally done under the guidance of computer navigation as this allows for accurate measurement of difference between the medial and lateral gaps and the amount of residual limb deformity and helps execute precise, controlled and quantitative lengthening of the lateral soft-tissue structures (lateral collateral ligament and popliteus tendon) (Fig. 4.16). Another alternative for dealing with excessive laxity medially in a valgus knee is to shorten the medial soft-

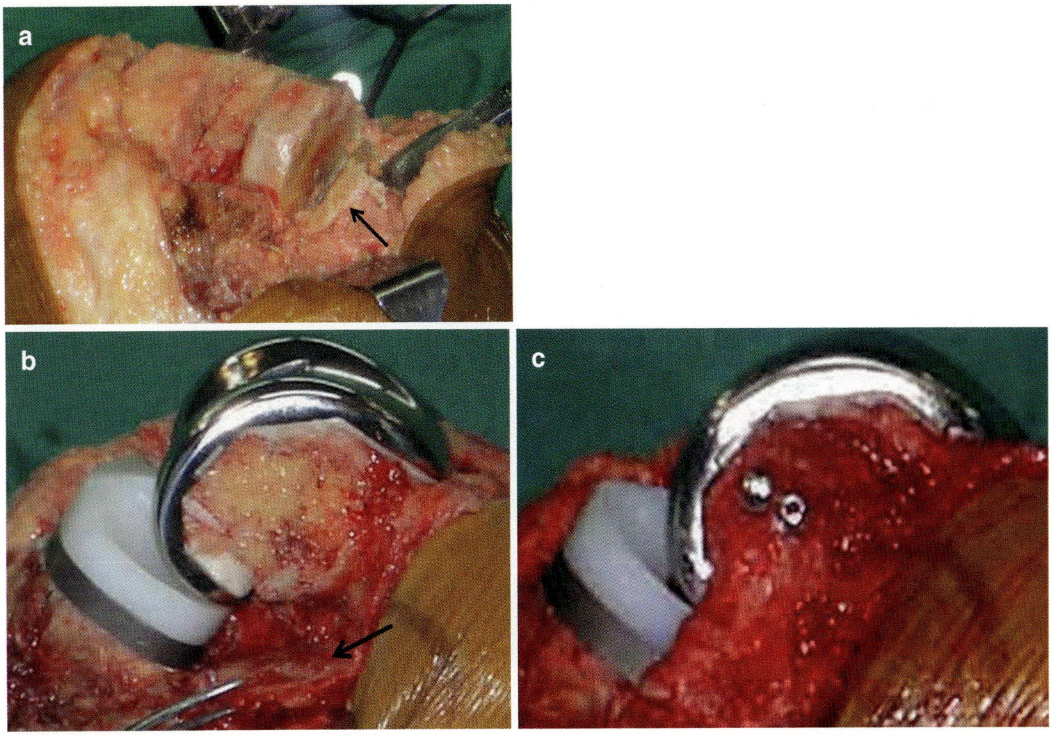

Fig. 4.15 Lateral epicondylar osteotomy (LEO). (**a**) Intraoperative photograph of the lateral epicondylar block (*arrow*) with its soft-tissue attachment separated from the lateral femoral condyle after all the femoral cuts have been performed. (**b**) Intraoperative photograph of the lateral epicondylar block (*arrow*) held with a towel clip after the femoral component has been cemented. (**c**) Intraoperative photograph of the lateral epicondylar block fixed in position using cancellous screw

tissue structure. This can be performed using several methods. These include MCL advancement from the tibial side or midsubstance division and imbrication of MCL [6]. Both these procedures have the disadvantage of affecting ligament strength and isometricity. Healy et al. [15] described a technique of detaching the femoral origin of the MCL with an epicondylar bone block. This medial epicondylar osteotomy (MEO) has the advantage of not causing direct damage to the MCL. The authors perform a sliding medial condylar osteotomy (SMCO) in a valgus knee whenever necessary using the technique described in the Chap. 3. Similar to the LEO, the authors prefer using computer navigation for performing SMCO in all their cases (for complete description of both these osteotomies, see Chap. 11). However, these procedures are rarely indicated and most severe and rigid valgus knees can be dealt with using a graduated lateral release with or without a LEO. Under certain rare circumstances when the MCL is too incompetent and is a cause of significant instability, a constrained prosthesis (with a taller post and deeper box) may be needed. However, every attempt must be made to balance the soft tissues so as not to excessively load the post leading to post wear and fracture.

Severe valgus knees with associated flexion deformity carry a high risk of postoperative common peroneal nerve palsy. Although this may be transient due to stretching of the nerve on full correction of the valgus and flexion deformities, this may cause considerable disability and distress in the patient causing delay in postoperative recovery. In knees with profound valgus deformity with associated significant fixed flexion deformity (≥20°), the authors undercorrect the flexion deformity to approximately less than 10°, keep the knee in flexion over a pillow for the first 48 h postoperatively to avoid undue stretching of the nerve and gradually correct it postoperatively using physiotherapy and occasionally a push-knee splint.

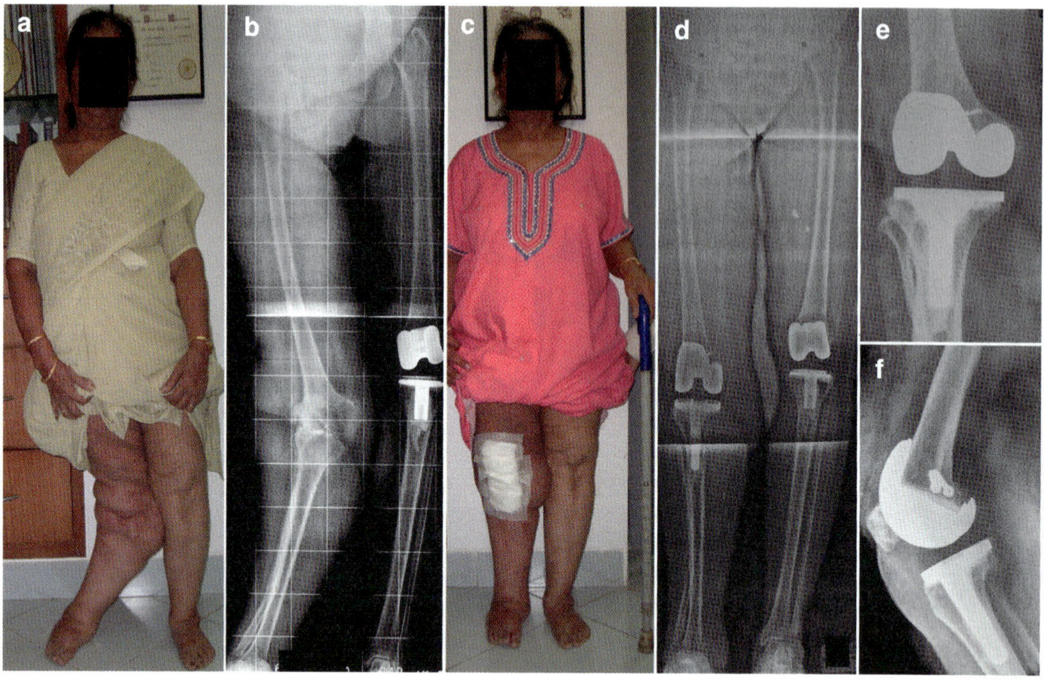

Fig. 4.16 Severe, rigid valgus deformity treated with computer-assisted TKA combined with lateral epicondylar osteotomy (LEO). (**a**) Preoperative clinical photograph of a patient showing severe valgus deformity of the right knee. (**b**) Preoperative standing hip-to-ankle radiograph of the same patient (**a**) showing severe valgus deformity of the right knee. (**c**) Postoperative clinical photograph of the same patient (**a**) at suture removal showing complete restoration of the right knee alignment. (**d**) Postoperative standing hip-to-ankle radiograph of the same patient (**a**) showing complete restoration of the right knee alignment after computer-assisted TKA combined with LEO. (**e**) Postoperative standing anteroposterior knee radiograph of the same patient (**a**) at 4 years follow-up showing complete restoration of the right knee alignment. (**f**) Postoperative lateral knee radiograph of the same patient (**a**) at 4 years follow-up showing cancellous screws used for LEO

Computer-Assisted Technique

The basic technique of computer-assisted TKA in valgus knees is similar to the one previously described for varus knees. Apart from assisting in performing precise bone cuts and graduated soft-tissue release and verification of limb alignment, bone cuts and soft-tissue tension, the optimised gap-balancing feature of the computer software helps in equalising the flexion gap to the extension gap by adjusting the level of distal femoral resection and the femoral component size and position. In limbs where an additional lateral epicondylar osteotomy (LEO) may be required, navigation allows for precise, controlled, quantitative lengthening of the tight lateral soft-tissue structures and proper restoration of limb alignment and soft-tissue balance [14].

References

1. Mullaji AB, Shetty GM, Kanna R, Vadapalli RC. The influence of preoperative deformity on valgus correction angle: an analysis of 503 total knee arthroplasties. J Arthroplasty. 2013;28:20–7.
2. Mullaji AB, Shetty GM, Lingaraju AP, Bhayde S. Which factors increase risk of malalignment of the hip-knee-ankle axis in TKA? Clin Orthop Relat Res. 2013;471:134–41.
3. Whiteside LA. Selective ligament release in total knee arthroplasty of the knee in valgus. Clin Orthop Relat Res. 1999;367:130–40.
4. Matsuda S, Miura H, Nagamine R, Mawatari T, Tokunaga M, Nabeyama R, Iwamoto Y. Anatomical

analysis of the femoral condyle in normal and osteoarthritic knees. J Orthop Res. 2004;22:104–9.

5. Whiteside LA, Arima J. The anteroposterior axis for femoral rotational alignment in valgus total knee arthroplasty. Clin Orthop Relat Res. 1995;321:168–72.
6. Favorito PJ, Mihalko WM, Krackow KA. Total knee arthroplasty in the valgus knee. J Am Acad Orthop Surg. 2002;10:16–24.
7. Mullaji A, Shetty GM. Persistent hindfoot valgus causes lateral deviation of weightbearing axis after total knee arthroplasty. Clin Orthop Relat Res. 2011;469:1154–60.
8. Chandler JT, Moskal JT. Evaluation of knee and hindfoot alignment before and after total knee arthroplasty: a prospective analysis. J Arthroplasty. 2004;19:211–6.
9. Ranawat AS, Ranawat CS, Elkus M, Rasquinha VJ, Rossi R, Babhulkar S. Total knee arthroplasty for severe valgus deformity. J Bone Joint Surg Am. 2005;87 Suppl 1:271–84.
10. Keblish PA. The lateral approach to the valgus knee. Surgical technique and analysis of 53 cases with over two-year follow-up evaluation. Clin Orthop Relat Res. 1991;271:52–62.
11. Sekiya H, Takatoku K, Takada H, Sugimoto N, Hoshino Y. Lateral approach is advantageous in total knee arthroplasty for valgus deformed knee. Eur J Orthop Surg Traumatol. 2014;24:111–5.
12. Bruzzone M, Ranawat A, Castoldi F, Dettoni F, Rossi P, Rossi R. The risk of direct peroneal nerve injury using the Ranawat "inside-out" lateral release technique in valgus total knee arthroplasty. J Arthroplasty. 2010;25:161–5.
13. Jia Y, Gou W, Geng L, Wang Y, Chen J. Anatomic proximity of the peroneal nerve to the posterolateral corner of the knee determined by MR imaging. Knee. 2012;19:766–8.
14. Mullaji AB, Shetty GM. Lateral epicondylar osteotomy using computer navigation in total knee arthroplasty for rigid valgus deformities. J Arthroplasty. 2010;25:166–9.
15. Healy WL, Iorio R, Lemos DW. Medial reconstruction during total knee arthroplasty for severe valgus deformity. Clin Orthop Relat Res. 1998;356:161–9.

Part III

Sagittal Plane Deformities

Flexion Deformity

5

Introduction

Knees with degenerative or rheumatoid arthritis may have associated intra-articular inflammation and effusion because of which they may assume a position of flexion in response to the pain and increased intra-articular pressure. Posterior femoral and tibial osteophytes along with those in the intercondylar notch in OA may enhance the deformity by tenting the posterior capsule or blocking full extension. This, in the long run, becomes a fixed flexion deformity, adding to the disability of the patient. Knee arthritis with a fixed flexion deformity interferes with ambulation causing increased energy expenditure, decreased stride length and velocity, decreased endurance and inability to stand for long periods [1–5]. Flexion deformities are commonly encountered in knees with varus or valgus deformities. Isolated flexion deformities in knee arthritis are rare, although in some knees fixed flexion deformity may be the predominant deformity when compared to coronal plane deformities. It is estimated that flexion contractures may occur in up to 60 % of knees undergoing TKA [4]. Griffin et al. [6] reported the incidence of flexion contractures as 62 % in varus knees, 31 % in valgus knees and 26 % in neutral knees. This chapter aims to discuss the management of fixed flexion deformities in TKA.

Pathoanatomy

Flexion deformities in arthritic knees may result from intercondylar notch osteophytes which act as a mechanical block preventing full extension [7], whereas posterior osteophytes cause tenting of the posterior capsule which can enhance this deformity (Fig. 5.1). In long-standing cases, these osteophytes are associated with secondary contracture and shortening of soft-tissue structures such as the posterior capsule, posterior oblique ligament, semimembranosus (in varus knee) and popliteofibular ligament (in valgus knee) which add to the deformity. In severe cases, the hamstrings and gastrocnemius may also be affected. Rarely in patients with inflammatory arthritis, neuromuscular disorders, haemophilia or long-standing immobility, flexion deformity is primarily the result of isolated soft-tissue contractures, and minimal osteophytes may be present (Fig. 5.2).

Consequences of long-standing flexion deformities in arthritic knees include bone loss on the posterior aspect of the tibial plateau and reduction of quadriceps strength leading to persistent extensor lag postoperatively. The latter is typically masked preoperatively due to the flexion deformity and becomes obvious once the flexion deformity has been fully corrected with TKA. It is necessary to keep this in mind and inform the patient regarding the possible need for extensive

A.B. Mullaji, G.M. Shetty, *Deformity Correction in Total Knee Arthroplasty*,
DOI 10.1007/978-1-4939-0566-9_5,

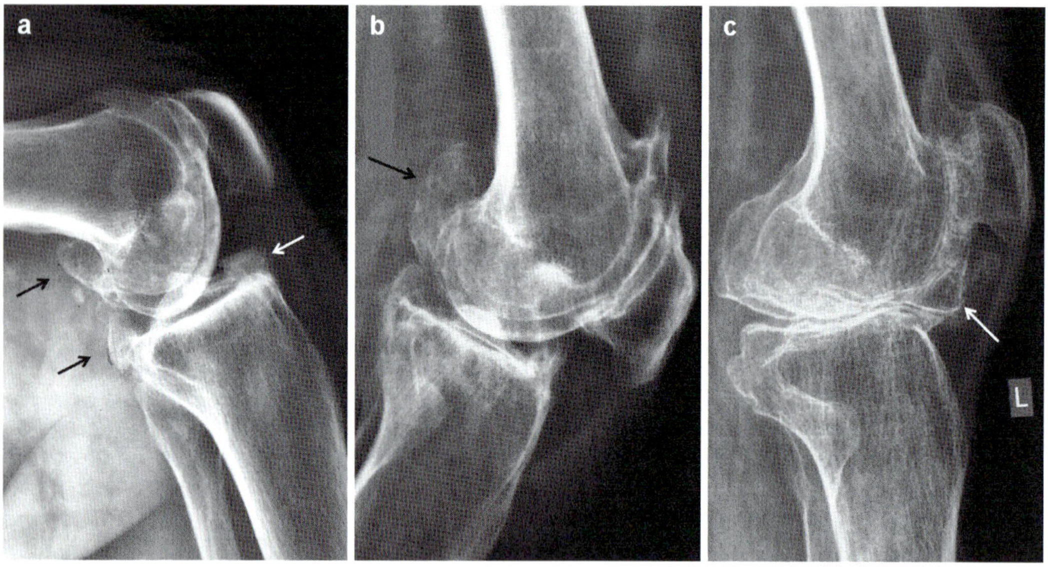

Fig. 5.1 Osteophytes in knees with flexion deformity undergoing TKA. (**a**) Lateral radiograph of the knee showing anterior tibial or "anvil" osteophyte (*white arrow*) and posterior tibial and femoral osteophytes (*black arrows*). Osteophytes at all these three locations can contribute to flexion deformity, anterior tibial osteophyte by mechanically blocking knee extension and posterior osteophytes by tenting soft-tissue structures. (**b**) Lateral radiograph of the knee showing a large posterior femoral osteophyte (*arrow*) which should be completely removed to not only achieve correction of flexion deformity but also prevent postoperative restriction of terminal flexion. (**c**) Lateral radiograph of the knee showing large osteophytes all around the knee joint including large, multiple osteophytes in the patellofemoral joint (*arrow*)

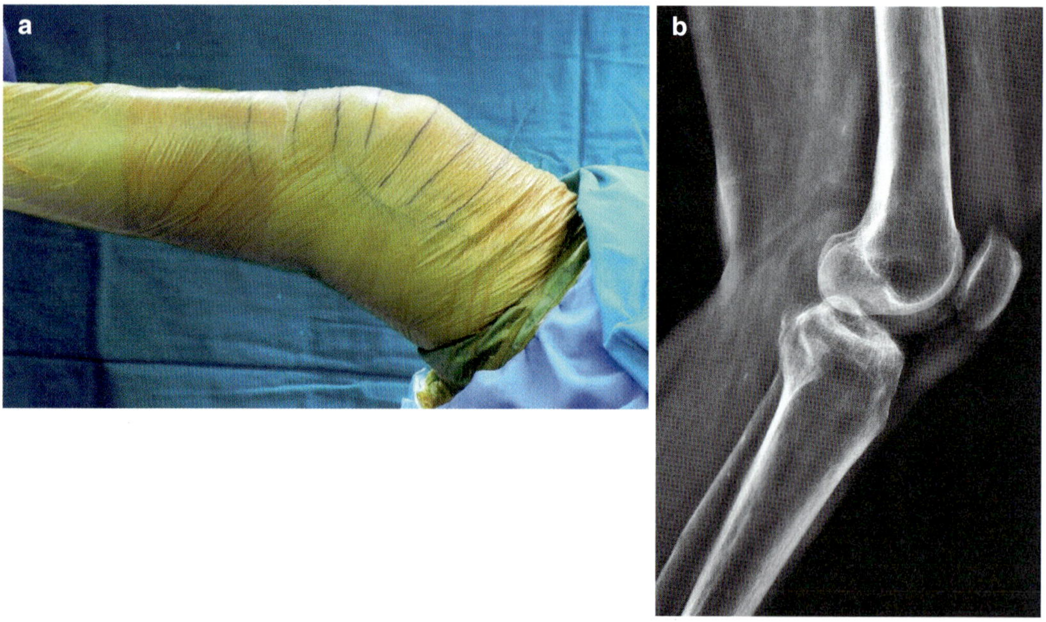

Fig. 5.2 Fixed flexion deformity of the knee due to contracture of soft-tissue structures. (**a**) Intraoperative clinical photograph of a patient showing fixed flexion deformity of almost 30°. (**b**) Lateral knee radiograph of the same patient showing absence of osteophytes around the knee joint. The flexion deformity in this patient with rheumatoid arthritis was purely due contracture of soft-tissue structures

Table 5.1 Classification of flexion contractures

Grade 1: <10°
Grade 2: 10°–30°
Grade 3: >30°

postoperative physiotherapy not only to maintain correction of the flexion deformity but also to strengthen the quadriceps. Lombardi et al. [8] have divided flexion deformities encountered in patients undergoing TKA into three grades based on the severity of deformity (Table 5.1). The primary step in correcting flexion deformity is to remove all osteophytes whenever present in order to remove their tenting effect on soft tissues. This usually takes care of most mild to moderate deformities. However, severe deformities may require an additional soft-tissue release posteriorly.

The flexion gap is much larger than the extension gap in an arthritic knee with flexion deformity. This mismatch is further increased when there is an associated severe coronal plane deformity requiring extensive medial or lateral soft-tissue release. This mismatch can be addressed to a certain extent with a posterior soft-tissue release. However, if the extension gap continues to be small, 2 mm of additional bone may need to be resected from the distal femur. Another method is to upsize the femoral component so as to close the flexion gap relative to the extension gap.

Surgical Technique

The first step, after exposure, to deal with flexion deformity is to remove all osteophytes. The medial and posteromedial tibial and medial femoral osteophytes need to be excised first followed by posterior femoral osteophytes. These posterior osteophytes can be approached and removed using a curved osteotome after subluxating the tibia forwards and placing the osteotome between the posteromedial corner of the tibia and the medial femoral condyle. The osteotome can also be inserted through the intercondylar notch at an oblique or transverse angle around the lateral edge of the medial femoral condyle. However, sometimes when the posterior osteophytes are too large, these can be better accessed and removed only after the tibial cut has been performed or by performing a preliminary freehand resection of the posterior femoral condyle. Removal of the posterior osteophytes prior to performing the distal femoral resection is important; it reduces the need for excess distal femoral resection and obviates or minimises the need for soft-tissue release thereby reducing the likelihood of mid-flexion instability.

The tibial cut needs to be adequate since the extension gap in arthritic knees with associated flexion deformity tends to be smaller when compared to the flexion gap. This discrepancy will get more pronounced after a medio-lateral soft-tissue release is performed to address an associated varus/valgus deformity or if an additional posterior release is performed for the flexion deformity. The authors typically remove 8–10 mm of the proximal tibia with reference to the unaffected side (Fig. 5.3). Before assessing medio-lateral gap balance in full extension, the surgeon needs to make sure that all posterior osteophytes and loose bodies have been removed so that the extension gap can be accurately judged. Any retained posterior osteophytes will result in an underestimation of the extension gap (Fig. 5.4). Rarely, if the flexion deformity persists despite complete posterior clearance, a posterior soft-tissue (posterior capsule, medial and lateral head of gastrocnemius) release is required. The authors perform this using a broad gouge which is applied flush to the femoral condyles and the soft tissues are gently stripped from their femoral attachment (Fig. 5.5). In severe cases, the capsule is divided with cautery midway between the femoral and tibial attachments on either side of the midline (so as not to damage the neurovascular bundle) with the knee held distracted with laminar spreaders in extension. The amount of distal femoral cut is decided based on the severity of associated coronal plane deformity and soft-tissue laxity. If there is an associated severe varus or valgus deformity, less bone may need to be resected from the distal femur. Leaving the pins that hold the distal cutting block behind till after the extension gap has been assessed allows one to revisit the cut if inadequate.

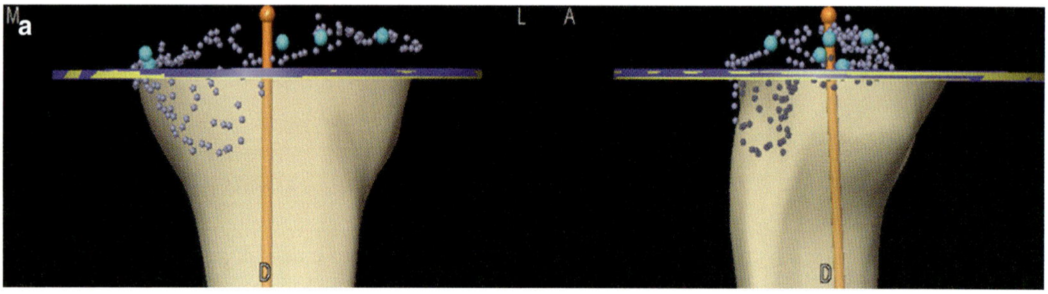

	Varus/Valgus	Resect High	Resect Low	Slope
Planned	0.0° Var	8.5 mm	2.0 mm	3.0° Post
Verified	0.5° Var	8.5 mm	2.0 mm	3.5° Post
Deviation	0.5° Var	0.0 mm	0.0 mm	0.5° Post

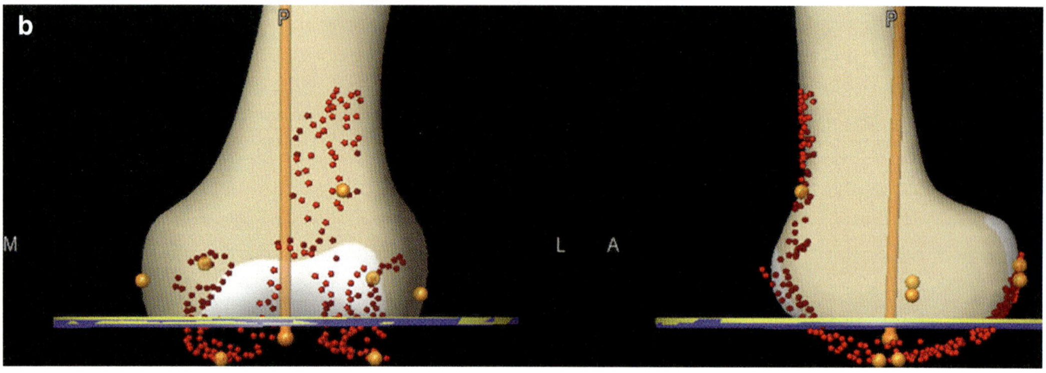

	Varus/Valgus	Resection	Flexion/Extension
Planned	0.0° Var	10.0 mm	1.5° Flex
Verified	0.5° Var	9.5 mm	1.5° Flex
Deviation	0.5° Valg	-0.5 mm	0.0° Flex

Fig. 5.3 Intraoperative computer screen snapshots of TKA performed in a patient with flexion deformity. The proximal tibial and distal femoral cuts need to be adequate since the extension gap in arthritic knees with associated flexion deformity tends to be smaller when compared to the flexion gap. (**a**) Thickness of proximal tibial resection is 8.5 mm. (**b**) Thickness of distal femoral resection is 9.5 mm

Subsequent assessment of the flexion gap usually shows that the extension gap previously achieved is much smaller than the flexion gap (Fig. 5.6a, b). This mismatch is addressed by adjusting the size and position of the femoral component. Upsizing, posteriorly shifting and slightly flexing the femoral component usually help in closing the large flexion gap and equalising it to the extension gap (Fig. 5.6c). Rarely, slight flexion deformity may persist despite all the above measures when the limb is assessed using trial components. We address this by resecting 2–3 mm from the distal femur. However, this should be performed cautiously as

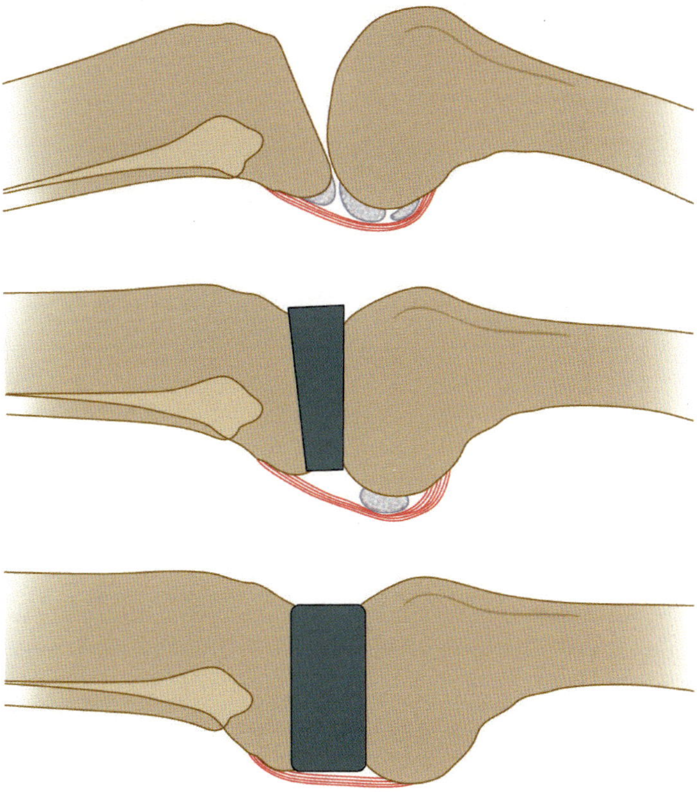

Fig. 5.4 Effect of posterior osteophytes on the extension gap during TKA. (**a**) Posterior tibial and femoral osteophytes cause tenting of posterior soft-tissue structures adding to the flexion deformity. (**b**) Incomplete removal of these posterior osteophytes can cause underestimation of the extension gap and may lead to error in flexion-extension gap balancing. (**c**) Complete posterior clearance (of osteophytes and loose bodies) is necessary with or without additional posterior soft-tissue release to ensure accurate assessment of the extension gap

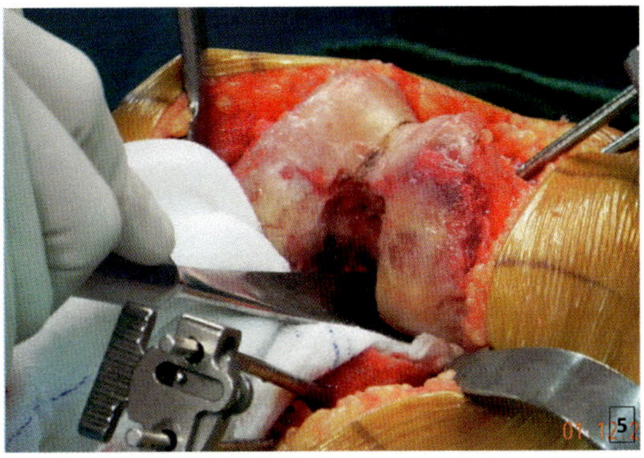

Fig. 5.5 Posterior soft-tissue release. Whenever required, this can be performed using a broad gouge (padded by a sponge) applied flush to the femoral condyles to gently strip soft tissue from their femoral attachment. Note that this is best performed after the tibial cut to allow easy access posteriorly

excessive resection from the distal femur may cause elevation of the joint line and mid-flexion instability.

Although seen very rarely, long-standing flexion deformities may be sometimes associated with severe contracture and shortening of the hamstring tendons. These shortened tendons can be felt on the posteromedial aspect of the knee joint as chords which typically get taut when the knee is extended. We usually address this after the trial implants are in place by doing a fractional lengthening of the contracted tendons using a separate incision on the posterior aspect of the knee directly over the taut, palpable tendon. Postoperative management is based on the degree of correction achieved and the amount of residual flexion contracture at the end of the procedure. A postoperative residual flexion contracture of $<5°$ can be managed with routine physiotherapy (Fig. 5.7). However, any correctible residual contracture between 5° and 10° at the end of the procedure, especially in patients where the flexion deformity was long-standing or exceeding 15–20°, will require application of an

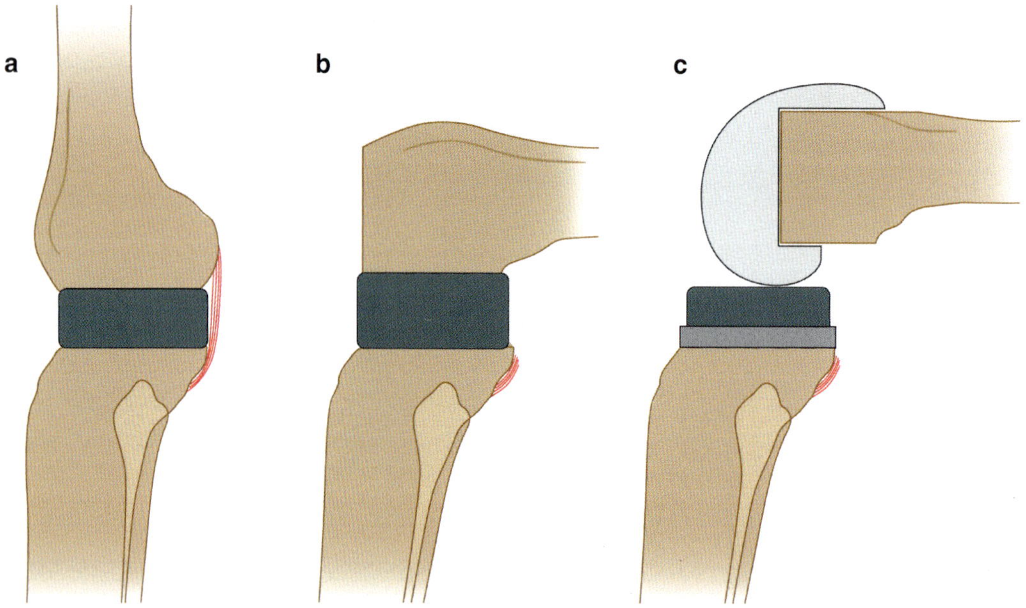

Fig. 5.6 Flexion-extension gap balancing during TKA in a patient with flexion deformity. (**a**) The extension gap tends to be smaller in knees with flexion deformity due to tautness of the posterior soft-tissue structures. Posterior release and additional resection of 2 mm from distal femur helps to increase this gap. (**b**) The flexion gap tends to be much larger compared to the extension gap in knees with flexion deformity. This difference is further increased when there is an associated severe coronal plane deformity requiring extensive medial or lateral soft-tissue release. (**c**) Upsizing, posteriorly shifting and slightly flexing the femoral component usually help in closing the large flexion gap and equalising it to the extension gap

above-knee plaster splint for 48 h postoperatively in order to maintain the knee in maximum correction. These patients may subsequently require a push-knee splint or a long knee brace while walking in order to maintain correction of the flexion contracture. However, irrespective of the amount of residual flexion contracture at the end of the procedure, these patients need careful surveillance during the postoperative rehabilitation period for signs of recurrence of flexion contracture which needs to be addressed aggressively using appropriate splints and physiotherapy.

Another common feature in patients with long-standing flexion contracture is an associated significant quadriceps weakness. This is usually not obvious preoperatively and gets unmasked postoperatively after the flexion contracture has been corrected. This may require prolonged physiotherapy in order to strengthen the quadriceps. Most patients with >20° of FFD preoperatively are given a push-knee splint for 30 min three times a day and while walking in the initial 2–4 weeks along with electrical stimulation of the quadriceps to strengthen them.

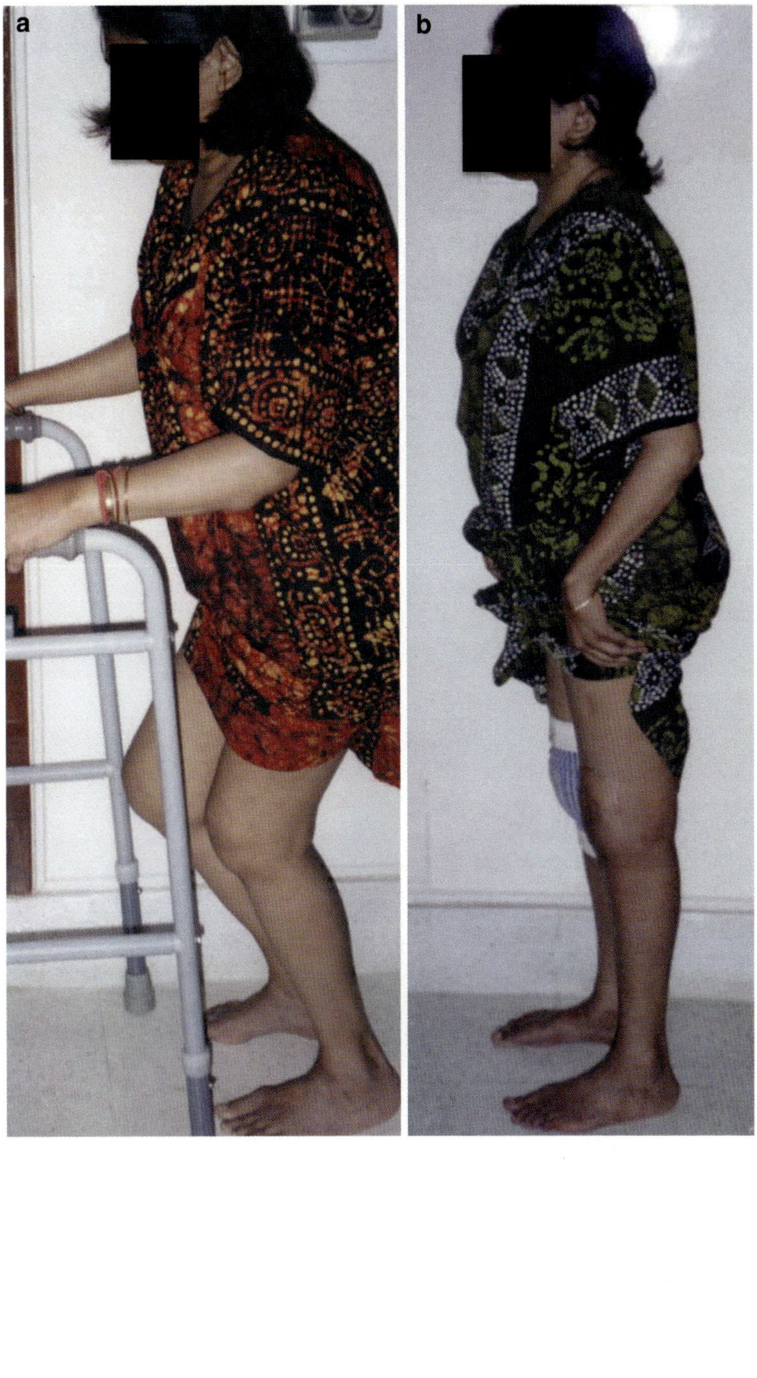

Fig. 5.7 Severe flexion deformity. (**a**) Preoperative clinical photograph of a patient showing severe bilateral flexion deformity. (**b**) Postoperative clinical photograph of the same patient (**a**) at suture removal showing complete correction bilateral flexion deformities with TKA and routine postoperative physiotherapy

Computer-Assisted Technique

The basic surgical technique for computer-assisted TKA in knees with flexion contractures is similar to the one previously described for conventional TKA. As previously described, adequate bone needs to be resected from both the proximal tibia and distal femur. Complete posterior clearance of osteophytes and loose bodies is necessary before assessing and recording the extension gap. The flexion gap is expected to be greater than the extension gap, especially in knees with severe flexion deformity. The *optimised gap-balancing* feature of the computer software can be used to simulate equalisation of flexion gap to the extension gap by simultaneously adjusting the level of distal femoral resection and the femoral component size and position (Fig. 5.8). Commonly, upsizing, posteriorly shifting (by 2–3 mm) and slightly flexing (usually 3–5°) the femoral component may be required to close the larger flexion gap and equalise it to the extension gap.

Navigation, as always, allows for measured and controlled soft-tissue release and bone cuts as per the amount of deformity and soft-tissue imbalance present in each knee. Navigation also helps the surgeon quantify the final extension alignment of the limb in the sagittal plane and ensure that the limb is not left in residual flexion deformity at the end of the procedure which may persist and then limit patient function and satisfaction postoperatively.

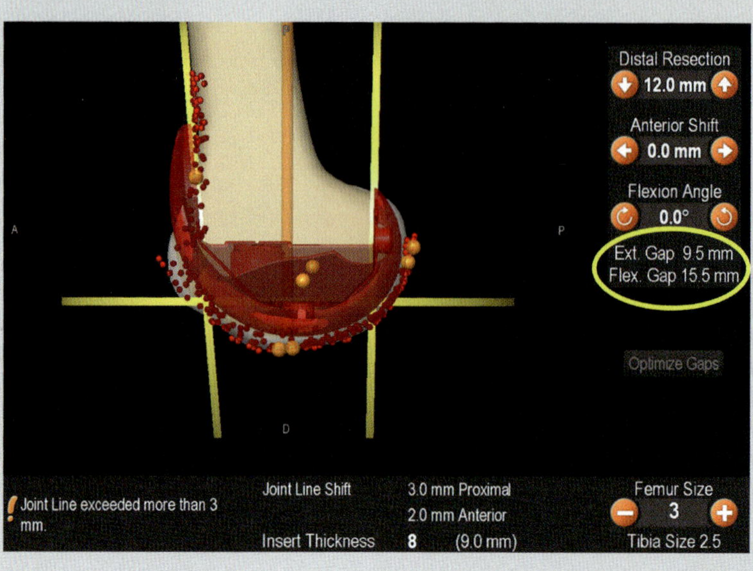

Fig. 5.8 Intraoperative computer screen snapshot showing the optimised gap-balancing feature of the navigation software. This can be used to simulate equalisation of flexion gap to the extension gap by simultaneously adjusting the level of distal femoral resection and the femoral component size and position. Note the large discrepancy between the flexion and the extension gap typically seen in arthritis knees with flexion deformity

References

1. Perry J, Antonelli D, Ford W. Analysis of knee-joint forces during flexed-knee stance. J Bone Joint Surg Am. 1975;57:961–7.
2. Harato K, Nagura T, Matsumoto H, Otani T, Toyama Y, Suda Y. Knee flexion contracture will lead to mechanical overload in both limbs: a simulation study using gait analysis. Knee. 2008;15:467–72.
3. Harato K, Nagura T, Matsumoto H, Otani T, Toyama Y, Suda Y. A gait analysis of simulated knee flexion contracture to elucidate knee-spine syndrome. Gait Posture. 2008;28:687–92.
4. Su EP. Fixed flexion deformity and total knee arthroplasty. J Bone Joint Surg Br. 2012;94(11 Suppl A):112–5.
5. Krych AJ, Pagnano MW. Flexion contractures: getting it straight. Semin Arthroplasty. 2009;20:38–9.
6. Griffin FM, Insall JN, Scuderi GR. Accuracy of soft tissue balancing in total knee arthroplasty. J Arthroplasty. 2000;15:970–3.
7. León HO, Blanco CE, Guthrie TB, Martínez OJ. Intercondylar notch stenosis in degenerative arthritis of the knee. Arthroscopy. 2005;21:294–302.
8. Lombardi AJ, Mallory T, Adams J. A stepwise algorithmic approach to flexion contractures in total knee arthroplasty. Arch Am Acad Orthop Surg. 1997;1:1–8.

6 Hyperextension Deformity

Introduction

Hyperextension deformity is uncommon in arthritic knees undergoing total knee arthroplasty (TKA), occurring in less than 5 % of patients [1–3]. In a recent study by the authors [3], the overall incidence of hyperextension in arthritic knees undergoing TKA was 3.9 % (45/1,150 limbs). Hyperextension can be encountered in patients with valgus deformities and excessive ligamentous laxity, in patients with rheumatoid arthritis (RA), in patients post high tibial osteotomy (HTO) and in patients with neuromuscular disorders such as poliomyelitis [4–6]. The results of our study indicated that the majority of patients with hyperextending, arthritic knees suffered from primary osteoarthritis (78 %) and 58 % of the limbs had an associated preoperative varus deformity compared to 42 % which had a valgus deformity [3].

Treating a hyperextending, arthritic knee with TKA could be challenging due to associated coronal plane deformities (varus or valgus), bony abnormalities such as reverse sloping of the tibial plateau and significant medio-lateral instability which may lead to difficulty in achieving a stable, well-balanced knee and the possibility of recurrence postoperatively [1–3]. Surgical techniques to deal with hyperextension during TKA includes posterior capsular plication, proximal and posterior transfer of the collateral ligaments, tightening the extension gap using thicker inserts, under-resecting the bone, undersizing the femoral component, using distal femoral augmentation blocks and using a constrained prosthesis [1–3, 7]. However, the technique of under-resection of tibia and femur, over-resection of the posterior surfaces of the femur, using a smaller femoral size with bone resection being done first and ligaments being balanced later will usually result in a stable, well-balanced knee [2, 3]. This chapter aims to outline the means of tackling hyperextension deformity during TKA.

Pathoanatomy

Arthritic knees with hyperextension have certain characteristic pathoanatomic features which need to be considered while performing a TKA. These are typically soft-tissue and bony abnormalities. Among the soft tissues, the posterior capsule is usually overstretched, causing hyperextension at the knee joint. This is associated with attenuation of the cruciate and collateral ligaments. These structural changes convert the posterior soft-tissue structures of the knee joint into a "hammock" (Fig. 6.1a) which needs to be made taut in order to correct this sagittal plane deformity and restore soft-tissue balance. In knees with associated valgus deformities, the iliotibial band may be contracted and anteriorly displaced which may accentuate the hyperextension deformity.

Owing to this attenuation of posterior soft-tissue structures, the resultant extension gap is much larger compared to the flexion gap in hyperextension deformities (Fig. 6.1b). Hence,

A.B. Mullaji, G.M. Shetty, *Deformity Correction in Total Knee Arthroplasty*,
DOI 10.1007/978-1-4939-0566-9_6,

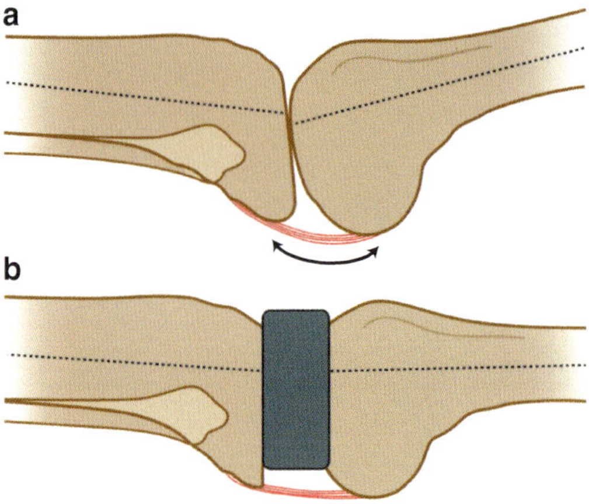

Fig. 6.1 Effect of posterior soft-tissue laxity and attenuation (posterior capsule particularly) in hyperextension deformity. (**a**) Overstretching and attenuation of the posterior capsule of the knee joint converts the posterior soft-tissue structures into a "hammock" in hyperextension deformities. (**b**) Owing to this attenuation of posterior soft-tissue structures, the resultant extension gap is much larger (compared to the flexion gap) in hyperextension deformity. Note that the tibial and the distal femoral bone cuts if too thick will significantly add to the already large extension gap

standard resections of proximal tibia and distal femur will further widen this extension gap, resulting in severe extension-flexion gap mismatch and an excessively large extension gap requiring a very thick insert. Hence, one of the basic principles of treating hyperextension deformity during TKA is to resect minimal bone from both proximal tibia and distal femur and strictly avoid release of posterior soft-tissue structures. Apart from these soft-tissue changes, hyperextension may be accentuated by bony abnormalities such as decreased posterior slope or anterior sloping of the tibia or significant wear or bone loss on the anterolateral or medial aspect of the tibial plateau (Fig. 6.2a). In patients who have undergone a previous high tibial osteotomy, impaction of the anterior tibial cortex may also result in an anterior slope (Fig. 6.2b). In either scenario, the surgeon needs to be careful to not aggravate the bony abnormality by resecting the proximal tibia with a neutral slope or, worse, an anterior slope.

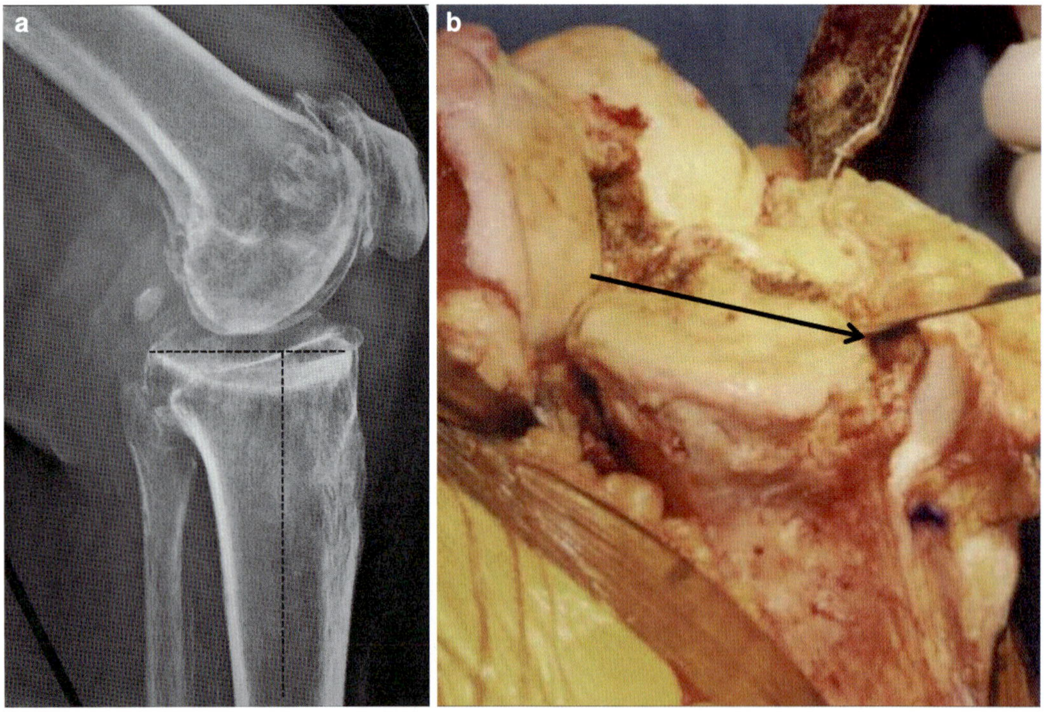

Fig. 6.2 Tibial slope in hyperextension deformity. (**a**) Lateral radiograph of the knee in a patient with hyperextension deformity shows an almost neutral tibial slope (*dotted line*). (**b**) Intraoperative photograph showing significant anterior sloping of the tibia (*arrow*). This patient was a case of post high tibial osteotomy TKA where significant anterior sloping of the tibia caused hyperextension at the knee joint

Rarely, hyperextension may be the consequence of a neuromuscular disorder such as poliomyelitis with associated bony deformities and muscular degeneration. These patients need to be thoroughly evaluated to assess the degree of neuromuscular deficit as they are at a higher risk for poor surgical outcome after TKA due to postoperative recurrence of hyperextension and instability with a standard posterior cruciate-substituting prosthesis or even one that is more constrained. Such cases may require a linked (hinged) device. We believe however that most of our cases are due to weak quadriceps where patients extend their knee to lock it by an altered posture and gait pattern.

Surgical Technique

The amount of bony resection is governed by the severity of the deformity: The greater the recurvatum, the less should be the resection. As per results of the retrospective study conducted by the authors on 45 computer-assisted TKAs done on arthritic knees with recurvatum deformity, the mean amount of proximal tibial and distal femoral bone resection was approximately 6.5 mm with respect to the good side [3]. Hence, the authors are careful not to resect more than 6–7 mm from the tibia and femur at the start of the procedure (Fig. 6.3). By retaining the pins that hold the cutting block in position, further resection is possible if needed to accommodate the thinnest spacer. Using the gap-balancing technique, the degree of soft-tissue release is decided by the amount of soft-tissue tightness assessed using a tensioning device. Generally these knees are quite lax and guarded releases have to be performed. Medial release for varus knees and lateral release for valgus knees is performed to restore the mechanical axis to 180°. Care is taken to perform no capsular release posteriorly. After the distal femoral and proximal tibial resections, a spacer block is used to confirm medio-lateral soft-tissue stability in full extension as well as the coronal alignment. A non-slotted AP cutting block is then positioned on the distal femur and the flexion gap is assessed with the same thickness spacer block that gave a satisfactory extension gap. Rotation is assessed based on the standard landmarks. A stylus or "angel wing" is used to ensure that no anterior notching occurs. If the flexion gap is found to equal the extension gap, the femoral size corresponding to the size of the AP block is confirmed. Slight alterations in position of the block can be made if 1–2 mm disparity exists in the gaps (provided that notching will not occur). Large disparities will need upsizing or, more likely, downsizing of the AP block. Once gaps are balanced, the AP cuts are completed; limb alignment and flexion-extension gap balancing are rechecked with the knee in full extension and 90° flexion using trial components. By following these basic principles, the vast majority of hyperextending knees can be managed with a regular cruciate-substituting implant without the need for a constrained prosthesis. From the analysis of our data of 45 TKAs done for hyperextending knees, most of the knees (92 %) were managed using inserts of thickness 12.5 mm or less and the remaining 8 % required inserts of thickness 15 mm [3]. None of the knees required inserts of thickness greater than 15 mm or constrained prostheses. The aim was to achieve a slight amount of flexion (2°–5°) at the end of the procedure [3].

The amount of proximal tibial and distal femoral resection, the extent of soft-tissue release, femoral sizing and the need for additional procedures (such as epicondylar osteotomy) were based on the degree of recurvatum deformity and the type of associated varus and valgus deformity. Postoperatively, the patient was allowed full weight-bearing walking and active knee flexion on the first postoperative day after drain removal. Patients were encouraged to keep a pillow below the knee for 2 weeks depending on the degree of recurvatum to allow tightening of the posterior soft-tissue structures. In cases with severe preoperative recurvatum where the recurvatum at the end of surgery was closer to 0°, a long-leg knee brace was used while walking for 2 weeks. No immobilisation was used routinely.

Hence, adhering to basic surgical principles of resecting less bone from the proximal tibia and distal femur and strictly refraining from performing a posterior release avoid the possibility of postoperative recurrence and ensure a successful outcome in these patients (Fig. 6.4).

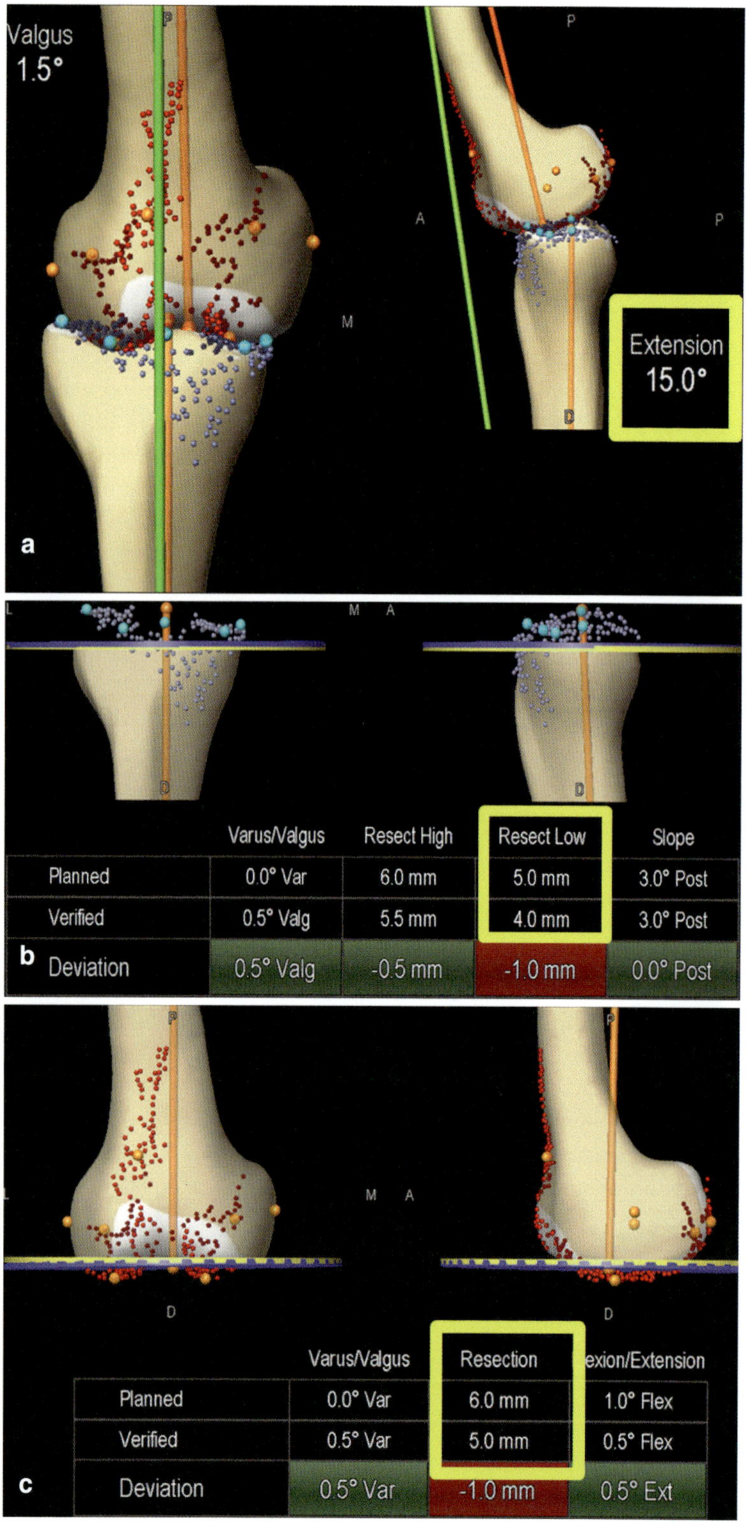

Fig. 6.3 Intraoperative computer screen snapshots of TKA performed in a patient with hyperextension deformity. (**a**) Patient has a combination of valgus (1.5°) and severe hyperextension deformity (15°). (**b**) Thickness of proximal tibial resection is limited to only 4 mm. (**c**) Thickness of distal femoral resection is limited to only 5 mm. (**d**) The knee has a final alignment of 1° varus and 6.5° flexion after components are cemented in place. (**e**) Intraoperative kinematics shows well-balanced medio-lateral gaps throughout the knee range of motion

Fig. 6.3 (continued)

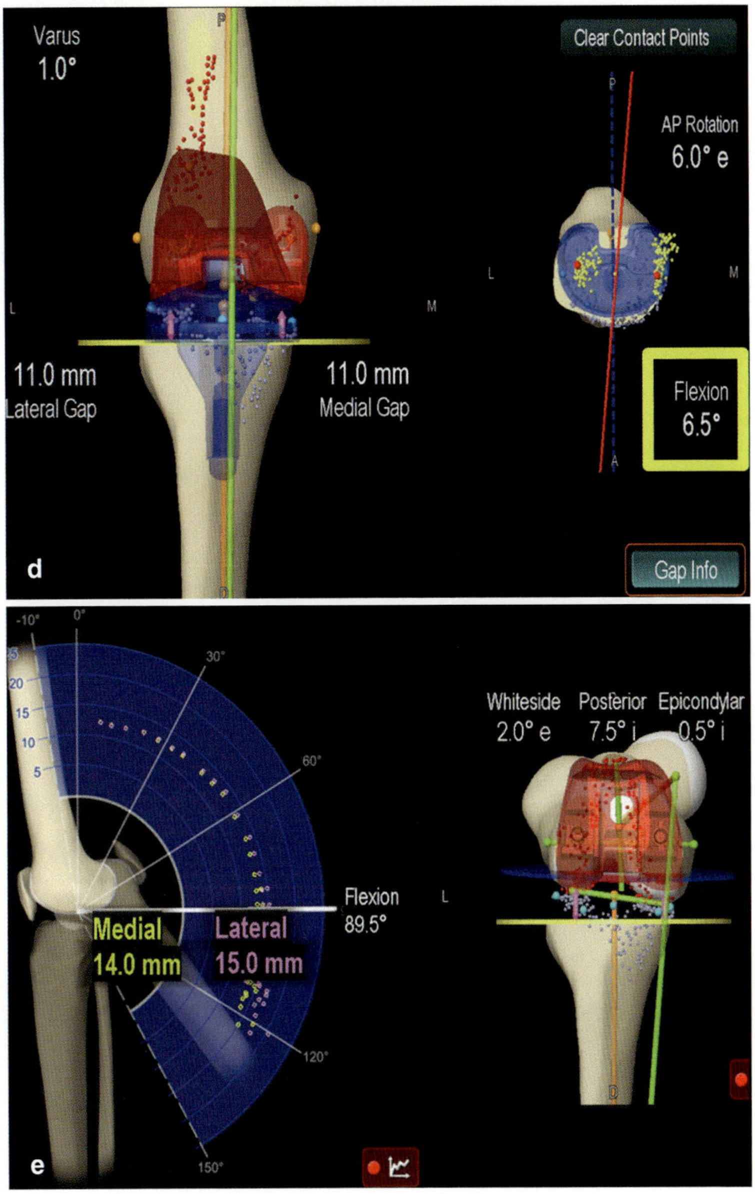

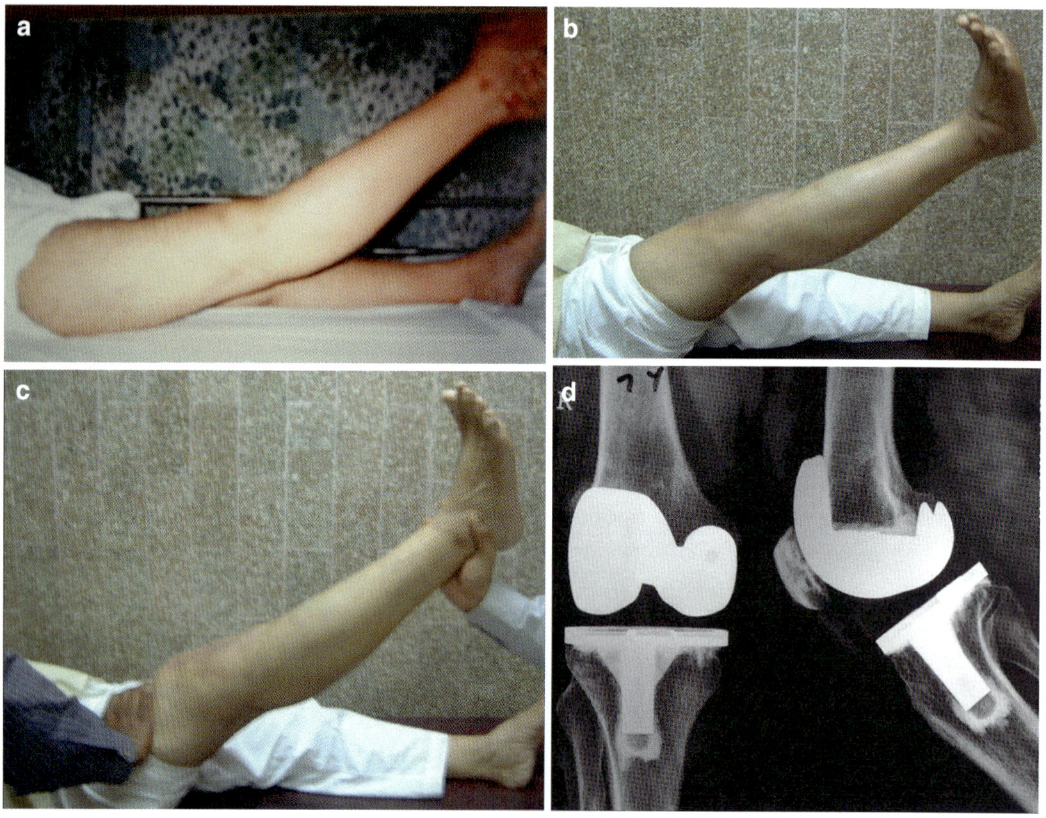

Fig. 6.4 Outcome of TKA in a patient with hyperextension deformity. (**a**) Preoperative clinical photograph showing severe hyperextension deformity (approximately 20°). (**b**) Clinical photograph of the same patient at 7 years post TKA showing no recurrence of hyperextension on straight leg raising. (**c**) Clinical photograph of the same patient at 7 years post TKA showing no recurrence of hyperextension on passive extension of the knee by the examiner. (**d**) Standing anteroposterior and lateral knee radiograph of the same patient at 7 years post TKA showing excellent alignment and fixation of the components. Note that the patient was successfully treated with a simple, cruciate-substituting design with a tibial insert thickness of 12.5 mm despite the severe preoperative hyperextension deformity

Computer-Assisted Technique

Conventional TKA lacks quantitative standardisation of bone resection, soft-tissue release and gap measurements which may result in some unpredictability in outcome. Like in any type or degree of knee deformity during TKA, computer-assisted navigation system accurately quantifies the amount of bone resection and soft-tissue release during TKA which helps to achieve optimum restoration of limb and component alignment and flexion and extension gap balance. The femoral component planning feature of the software is particularly valuable in determining femoral component size and position to equalise gaps. In addition, CAS enables the surgeon to identify even few degrees of hyperextension early in the procedure (Fig. 6.3). This should immediately alert the surgeon to be cautious with resection and releases and perform both in an incremental fashion. Revisiting a cut is preferable to resecting more bone at the beginning.

CAS also enables the surgeon to "fine-tune" the final extension alignment of the knee to ensure a few degrees (2°–5°) of flexion at the end of the procedure (Fig. 6.3). This may be difficult to discern by "eye balling" especially in obese patients. Using an algorithmic approach along with computer navigation help in successfully correcting recurvatum without resorting to constrained implants and excessively thick inserts (Fig. 6.5).

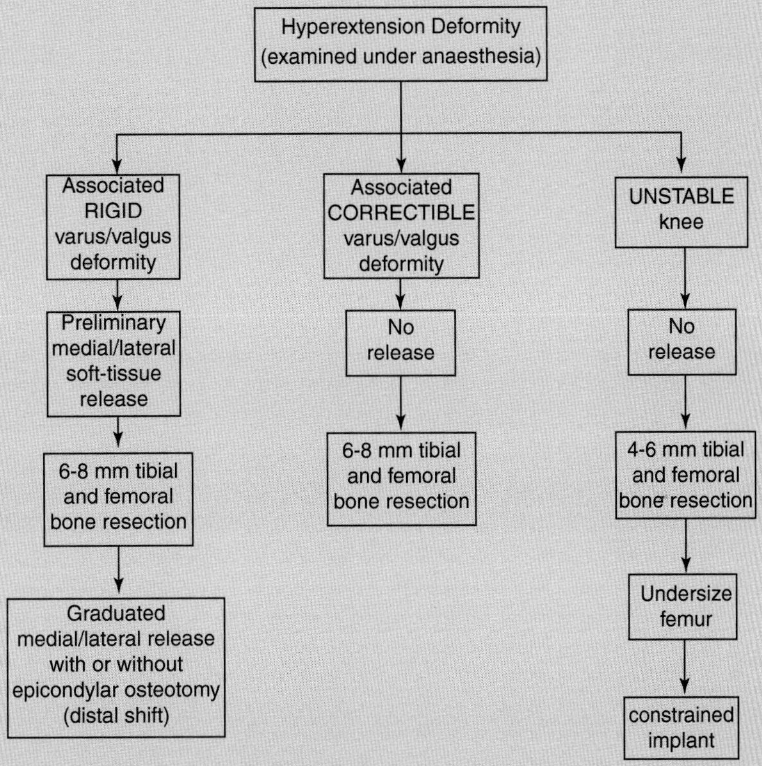

Fig. 6.5 Algorithm used by the authors to treat hyperextension deformity during TKA

References

1. Meding JB, Keating EM, Ritter MA, Faris PM, Berend ME. Genu recurvatum in total knee replacement. Clin Orthop Relat Res. 2003;416:64–7.
2. Whiteside LA, Mihalko WM. Surgical procedure for flexion contracture and recurvatum in total knee arthroplasty. Clin Orthop Relat Res. 2002;404:189–95.
3. Mullaji A, Lingaraju AP, Shetty GM. Computer-assisted total knee replacement in patients with arthritis and a recurvatum deformity. J Bone Joint Surg Br. 2012;94:642–7.
4. Insall JN, Haas SB. Complications of total knee arthroplasty. In: Insall JN, Windsor RE, Scott WN, Kelly MA, Aglietti P, editors. Surgery of the knee. New York: Churchill Livingstone; 1993. p. 891–934.
5. Insall JN. Surgical techniques and instrumentation in total knee arthroplasty. In: Insall JN, Windsor RE, Scott WN, Kelly MA, Aglietti P, editors. Surgery of the knee. New York: Churchill Livingstone; 1993. p. 739–804.
6. Giori NJ, Lewallen DG. Total knee arthroplasty in limbs affected by poliomyelitis. J Bone Joint Surg Am. 2002;84:1157–61.
7. Parratte S, Pagnano MW. Instability after total knee arthroplasty. J Bone Joint Surg Am. 2008;90:184–94.

Part IV

Complex Deformities

Rotational Deformity

7

Introduction

The rotational alignment of femoral and tibial components in TKA is based on various bony landmarks and reference axes around the knee joint. However, most of these landmarks and reference axes have been derived from normal unaffected knees. In knees with arthritis, these landmarks and axes may get distorted due to significant cartilage wear, bone loss, soft-tissue contracture and additional extra-articular bony deformities frequently associated with severe knee deformity [1].

Varus arthritic deformities of the knee are typically associated with increased external rotation of the tibia [2]. Similarly, severe arthritis and deformity are associated with excessive wear of the femoral condyles, and excessive medial or lateral soft-tissue contracture leading to increased internal or external rotation of the distal femur [3]. These pathological changes cause distortion of standard reference axes and landmarks such as the tibial tubercle, posterior condyle angle, epicondylar axis and anteroposterior axis. Hence, if such torsional deformities are not taken into account during TKA, it may result in rotational malalignment of components which will lead to patellar maltracking, abnormal gait, postoperative pain, poor function and early wear [4–8]. This chapter aims to address rotational deformities in arthritic knees undergoing TKA.

Pathoanatomy

The lower extremity from an *in utero* position of internal rotation slowly undergoes lateral or external rotation throughout the growth phase of the child till skeletal maturity [9]. Staheli and Engel [10] in their study of tibial torsion in children estimated tibial torsion at 15° of external rotation at skeletal maturity. Based on the orientation of the bimalleolar axis with respect to the flexion-extension axis of the knee joint, the tibia shows dynamic internal rotation when the knee is flexed [11, 12]. During gait, the tibia shows dynamic internal rotation with respect to the femur at mid and terminal stance and dynamic external rotation from toe off until slightly before heel strike [12]. In normal subjects, the tibia is typically in external rotation with Caucasian limbs showing greater external rotation compared to Asian limbs [13].

Whether abnormal torsion is a cause or a consequence of knee osteoarthritis is still unclear. Nagamine et al. [14] in their CT scan analysis of normal and osteoarthritic tibiae in Japanese subjects had suggested that the traditional way of sitting on the floor with the foot internally rotated (tatami position) since childhood may cause growth disturbance at the proximal tibial meta physis, causing tibia vara and medial torsion of the tibia. Krackow et al. [15] in a recent study to quantify the association between medial knee

A.B. Mullaji, G.M. Shetty, *Deformity Correction in Total Knee Arthroplasty*,
DOI 10.1007/978-1-4939-0566-9_7, © Springer Science+Business Media New York 2014

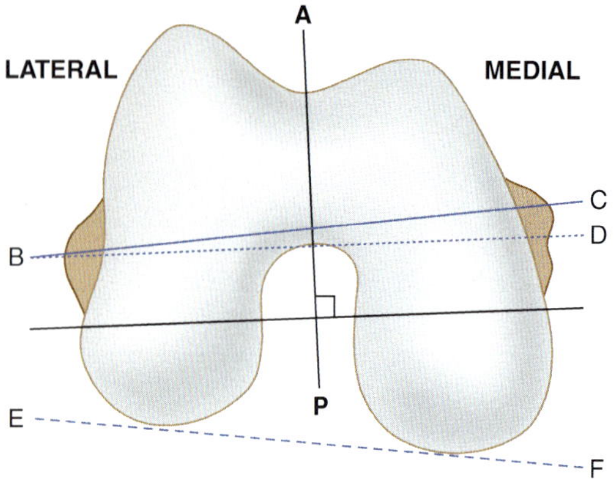

Fig. 7.1 Distal femoral bony landmarks frequently used to determine rotation of the femoral component. Line *AP* – Anteroposterior axis or the Whiteside's line drawn along the deepest part of the trochlear sulcus. The femoral component is placed perpendicular to this axis. Line *BC* – Anatomic transepicondylar axis connecting the lateral epicondyle (point *B*) and the medial epicondyle (point *C*). Line *BD* – Clinical transepicondylar axis connecting the lateral epicondyle (point *B*) and the medial sulcus (point *D*). Line *EF* – Posterior condylar line drawn tangent to the posterior-most point of the medial and lateral posterior femoral condyles

loading and tibial torsion reported that subjects with medial OA and associated tibial intorsion walked with significantly greater knee loading compared to controls. Hence, the incidence and pattern of torsional deformity in patients with knee OA shows wide variation depending on the ethnicity of the population and severity of deformity.

Several techniques are used to determine the rotational position of the femoral component during TKA. These include using bony landmarks on the distal femur, soft-tissue tension and flexion gap (gap balancing) and computer navigation [16]. However, no single technique has emerged as a clear winner [17], and most surgeons use a combination of two or more techniques. Distal femoral bony landmarks are most frequently and principally used to determine rotation of the femoral component (Fig. 7.1). However, several reports have underlined the fact that such bony landmarks show wide variation not only among arthritic knees but even among normal subjects [2, 18–22]. Furthermore, use of one specific bony landmark may be unreliable to determine femoral component rotation and may be affected by severity and type of underlying arthritic knee deformity. For example, the anteroposterior axis (Whiteside's line) may not be reliable in cases with severe patellofemoral arthritis which may cause significant trochlear wear and distortion [23, 24], and the posterior condylar angle (PCA) may not be reliable in knees with severe wear and bone loss of the posterior condyles [25]. Hence, in such cases some other technique must be used to determine femoral rotation. The gap-balancing technique involves rotating the femoral component so as to achieve medio-lateral flexion gap symmetry (with the help of a tensioning device such as laminar spreaders) after having achieved a balanced and symmetric extension gap. However, the femoral rotation required may vary depending on the amount of distal femoral bony loss or distortion and the extent of medio-lateral flexion gap asymmetry. Although computer navigation has proven to improve limb and component alignment during TKA, studies have reported malrotation of the femoral component during CAS TKA when a single anatomic landmark is used as reference [26, 27]. For example, using only the epicondylar axis as reference may lead to excessive external rotation of the femoral component. However, using a combination of anatomic and kinematic data has been reported to improve accuracy of rotational alignment of the femoral component [27].

On the tibial side, options to determine tibial component rotation include using bony landmarks and putting the knee through an arc of flexion and extension and positioning the tibial tray vis-à-vis the femoral component (the "self-positioning" method) [16]. Traditionally, the tibial tubercle (junction of the middle and medial one-third) has been used as a fixed bony landmark to determine the rotational alignment of the tibial tray. However, similar to distal femoral bony landmarks, the tibial tubercle may show wide variations among patients depending on the severity of knee deformity and ethnicity [2, 28–30]. Sun et al. [29] in a CT scan-based study of Chinese osteoarthritic knees reported that the tibial component has a tendency to be placed in greater external rotation when the medial one-third of the tibial tuberosity is used as a landmark in arthritic knees with varus or valgus deformities. Hence, they concluded that the tibial tuberosity is an unreliable rotational landmark for tibial tray in Asian patients with deformed, arthritic knees [29]. In a similar study on European subjects, Bonnin et al. [31] reported significant variation in the position of the tibial tuberosity which caused not only excessive external rotation of the tibial component but also deficient coverage of the tibial cut surface by the tibial tray.

Surgical Technique

Femur

The severity and type of knee deformity and the presence of an extra-articular rotational deformity must be taken into account before deciding on the rotational alignment of the femoral component during TKA. Matsui et al. [2] in a CT scan study of 150 arthritic knees and 31 normal controls reported progressive external rotation of the distal femur with increasing severity of varus deformity when compared to rotation in normal controls. However, this difference was significant only when the epicondylar axes (either surgical or clinical) were compared, whereas there was no difference when the posterior condylar axes were compared. Therefore, the distal femoral rotation in an arthritic knee with varus <10° is similar to a normal knee, whereas the distal femur may be in excessive external rotation when the varus deformity is 20° or more. In valgus knees, Matsuda et al. [3] using MRI analysis of the distal femur reported that the posterior condylar line with respect to the transepicondylar axis was in 11.5° internal rotation compared to 6.4° internal rotation in normal knees and 6.1° internal rotation in varus knees. This is probably due to significant distortion and wear of the lateral femoral condyle in valgus knees.

Owing to wide variations in bony landmarks in arthritic knees, the authors use the combined referencing technique to determine femoral component position during TKA. Using a soft-tissue tensioner, the medio-lateral gap is first assessed with the knee in 90° flexion, and the tentative posterior cut is marked (parallel to the cut tibial surface) on the distal femur surface based on soft-tissue tension. We use the AP axis as the preliminary reference to position the AP cutting block equivalent to the femoral component size estimated. In cases where the femoral trochlea shows significant wear, the epicondylar axis is used as the preliminary reference. The surgeon then references the anterior cortex of the distal femur (using a stylus or angel wing) to avoid notching and the previously made mark on the posterior aspect of the distal femoral cut surface based on soft-tissue tension. The AP cutting block should be generally parallel to the epicondylar axis and perpendicular to the AP axis (Whiteside's line). Appropriate soft-tissue releases are performed if required to achieve medio-lateral gap balance. In valgus knees there may be excessive tightness laterally, and medially in varus knees. This becomes evident if the cutting block position deviates significantly from any of the chosen references. After pinning the AP cutting block to the distal femur, the flexion gap balance is assessed using a spacer block. If the flexion gap seems too tight either medially or laterally, the AP block may be slightly externally or internally rotated.

Rarely, in cases with severe femoral EAD where there is also a significant rotational component (Fig. 7.2), the malrotation may have to be corrected while performing a corrective osteotomy [32].

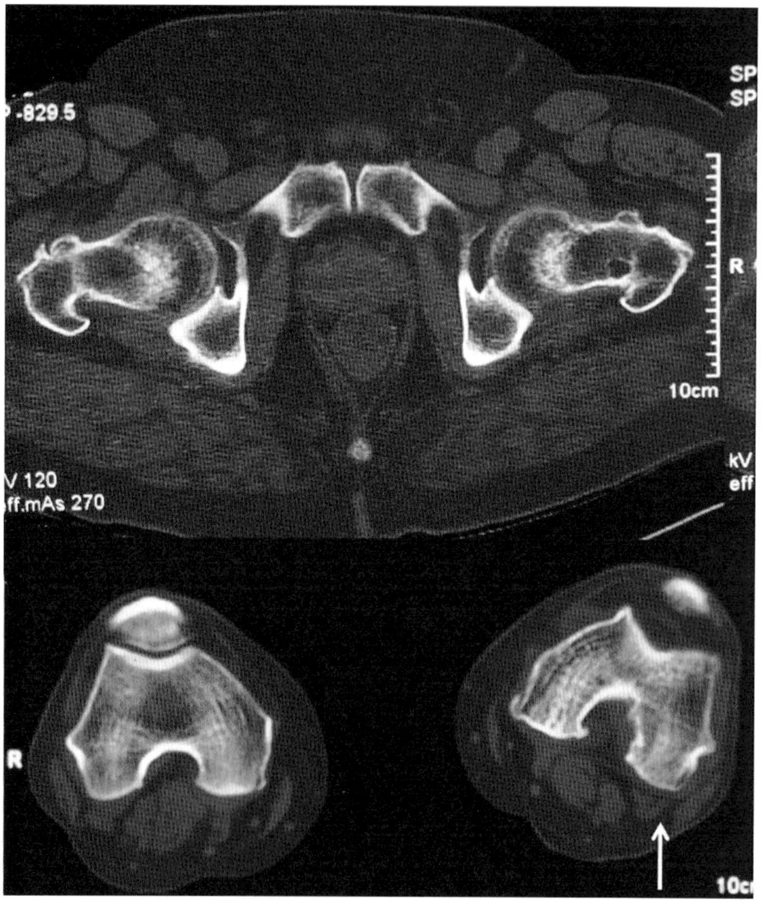

Fig. 7.2 Preoperative CT scan of a patient showing external rotation deformity of the distal femur on the left side (*arrow*) secondary to a malunited fracture at the distal femoral shaft

Tibia

Similar to the femur, the rotational profile of the tibia changes with the severity and type of knee deformity. Greater varus knee deformity may be associated with increasing internal rotation of the tibia (Fig. 7.3). In view of variation in the position of tibial tubercle among patients, the "self-positioning" technique to determine tibial tray rotation minimises femorotibial rotational mismatch and maximises coverage of the bony tibial surface by the tibial tray [33]. The authors note the position of both malleoli after the tibial tray position is finalised using the self-positioning technique. In cases where significant malrotation of the tibia (which may be due to an associated tibial extra-articular deformity) is present, a mobile-bearing design is used to prevent femoro-tibial rotational mismatch and postoperative gait abnormality. If only a few degrees of intorsion of the tibia is present, the tibial tray is internally rotated by the same amount. This is important else the patient may walk with a marked intoeing gait.

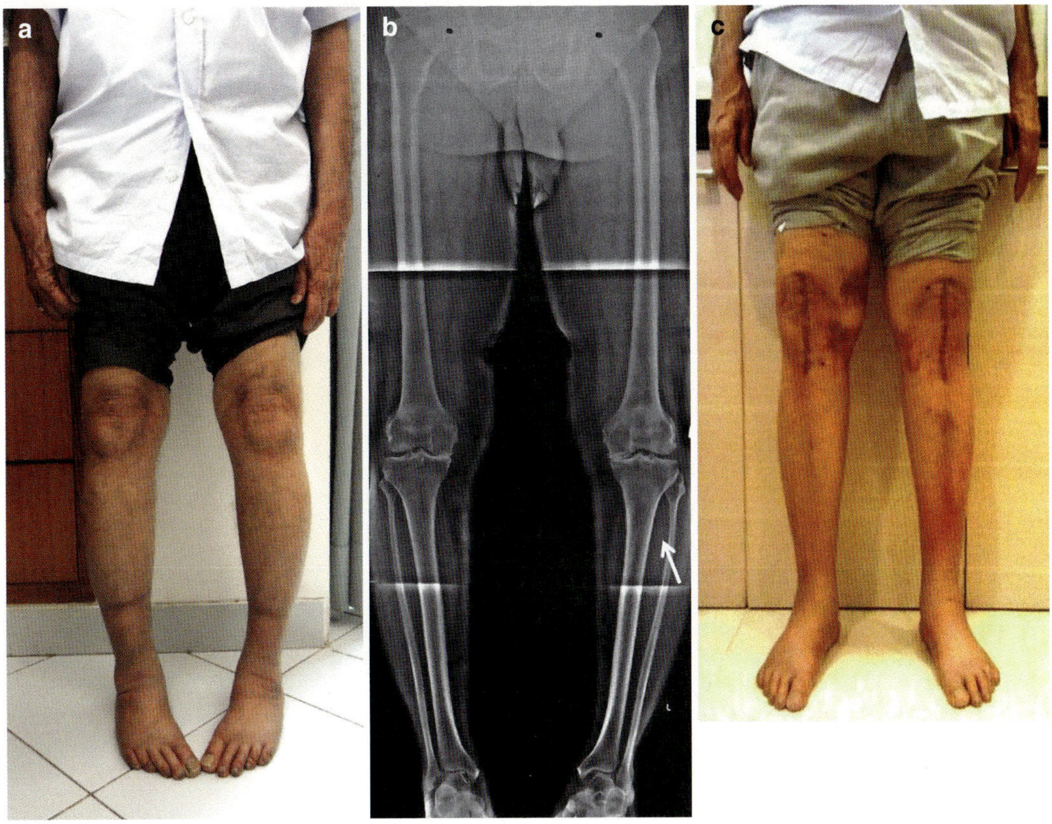

Fig. 7.3 Tibial torsion seen preoperatively in patients undergoing TKA. (**a**) Preoperative clinical photograph showing significant bilateral tibial intorsion. (**b**) Preoperative standing, full-length hip-to-ankle radiograph of the same patient (a) showing significant tibial intorsion (left more than the right). Note that the complete profile of the fibula is well seen and the gap between the tibia and the fibula is prominent (*arrow*), implying significant intorsion of the leg when the patient is standing with both patella facing forwards. (**c**) Postoperative clinical photograph of the same patient showing restoration of rotational alignment of the lower limb

References

1. Mullaji AB, Shetty GM, Lingaraju AP, Bhayde S. Which factors increase risk of malalignment of the hip-knee-ankle axis in TKA? Clin Orthop Relat Res. 2013;471:134–41.
2. Matsui Y, Kadoya Y, Uehara K, Kobayashi A, Takaoka K. Rotational deformity in varus osteoarthritis of the knee: analysis with computed tomography. Clin Orthop Relat Res. 2005;433:147–51.
3. Matsuda S, Miura H, Nagamine R, Mawatari T, Tokunaga M, Nabeyama R, Iwamoto Y. Anatomical analysis of the femoral condyle in normal and osteoarthritic knees. J Orthop Res. 2004;22:104–9.
4. Nicoll D, Rowley DI. Internal rotational error of the tibial component is a major cause of pain after total knee replacement. J Bone Joint Surg Br. 2010;92:1238–44.
5. Ghosh KM, Merican AM, Iranpour F, Deehan DJ, Amis AA. The effect of femoral component rotation on the extensor retinaculum of the knee. J Orthop Res. 2010;28:1136–41.
6. Malo M, Vince KG. The unstable patella after total knee arthroplasty: etiology, prevention, and management. J Am Acad Orthop Surg. 2003;11:364–71.
7. Sternheim A, Lochab J, Drexler M, Kuzyk P, Safir O, Gross A, Backstein D. The benefit of revision knee arthroplasty for component malrotation after primary total knee replacement. Int Orthop. 2012;36:2473–8.
8. Bell SW, Young P, Drury C, Smith J, Anthony I, Jones B, Blyth M, McLean A. Component rotational alignment in unexplained painful primary total knee arthroplasty. Knee. 2014;21:272–7.
9. Badelon O, Bensahel H, Folinais D, Lassale B. Tibiofibular torsion from the fetal period until birth. J Pediatr Orthop. 1989;9:169–73.

10. Staheli LT, Engel GM. Tibial torsion: a method of assessment and a survey of normal children. Clin Orthop Relat Res. 1972;86:183–6.
11. Iwaki H, Pinskerova V, Freeman MA. Tibiofemoral movement 1: the shapes and relative movements of the femur and tibia in the unloaded cadaver knee. J Bone Joint Surg Br. 2000;82:1189–95.
12. Davids JR, Davis RB. Tibial torsion: significance and measurement. Gait Posture. 2007;26:169–71.
13. Mullaji AB, Sharma AK, Marawar SV, Kohli AF. Tibial torsion in non-arthritic Indian adults: a computer tomography study of 100 limbs. Indian J Orthop. 2008;42:309–13.
14. Nagamine R, Miyanishi K, Miura H, Urabe K, Matsuda S, Iwamoto Y. Medial torsion of the tibia in Japanese patients with osteoarthritis of the knee. Clin Orthop Relat Res. 2003;408:218–24.
15. Krackow KA, Mandeville DS, Rachala SR, Bayers-Thering M, Osternig LR. Torsion deformity and joint loading for medial knee osteoarthritis. Gait Posture. 2011;33:625–9.
16. Scott RD. Femoral and tibial component rotation in total knee arthroplasty: methods and consequences. Bone Joint J. 2013;95-B(11 Suppl A):140–3.
17. Siston RA, Patel JJ, Goodman SB, Delp SL, Giori NJ. The variability of femoral rotational alignment in total knee arthroplasty. J Bone Joint Surg Am. 2005;87:2276–80.
18. Mullaji AB, Sharma AK, Marawar SV, Kohli AF, Singh DP. Distal femoral rotational axes in Indian knees. J Orthop Surg (Hong Kong). 2009;17:166–9.
19. Matsuda S, Miura H, Nagamine R, Urabe K, Mawatari T, Iwamoto Y. A comparison of rotational landmarks in the distal femur and the tibial shaft. Clin Orthop Relat Res. 2003;414:183–8.
20. Yau WP, Chiu KY, Tang WM. How precise is the determination of rotational alignment of the femoral prosthesis in total knee arthroplasty: an in vivo study. J Arthroplasty. 2007;22:1042–8.
21. Moon YW, Seo JG, Lim SJ, Yang JH. Variability in femoral component rotation reference axes measured during navigation-assisted total knee arthroplasty using gap technique. J Arthroplasty. 2010;25:238–43.
22. Luyckx T, Zambianchi F, Catani F, Bellemans J, Victor J. Coronal alignment is a predictor of the rotational geometry of the distal femur in the osteoarthritic knee. Knee Surg Sports Traumatol Arthrosc. 2013;21:2331–7.
23. Lingaraj K, Bartlett J. The femoral sulcus in total knee arthroplasty. Knee Surg Sports Traumatol Arthrosc. 2009;17:499–502.
24. Poilvache PL, Insall JN, Scuderi GR, Font-Rodriguez DE. Rotational landmarks and sizing of the distal femur in total knee arthroplasty. Clin Orthop Relat Res. 1996;331:35–46.
25. Fujii T, Kondo M, Tomari K, Kadoya Y, Tanaka Y. Posterior condylar cartilage may distort rotational alignment of the femoral component based on posterior condylar axis in total knee arthroplasty. Surg Radiol Anat. 2012;34:633–8.
26. Piriou P, Peronne E, Ouanezar H. Rotational alignment of the femoral component using trochlear navigation during total knee arthroplasty: a dual-center study of 145 cases. J Arthroplasty. 2013;28:1107–11.
27. Siston RA, Cromie MJ, Gold GE, Goodman SB, Delp SL, Maloney WJ, Giori NJ. Averaging different alignment axes improves femoral rotational alignment in computer-navigated total knee arthroplasty. J Bone Joint Surg Am. 2008;90:2098–104.
28. Sahin N, Atıcı T, Öztürk A, Özkaya G, Özkan Y, Avcu B. Accuracy of anatomical references used for rotational alignment of tibial component in total knee arthroplasty. Knee Surg Sports Traumatol Arthrosc. 2012;20:565–70.
29. Sun T, Lu H, Hong N, Wu J, Feng C. Bony landmarks and rotational alignment in total knee arthroplasty for Chinese osteoarthritic knees with varus or valgus deformities. J Arthroplasty. 2009;24:427–31.
30. Howell SM, Chen J, Hull ML. Variability of the location of the tibial tubercle affects the rotational alignment of the tibial component in kinematically aligned total knee arthroplasty. Knee Surg Sports Traumatol Arthrosc. 2013;21:2288–95.
31. Bonnin MP, Saffarini M, Mercier PE, Laurent JR, Carrillon Y. Is the anterior tibial tuberosity a reliable rotational landmark for the tibial component in total knee arthroplasty? J Arthroplasty. 2011;26:260–7.
32. Drexler M, Dwyer T, Marmor M, Reischl N, Attar F, Cameron J. Total knee arthroplasty in patients with excessive external tibial torsion >45° and patella instability–surgical technique and follow up. J Arthroplasty. 2013;28:614–9.
33. Berhouet J, Beaufils P, Boisrenoult P, Frasca D, Pujol N. Rotational positioning of the tibial tray in total knee arthroplasty: a CT evaluation. Orthop Traumatol Surg Res. 2011;97:699–704.

8 Extra-Articular Deformity

Introduction

In most total knee arthroplasties (TKAs) for arthritic knees with intra-articular varus or valgus deformity, both alignment and ligament balance can be achieved with appropriate bone cuts and soft-tissue releases. However, TKA becomes technically challenging when knee arthritis is associated with an extra-articular deformity (EAD) of either the femur or the tibia. Such deformities are secondary to trauma (malunion or non-union), previous osteotomy, metabolic causes such as osteomalacia or osteoporosis causing excessive bowing or stress fractures and congenital causes (Fig. 8.1) [1–4]. Stress fracture although uncommon is a frequent cause of tibial EAD in patients with knee arthritis.

Options for dealing with such EADs during TKA include intra-articular correction along with bone resection and extensive soft-tissue release and staged or simultaneous corrective osteotomy at the apex of the EAD along with intra-articular correction. Conventional techniques, although effective in majority of such cases, may not be appropriate in selected limbs where the presence of hardware or excessive distortion of the femoral canal due to deformity may make the use of an intramedullary femoral guide difficult (Fig. 8.2) [4]. Recent reports describing the use of navigated TKA for knee arthritis with EADs have indicated good results with appropriate bone cuts and soft tissue releases [1, 5–8]. Navigation systems use the centre of the femoral head, the centre of the knee joint and the centre of the ankle to calculate the mechanical axis; help in avoiding excess bone resection; allow graduated measured soft-tissue release; and align the femoral component based on the mechanical axis derived from the femoral head centre and knee centre, bypassing the femoral extra-articular deformity. Hence, femoral EAD with distortion of the femoral canal and the presence of hardware especially in the distal half of the femur may be an appropriate indication for computer-assisted surgery in this subgroup of patients undergoing TKA. This chapter aims to outline the means of dealing with EADs during TKA.

Pathoanatomy

Extra-articular deformities in knees which undergo TKA complicate the procedure in a number of ways. First, an EAD either in the tibia or the femur adds to the overall deformity in a limb already deformed due to knee arthritis (Fig. 8.3). Hence, realignment in such limbs will require extensive soft-tissue release and achieving medio-lateral balance will be challenging especially if there is a dearth of osteophytes and excessive lateral laxity (in a varus knee, or vice versa) at the knee. Such limbs are therefore cases which may require additional procedures such as lateral epicondylar or sliding medial condylar osteotomy to achieve optimum limb alignment and soft-tissue balance [9, 10]. Second, some of these limbs with associated EAD especially secondary to a previous surgical procedure (high tibial osteotomy or fracture

A.B. Mullaji, G.M. Shetty, *Deformity Correction in Total Knee Arthroplasty*,
DOI 10.1007/978-1-4939-0566-9_8,

fixation) have hardware in situ which makes use of conventional intramedullary alignment jigs challenging and may require hardware removal before the start of TKA (Fig. 8.2). Third, an EAD close to the knee joint may distort local bony anatomy and make optimum component alignment challenging to achieve. Finally, severe EADs, especially in the proximal tibia or distal femur, may require an additional corrective osteotomy performed either simultaneously with TKA or in a staged manner [1].

The most common EAD encountered during TKA is excessive coronal bowing of the femoral shaft [1] (Fig. 8.3). A study published by the senior author reports the incidence of excessive coronal bowing of the femoral shaft at 15 % in arthritic knees which undergo TKA in Indian study population [11]. Similar findings have been reported in

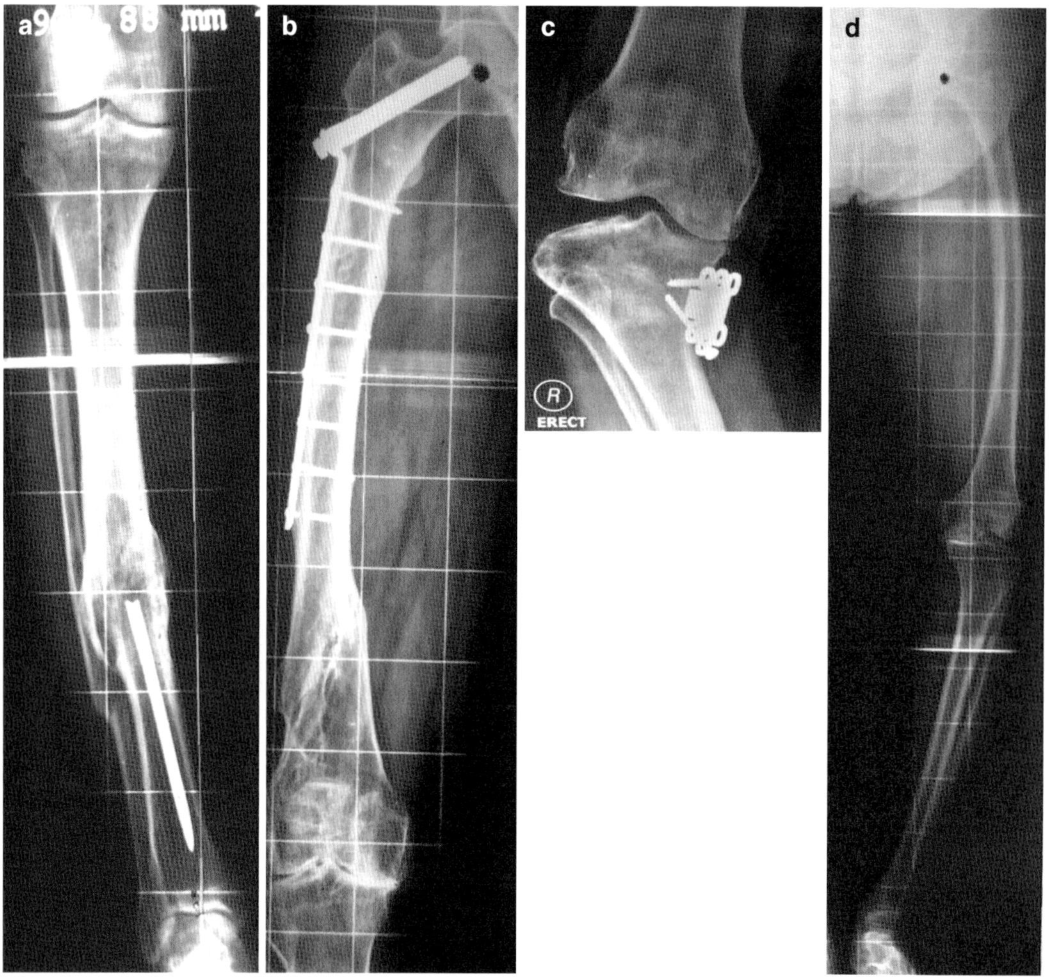

Fig. 8.1 Causes of extra-articular deformities in knees undergoing TKA. (**a**) Post-traumatic deformity in the distal ½ of the tibial shaft with broken nail in situ. (**b**) Post-traumatic deformity in the distal 1/3 of femur due to a malunited fracture with implant in the proximal ½ of femur. (**c**) Severe extra-articular deformity in the proximal end of the tibia secondary to high tibial osteotomy (HTO) with implant in situ. (**d**) Severe bowing of the femoral shaft probably secondary to osteopenia and/or osteomalacia compounding the knee deformity. (**e**) Stress fracture in the upper 1/3 of the tibial shaft causing varus deformity locally. (**f**) Proximal tibia varus. (**g**) Bowing of the proximal ½ of the femoral shaft secondary to probably a congenital cause

Fig. 8.1 (continued)

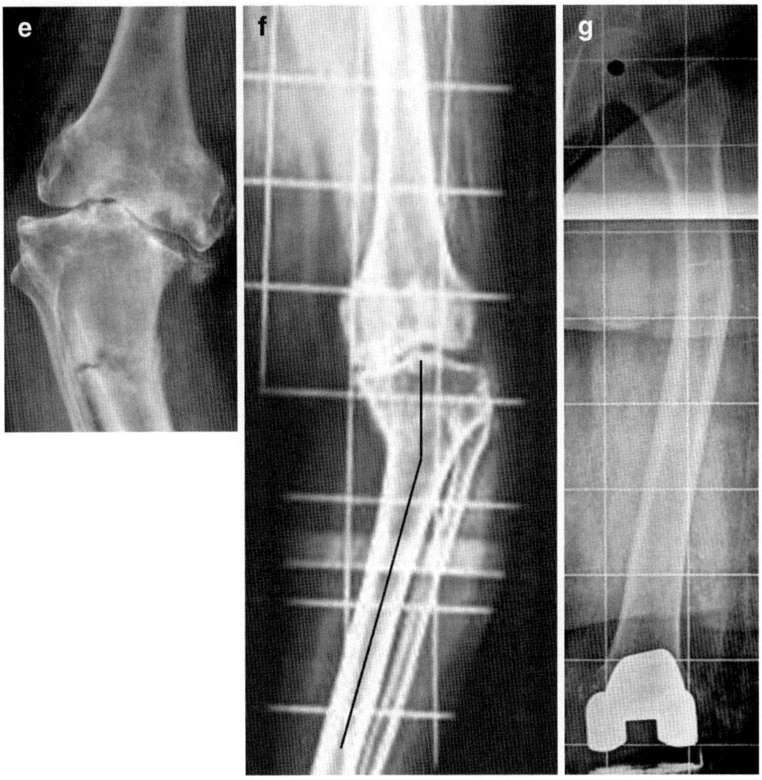

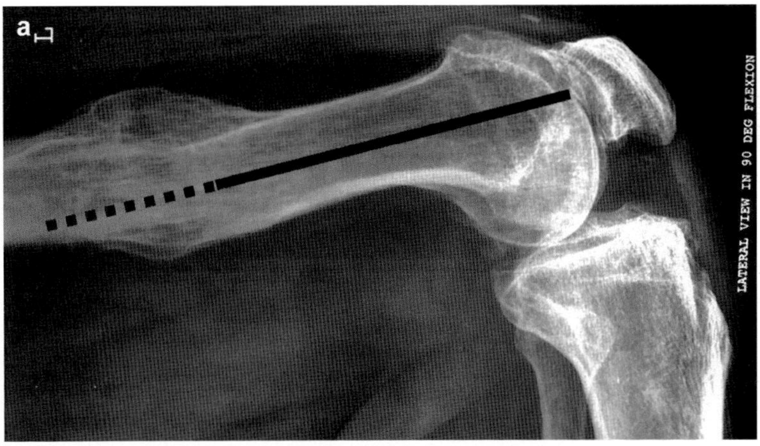

Fig. 8.2 Excessive distortion of the femoral canal due to extra-articular deformity or presence of hardware makes the use of an intramedullary femoral guide challenging during conventional TKA. (**a**) Extra-articular deformity at the distal 1/3 of the femur due to a malunited fracture caused an extension deformity of the distal fragment. Use of an intramedullary femur guide rod (*black line*) will cause it to go posteriorly within the distorted canal. (**b**) Extra-articular deformity at the distal 1/3 of the femur due to a malunited fracture caused a varus deformity of the distal fragment. Use of an intramedullary femur guide rod (*black line*) will cause it to go laterally within the distorted canal. (**c**) An intramedullary nail previously used to fix a distal femur shaft fracture. This nail will have to be removed if an intramedullary femur guide rod needs to be used during conventional TKA

Fig. 8.2 (continued)

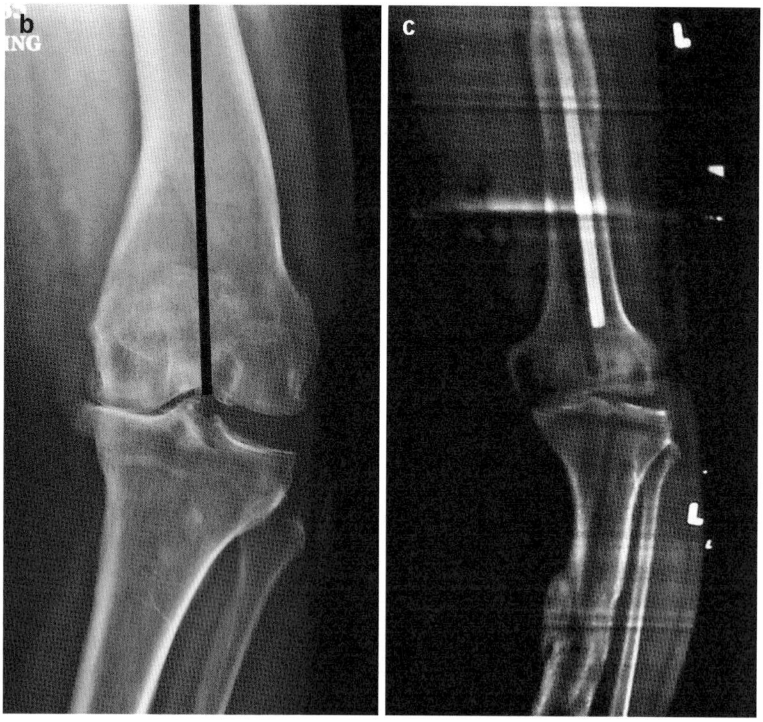

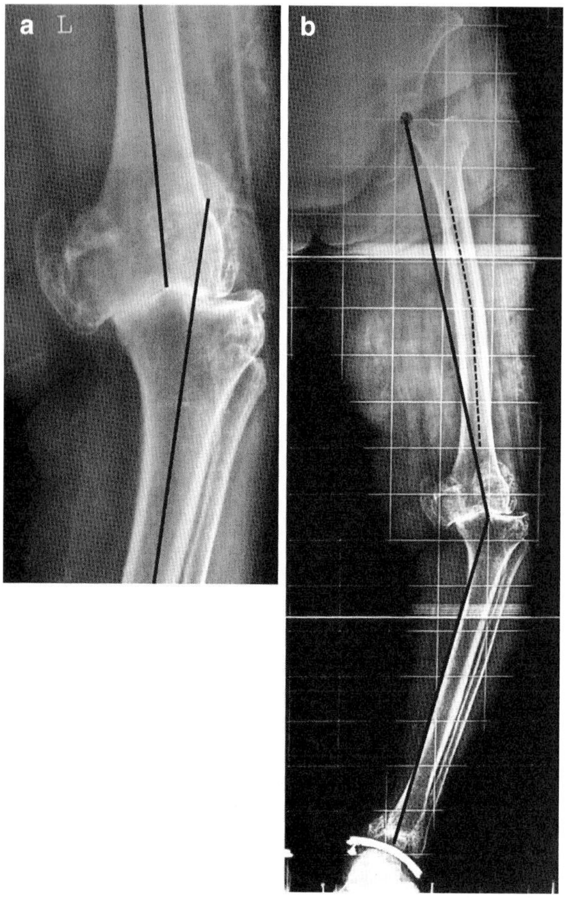

Fig. 8.3 A common cause of femoral extra-articular deformity in patients undergoing TKA – excessive coronal bowing of the femoral shaft. This adds to the overall deformity of the limb. (**a**) Standing knee anteroposterior radiograph showing a knee deformity of 15° varus (*black line*). (**b**) Standing, full-length hip-to-ankle radiograph of the same patient shows that the overall limb deformity (hip-knee-ankle angle) is actually 30° varus. Excessive coronal bowing of the femoral shaft (*dotted line*) at 12° in this case adds to the overall deformity of the limb which can be easily missed if only short knee films are used

Table 8.1 Classification of tibial stress fractures in patients undergoing TKA

I. Intra-articular
(A) Malunited
(B) Ununited
II. Extra-articular
(A) Impending
(B) Acute
(C) United
(D) Malunited
(E) Ununited

other study populations especially in Asians. Another common cause of EAD in the femur is a malunited fracture typically with hardware in situ. Similarly, in the tibia, the common causes of EAD include proximal tibia vara due to distortion and bony adaptation secondary to knee arthritis and/or metabolic causes, malunited fractures, stress fractures secondary to metabolic causes and deformity secondary to a previous high tibial osteotomy (HTO). As per the classification proposed by the authors (Table 8.1), tibial stress fractures in arthritic knees are primarily intra-articular or extra-articular type (Fig. 8.4) [2]. Based on the type of stress fractures, the surgical technique and implant used may vary during TKA.

Post-HTO is a special category of tibial EAD which brings its own challenges while performing TKA. The issues which need to be dealt with during a post-HTO TKA include a previous skin incision, periarticular bony distortion, soft-tissue changes, implant in situ and patellar changes such as maltracking and patella infera (Table 8.2). Periarticular bony distortion secondary to a previous HTO include medial tibial bone loss and lateral femoral condylar deficiency, excessive medial or lateral and/or posterior or anterior sloping of tibial plateau, excessive medial or lateral and/or anterior or posterior translation of the proximal tibia and internal or external torsion of the proximal tibia (Fig. 8.5) [12, 13].

Preoperative Planning

A full-length hip-to-ankle radiograph is necessary to plan for TKA in cases with femoral or tibial EAD. A thorough evaluation of soft-tissue balance under anaesthesia is also invaluable especially in knees which have been previously operated.

Femoral Extra-Articular Deformities

On preoperative standing, full-length hip-to-ankle radiographs, the proposed distal femoral cut is drawn perpendicular to the mechanical axis of the femur. If the EAD is close to the joint or is more than 20° in the coronal plane or if the plane of the distal cut is likely to compromise the attachment of the lateral collateral ligament on the lateral epicondyle, a corrective osteotomy is considered (Fig. 8.6) [1, 3]. In the presence of significant femoral bowing (as evidenced by an increase in the angle between the mechanical axis and the distal femoral anatomic axis), the distal femoral valgus resection angle should be measured preoperatively and proportionately increased during the procedure (Fig. 8.7) [14]. Severe femoral bowing with minimal osteophytes and severe lateral laxity with or without rigid medial soft-tissue contracture in varus arthritic knees should alert the surgeon that balancing and realignment may be difficult using only intra-articular correction and a sliding osteotomy of the medial condyle may be required (Fig. 8.8) [10].

Tibial Extra-Articular Deformities

On preoperative standing, full-length hip-to-ankle radiographs, the axis of the tibia distal to the deformity is drawn and extended proximally towards the knee joint. If the distal tibial axis does not pass through the tibial plateau or if the EAD is close to the joint or is more than 30° in the coronal plane, a corrective osteotomy is likely to be indicated (Fig. 8.9) [1, 3]. In cases where TKA is planned in a post-HTO knee, periarticular bony distortion of the proximal tibia and hardware (Fig. 8.5) which may interfere with fixation of the tibial component should be noted on radiographs, and surgical steps to tackle each issue need to be planned. Furthermore, the site of a previous skin incision should be noted and the TKA

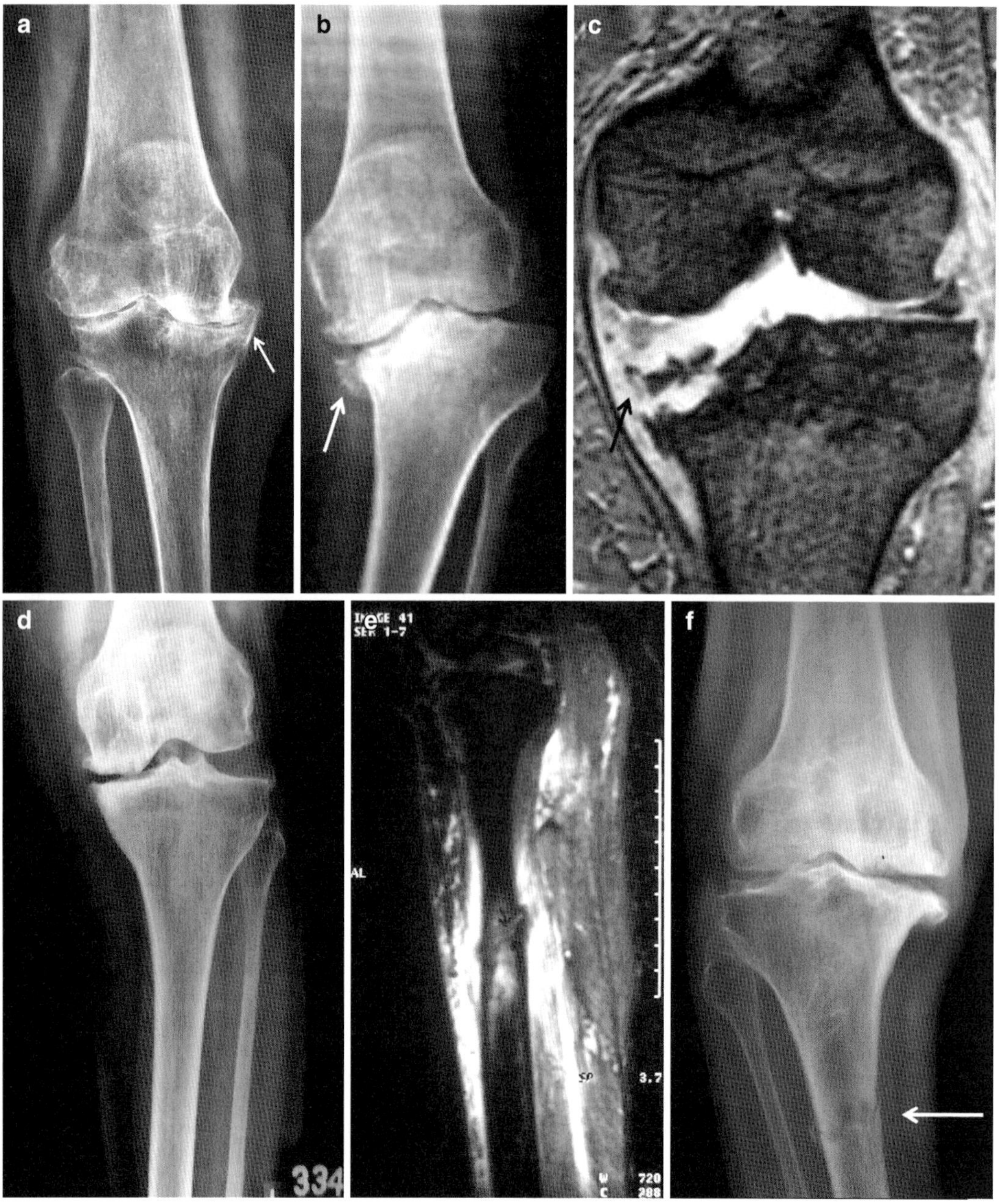

Fig. 8.4 Types of tibial stress fractures seen in knees undergoing TKA. (**a**) Type IA – Malunited intra-articular fracture (*arrow*). (**b**) Type IB – Ununited intra-articular fracture (*arrow*). (**c**) MRI of the same patient in (b) shows the extent of fracture and medial tibial bone defect (*black arrow*) caused by it. (**d**) Type IIA – Impending extra-articular fracture which is not obvious on plain knee radiograph. The patient had local tenderness on the anterior aspect of proximal 1/3 of the tibial shaft on clinical examination. (**e**) MRI of the same patient in (d) shows the stress fracture on proximal 1/3 of the tibial shaft (*black arrow*). Impending stress fractures can be diagnosed clinically and need an MRI for confirmation. (**f**) Type IIB – Acute extra-articular fracture of the proximal 1/3 of the tibial shaft (*arrow*). (**g**) Type IIC – United extra-articular fracture of the proximal 1/3 of the tibial shaft (*arrow*) which has healed without any local residual deformity. (**h**) Type IID – Malunited extra-articular fracture of the proximal 1/3 of the tibial shaft causing severe varus extra-articular deformity of approximately 37° at the fracture site. (**i**) Type IIE – Ununited extra-articular fracture of the proximal 1/3 of the tibial shaft

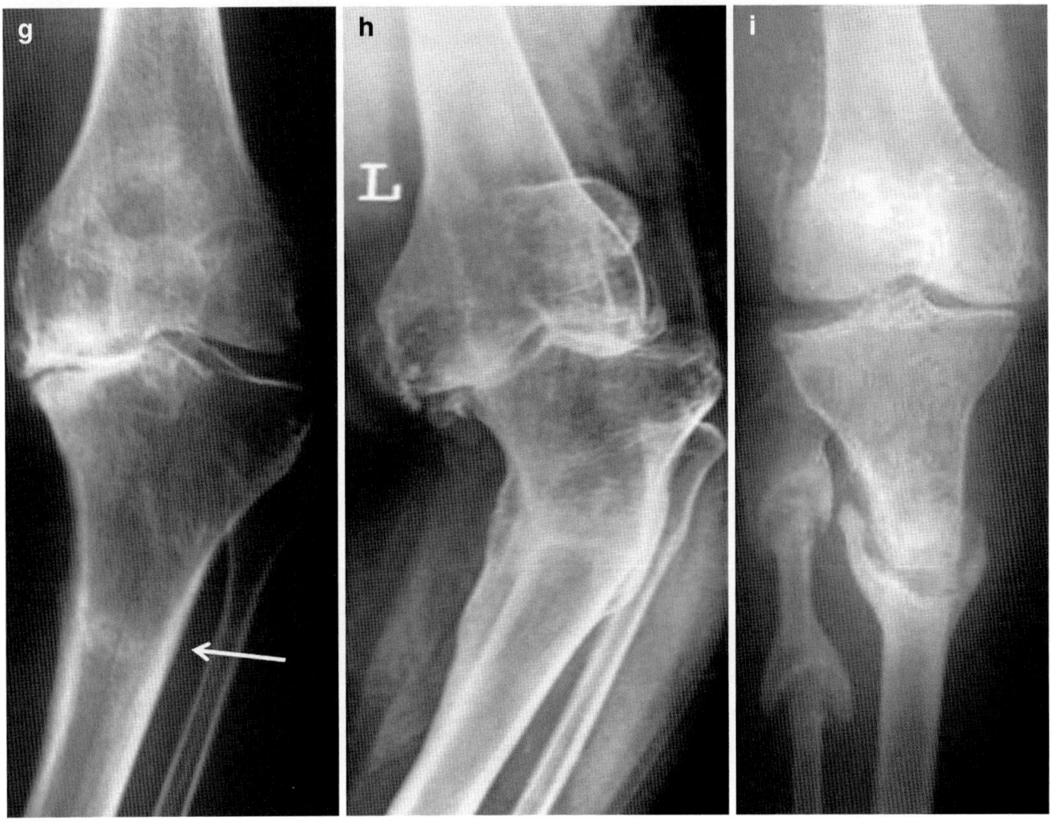

Fig. 8.4 (continued)

Table 8.2 Changes in the knee frequently encountered during post-high tibial osteotomy TKAs which can pose a challenge for the surgeon

Previous vertical skin incisions
Patella maltracking, fibrosis around patellar tendon insertion, patella infera
Implant in situ
Tibial bone loss
Decreased or increased tibial slope
Medial or lateral translation of proximal tibia
Anterior or posterior translation of the proximal tibia
Internal or external torsion of the proximal tibia
Medio-lateral soft-tissue imbalance
Excessive posterior soft-tissue laxity
Extra-articular deformity

incision should be planned such that it does not jeopardise blood supply of skin flaps.

Surgical Technique

Femoral Extra-Articular Deformities

The basic principles for intra-articular correction of the deformity remain the same as in any routine case of TKA. However, in order to accommodate the EAD, a conservative bone cut and an extensive soft-tissue release may be necessary. In case of deformity or hardware involving the distal half of the femoral canal, a shorter intramedullary

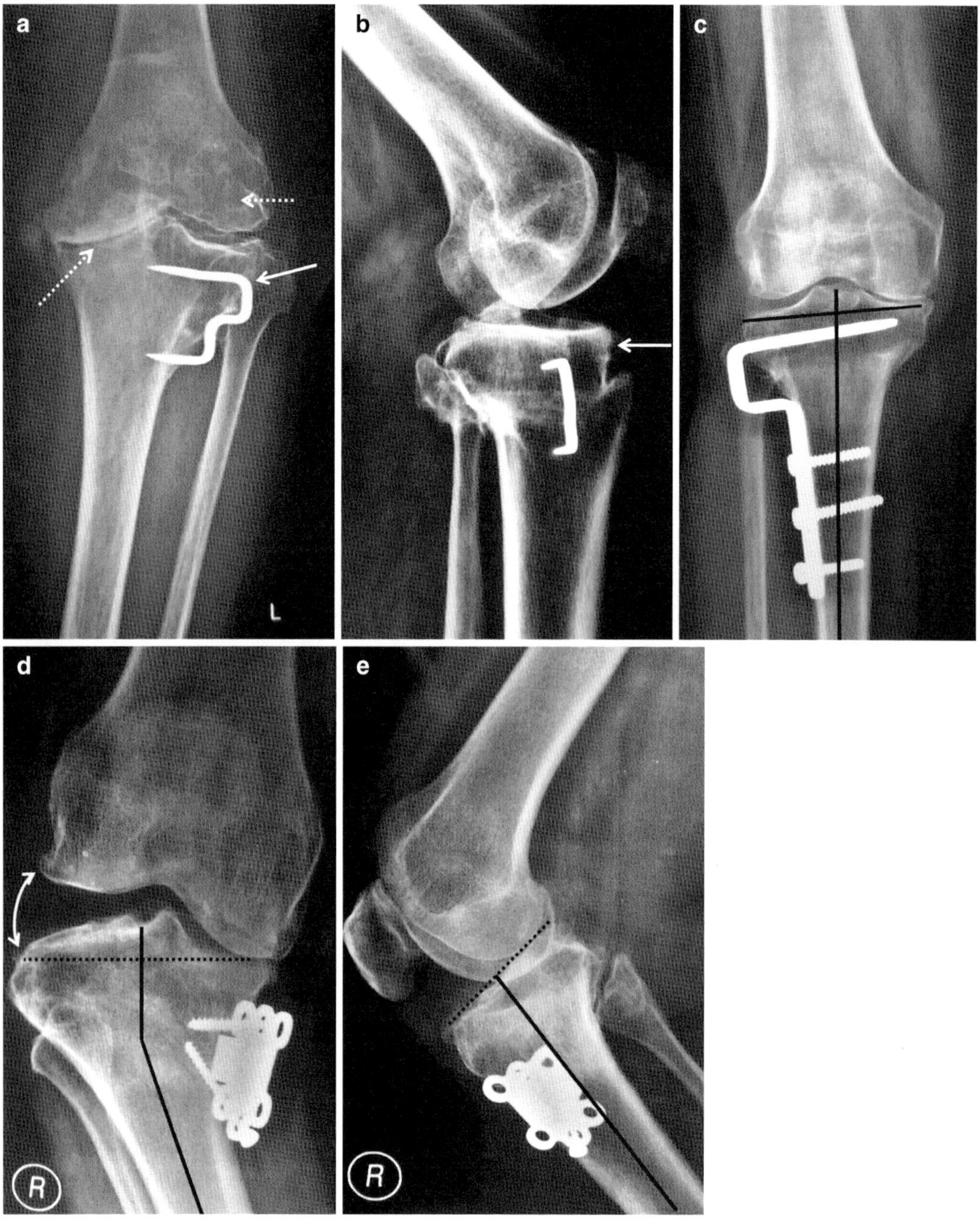

Fig. 8.5 Knee radiograph showing periarticular bony distortion secondary to a previous high tibial osteotomy (*HTO*). (**a**) Plain knee radiograph showing medial tibial bone loss (*dotted arrow*), lateral femoral condylar deficiency (*dotted arrow*) and bony overgrowth of the lateral tibia (*solid arrow*). (**b**) Posterior translation of the proximal end of the tibia (*arrow*). (**c**) Coronal angulation of the tibial plateau with implant in situ. (**d**) Severe extra-articular varus deformity of the proximal tibia with implant in situ. There is associated excessive lateral side soft-tissue laxity seen here as excessive opening of the lateral joint space (*curved arrow*). (**e**) Reverse sloping of the tibial plateau (*dotted line*)

femoral guide rod may be used to avoid malposition of the cutting block. However, if the implant or deformity interferes with use of the intramedullary guide rod (Fig. 8.2), either an extramedullary femoral guide rod or navigation must be used. An extensive soft-tissue release is performed in a graded, stepwise (subperiosteal elevation of the deep medial collateral ligament (MCL), posteromedial capsule and semimembranosus) manner [15, 16]. If medial extension gap tightness persists despite the extensive release (after assessment with a spacer block), a reduction osteotomy of the posteromedial aspect of the upper tibia is performed to reduce tenting of the superficial MCL [17]. The authors do not perform elevation of superficial MCL and release of pes anserinus insertion as part of the extensive release as these can lead to excessively large flexion and/or extension gaps medially. Femoral component upsizing may be necessary in order to

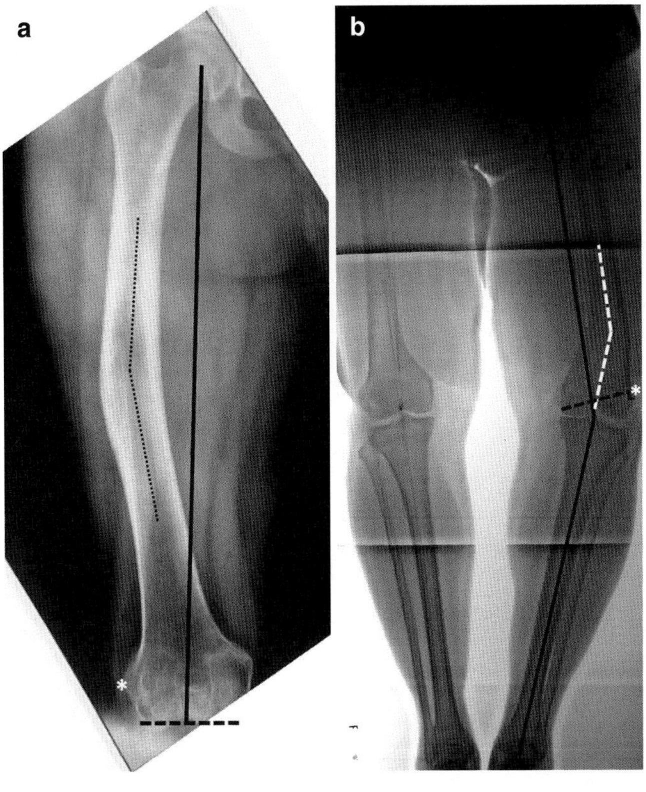

Fig. 8.6 Preoperative planning in a patient with a femoral extra-articular undergoing TKA. (**a**) Preoperative full-length anteroposterior radiograph of the femur showing extra-articular deformity of 15° secondary to malunited fracture of the femoral midshaft. Note that the proposed distal femoral cut (*dashed line*) drawn perpendicular to the mechanical axis of the femur will not compromise the attachment of the lateral collateral ligament (*LCL*) on the lateral epicondyle (*asterisk*) and a corrective osteotomy is not required here. (**b**) Preoperative standing, full-length hip-to-ankle radiograph of a patient with extra-articular deformity in the distal 1/3 femur due to malunited fracture. The limb deformity (hip-knee-ankle angle) in this patient was 22.5°, and the deformity in the distal 1/3 femur due to malunited fracture (*white dashed line*) was 12.5°. However, the proposed distal femoral cut (*black dashed line*) when drawn perpendicular to the mechanical axis of the femur showed that it would have compromised the attachment of the LCL on the lateral epicondyle (*asterisk*). (**c**) Standing knee radiograph of the same patient (b) showing excessive lateral side soft-tissue laxity seen here as excessive opening of the lateral joint space (*arrow*) and deficiency of osteophytes. Considering the severity and proximity of the extra-articular deformity (*dashed line*) to the knee joint, possibility of compromise of LCL with the distal femoral cut, significant lateral soft-tissue laxity and the deficiency of osteophytes, a lateral closing wedge corrective osteotomy at the distal femur will be required in this patient to restore limb alignment

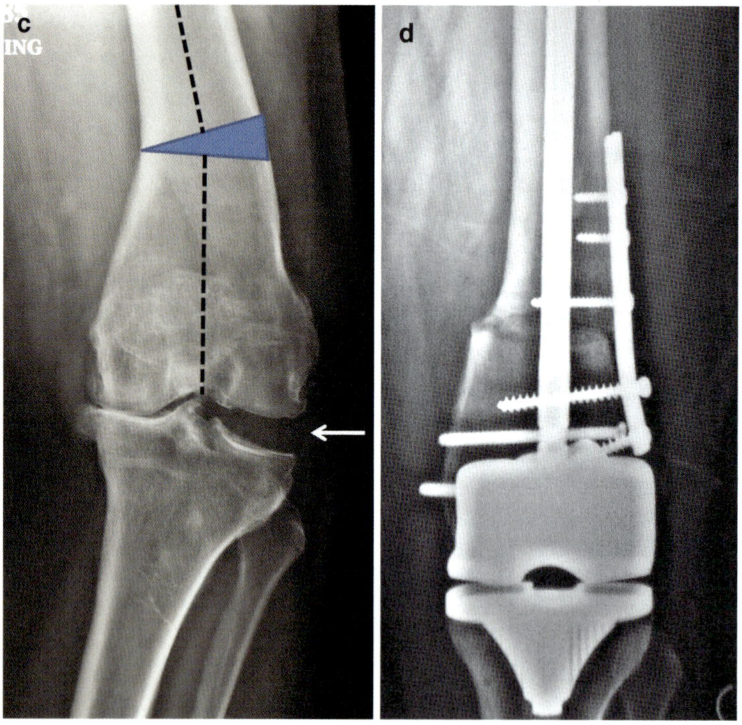

Fig. 8.6 (continued)

balance the larger flexion gap. In the majority of limbs with femoral EADs, the above technique of bone resection and soft-tissue release helps in achieving rectangular gaps and accurately restoring limb alignment (Fig. 8.10) [1].

However, in cases of varus knee osteoarthritis with severe femoral bowing throughout the femoral shaft (commonly due to osteopenia and/or osteomalacia) and with no or minimal osteophytes at the knee and excessive lateral soft-tissue laxity, a sliding medial condylar osteotomy (see Chap. 11 for description of the technique) may be required to achieve a well-balanced and well-aligned knee (Fig. 8.11). Rarely, in cases with severe deformities where the distal femoral cut may compromise the femoral attachment of the collateral ligaments, a simultaneous corrective osteotomy (see Chap. 11 for complete description of the technique) may be necessary at the apex of the EAD. An intramedullary interlocking nailing is appropriate for fixation for this osteotomy and a sleeve-stem construct may be useful in distal deformities.

Tibial Extra-Articular Deformities

Similar to femoral EADs, the basic principle of extensive soft-tissue release with or without a reduction osteotomy works well in restoring limb alignment and soft-tissue balance in most cases with associated tibial EADs. However, centralising the tibial component with respect to the tibial mechanical axis can be tricky in the presence of tibial EAD. While using a tibial component with a stem extender, the component needs to be properly placed so that the stem remains centrally within the medullary canal (in both coronal and sagittal plane) and there is no abutment of the stem on either cortex. Furthermore, the tibial tray should also be fixed perpendicular to the tibial mechanical axis in the coronal plane (so that the tibial tray stem is in line with the tibial mechanical axis). However, due to distortion of the tibia by an EAD, the mechanical axis and medullary axis of the proximal tibia will not overlap (Fig. 8.12a). Therefore, tibial tray placement must be individualised to achieve optimum placement in both

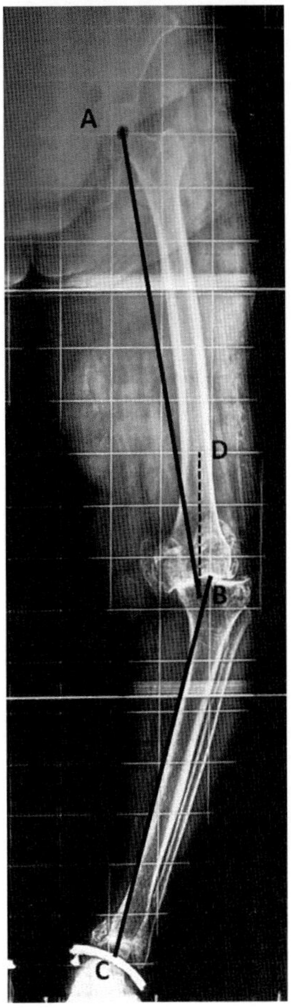

Fig. 8.7 Distal femoral valgus resection angle in the presence of significant femoral bowing measured on preoperative standing, full-length hip-to-ankle radiograph. In this patient the limb deformity (angle *ABC*) was 25° varus. Due to an associated femoral shaft bowing (7°), the distal femoral valgus resection angle in this patient was 9.5° (angle *ABD*). Hence, in the presence of significant femoral bowing (as evidenced by an increase in the angle between the mechanical axis and the distal femoral anatomic axis), the distal femoral valgus resection angle should be measured preoperatively and proportionately increased during the procedure

coronal and sagittal plane (Fig. 8.12b–e). On preoperative full-length hip-to-ankle radiographs, the surgeon needs to plan the placement of the tibial component vis-à-vis the tibial mechanical axis and the proximal medullary canal. The position of the tibial tray can be decided based on the position and severity of EAD. In cases where the mechanical axis is shifted medially (but still parallel to the medullary axis of the proximal tibia) due to EAD (such as malunited fractures, tibia vara or rarely coronal bowing of the shaft), the centre of placement of the tray should be lateralised (Fig. 8.12b–i). In cases where there is significant EAD and the tibial mechanical axis is angled away from the medullary axis of the proximal tibia, the tibial tray is best aligned to the mechanical axis preferably with a short-stem component which will minimise the risk of cortical abutment (Fig. 8.12j–k). Rarely a corrective osteotomy (see Chap. 11 for complete description of the technique) may be required if the extra-articular deformity is significant, close to the knee joint and where the distal tibial axis does not pass through the tibial plateau (Fig. 8.9c).

Among the extra-articular deformities encountered in the tibia, stress fractures are treated based on their type [2]. Malunited intra-articular fractures can be treated with routine TKA, whereas united intra-articular fractures may rarely cause severe medial tibial bone loss where either bone grafting (with resected bone from the TKA cuts) (Fig. 8.13a–b) or metal augments may be required. Impending and united extra-articular fractures can be treated with routine TKA, whereas acute fractures may need a tibial stem extender to improve stability and promote fracture healing (Fig. 8.13c–g). Ununited extra-articular fractures will require local debridement and a tibial stem extender in order to stabilise the fracture site (Fig. 8.13h–i). Malunited stress fractures can be usually treated by routine TKA, but rarely a corrective closing wedge osteotomy and a tibial stem extender may be required.

Post-HTO Deformities

A special category of knees with extra-articular tibial deformity which are undergoing TKA is the post-HTO knee. As previously discussed, it poses several challenges for the surgeon while performing TKA. Beginning with the skin incision, a previous horizontal skin incision is less problematic and goes well with a midline vertical incision for the TKA (Fig. 8.14a). However, a previous vertical skin incision especially if close to the midline may pose a challenge, and it is best to use the same incision with

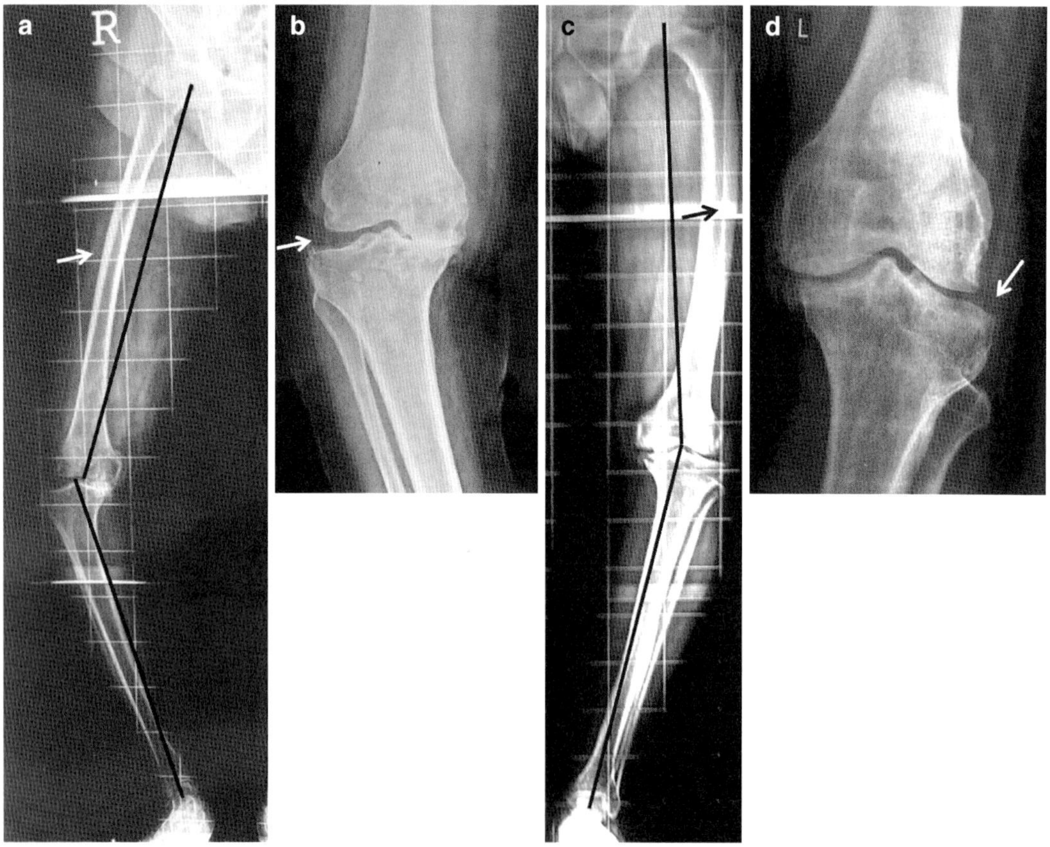

Fig. 8.8 Example of limbs with significant coronal bowing of the femoral shaft where balancing and realignment may be difficult using only intra-articular correction and a sliding osteotomy of the medial condyle (*SMCO*) is required. (**a**) Preoperative standing, full-length hip-to-ankle radiograph showing limb deformity (hip-knee-ankle angle) of 35° with associated significant coronal bowing (6°) of the femoral shaft (*arrow*). (**b**) Preoperative standing knee radiograph of the same patient (a) showing excessive lateral side soft-tissue laxity seen here as excessive opening of the lateral joint space (*arrow*) and lack of osteophytes. (**c**) Preoperative standing, full-length hip-to-ankle radiograph of another patient showing limb deformity (hip-knee-ankle angle) of 15° with associated significant coronal bowing (11°) of the femoral shaft (*arrow*). (**d**) Preoperative standing knee radiograph of the same patient (c) showing excessive lateral side soft-tissue laxity seen here as lateral translation of the tibia (*arrow*) and lack of osteophytes. This patient also had rigid contracture of the medial soft-tissue structures

proximal and distal extensions for TKA. In cases where a more extensive exposure is required for the removal of old implant, the new incision should be merged with the new one if possible so as to minimise damage to blood supply of the skin flap (Fig. 8.14b–c). Owing to scarring around the patellar tendon attachment, exposure and eversion of the patella may be difficult and will require release and excision of fibrous tissue to facilitate lateral displacement of the extensor mechanism and achieve adequate exposure of the tibial surface. Old hardware if present may require removal before the start of the TKA. If there is a possibility that the implant may interfere with fixation of the tibial tray (Fig. 8.14c), the hardware should be removed either through the same TKA incision if possible or through a small separate incision. A post-HTO knee may present with different combinations of coronal (varus or valgus) and sagittal (hyperextension or flexion) plane deformities. Based on the severity of deformity and soft-tissue balance, thickness of the tibial cut may have to be modified (less bone resected in cases with severe deformities and

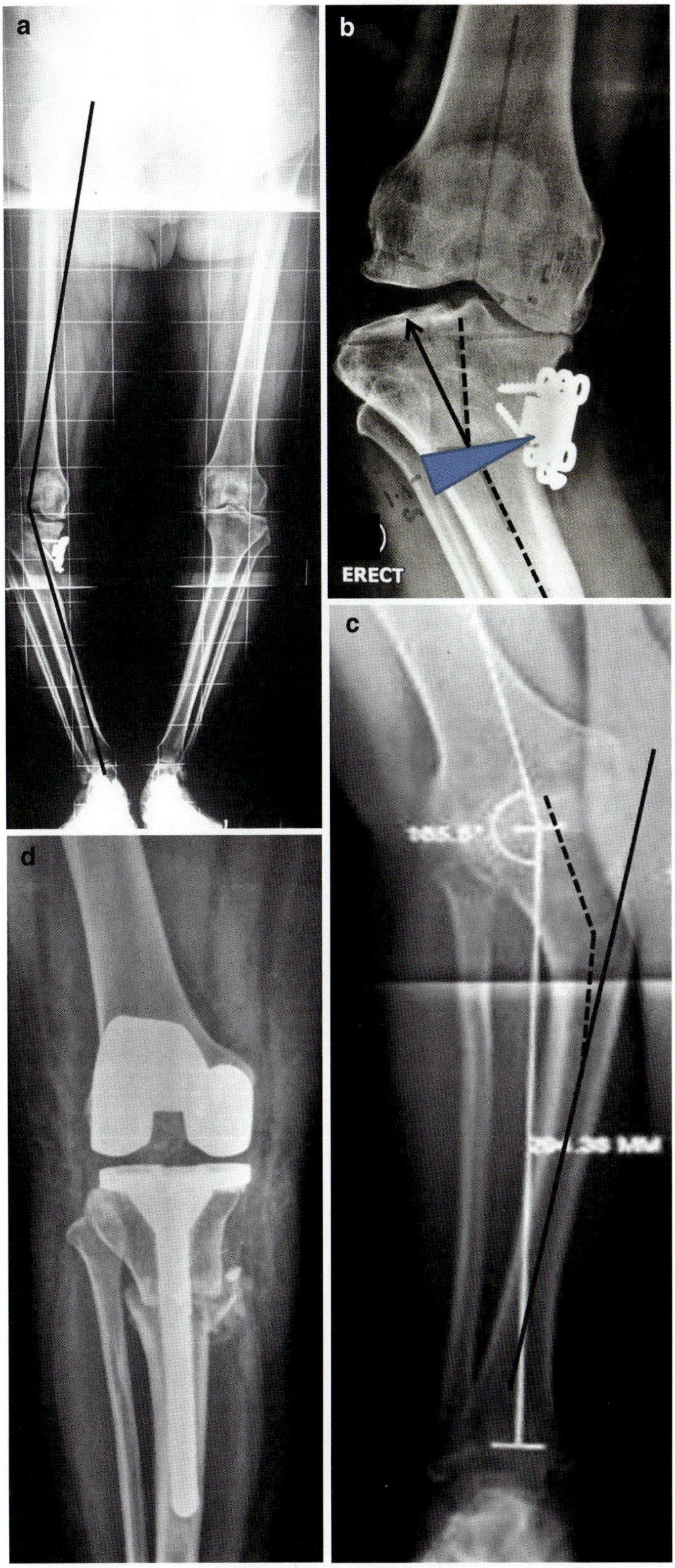

Fig. 8.9 Preoperative planning in a patient with a tibial extra-articular undergoing TKA. (**a**) Preoperative standing, full-length hip-to-ankle radiograph showing limb deformity (hip-knee-ankle angle) of 25° varus with associated post-HTO proximal tibial extra-articular deformity. (**b**) Preoperative standing knee radiograph of the same patient showing extra-articular deformity of the proximal tibia of 25° varus (*dashed line*). *Solid line* is proximal extension of tibial medullary axis. Considering the severity and proximity of the extra-articular deformity to the knee joint, significant lateral soft-tissue laxity and the deficiency of osteophytes, a corrective osteotomy will be required in this patient to restore limb alignment. (**c**) Preoperative full-length anteroposterior radiograph of the tibia showing extra-articular deformity of 20° (*dashed line*) secondary to malunited fracture of the proximal tibial shaft. Note that the distal tibial axis does not pass through the tibial plateau (*solid black line*) and the extra-articular deformity is severe and close to the knee joint, and hence, a corrective osteotomy is required here

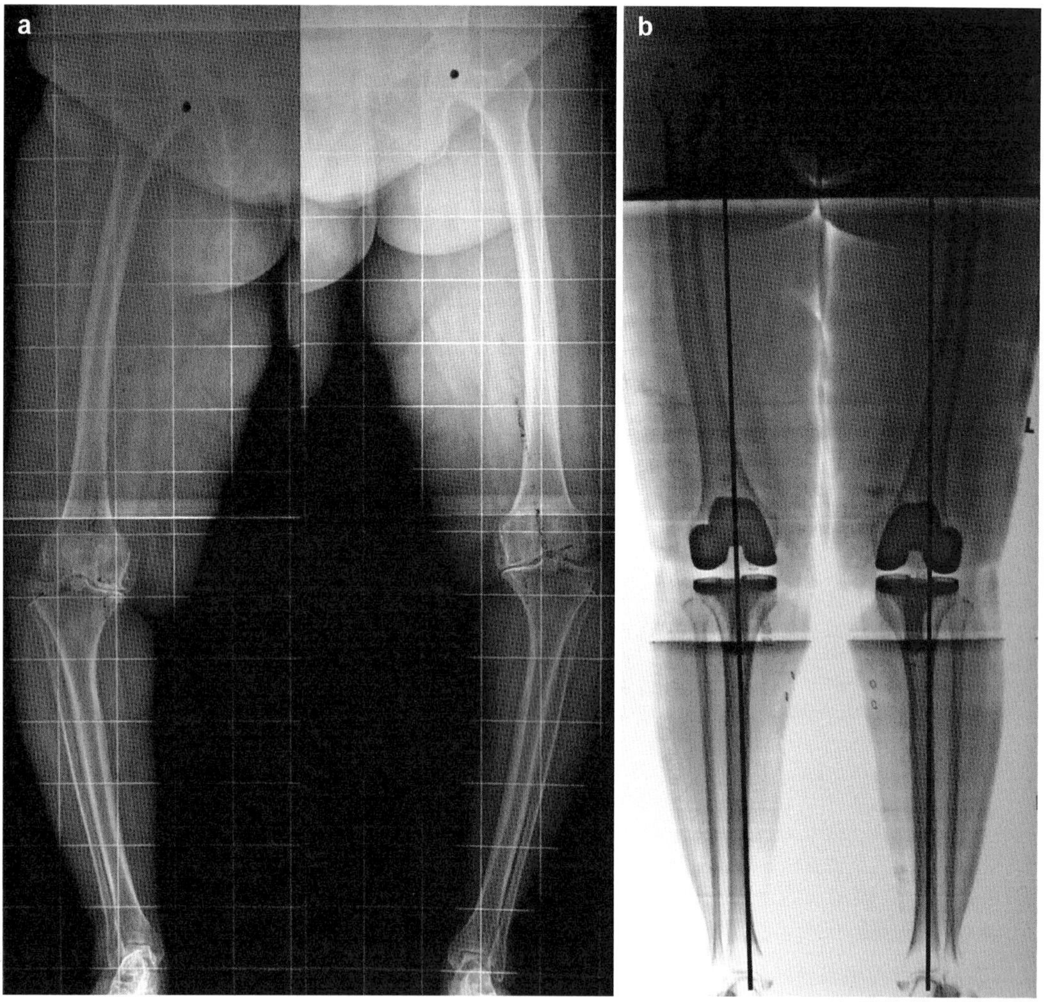

Fig. 8.10 Example of limbs with significant coronal bowing of the femoral shaft where balancing and realignment was performed using intra-articular corrective measures such as extensive soft-tissue releases and a reduction osteotomy. Note that in the majority of limbs with femoral extra-articular deformities, the above intra-articular technique helps in achieving rectangular gaps and accurately restored limb alignment. (**a**) Preoperative standing, full-length hip-to-ankle radiograph showing limb deformity (hip-knee-ankle angle) of 24° (*right side*) and 23° (*left side*) varus with associated significant coronal bowing of 6° (*right side*) and 10° (*left side*) of the femoral shaft. (**b**) Postoperative standing, full-length hip-to-ankle radiograph of the above patient showing restoration of limb alignment on both sides using only intra-articular measures

significant medio-lateral soft-tissue imbalance). Furthermore, the tibial slope may be decreased or increased due to the previous HTO which should be determined on preoperative lateral knee radiographs and care exercised not to be misled by the altered slope. A closing wedge HTO usually causes decrease in slope, whereas opening wedge may cause increase in slope [12]. Rarely, a knee will have an anterior slope with resulting hyperextension at the knee. Accordingly the surgeon needs to factor this in while determining the sagittal plane of the tibial cut.

The surgeon needs to be careful while positioning the tibial tray with respect to the tibial cut surface. Both preoperative planning on knee radiographs and intraoperative checking with trial components are crucial to get this right. In the presence of medial or lateral translation of the proximal tibia, it may be challenging to fully centralise the tibial component stem within the

Fig. 8.11 Example of a limb with significant coronal bowing of the femoral shaft where balancing and realignment was not possible using only intra-articular correction and a sliding osteotomy of the medial condyle (*SMCO*) was required. (**a**) Preoperative standing, full-length hip-to-ankle radiograph showing limb deformity (hip-knee-ankle angle) of 35° with associated significant coronal bowing (6°) of the femoral shaft. Note that the patient also has excessive lateral soft-tissue laxity (*arrow*) and the deficiency of osteophytes medially. (**b**) Postoperative standing, full-length hip-to-ankle radiograph of the above patient showing complete restoration of limb alignment after performing a SMCO. (**c**) Enlarged radiographic image of the SMCO site of the above patient where the condylar fragment has been fixed with cancellous screws. The condylar fragment is distalised and fixed (*dotted arrow*) in order to increase the medial joint space and equalise the medial gap to the lateral gap

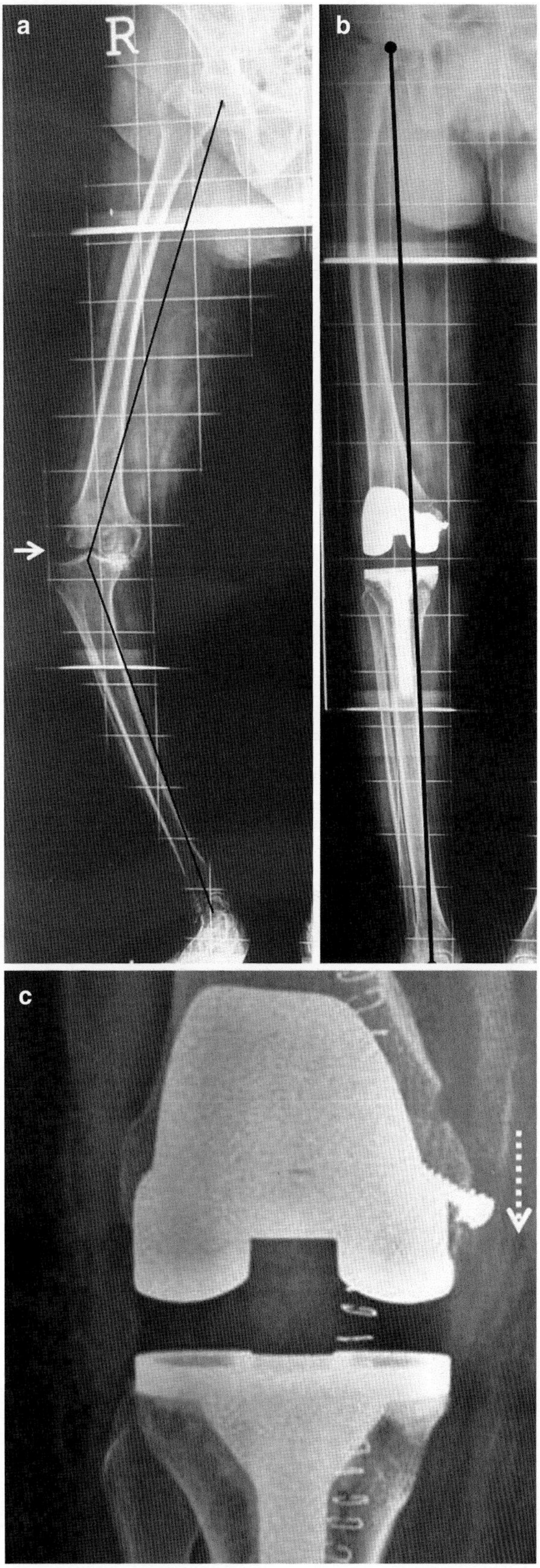

medullary canal and also align it with the mechanical axis of the tibia. In such cases it is best to place the component in line with the mechanical axis of the tibia to avoid cortical abutment of the stem, although a lateral or medial position of the stem within the medullary canal may be unavoidable (Fig. 8.15a–d). The surgeon may use tibial components with an offset stem if available in such situations. Rotational malunion of the proximal tibia may render the tibial tubercle an unreliable landmark to determine the rotational position of the tibial component. The surgeon therefore needs to verify the rotational position of the tray with respect to the distal tibia (malleoli) and also by putting the knee through an arc of flexion and extension. Few cases may present with a large medial tibial bone defect secondary to the osteotomy in which case medial build up with bone graft or augment may be necessary. Rarely, severe extra-articular deformity in

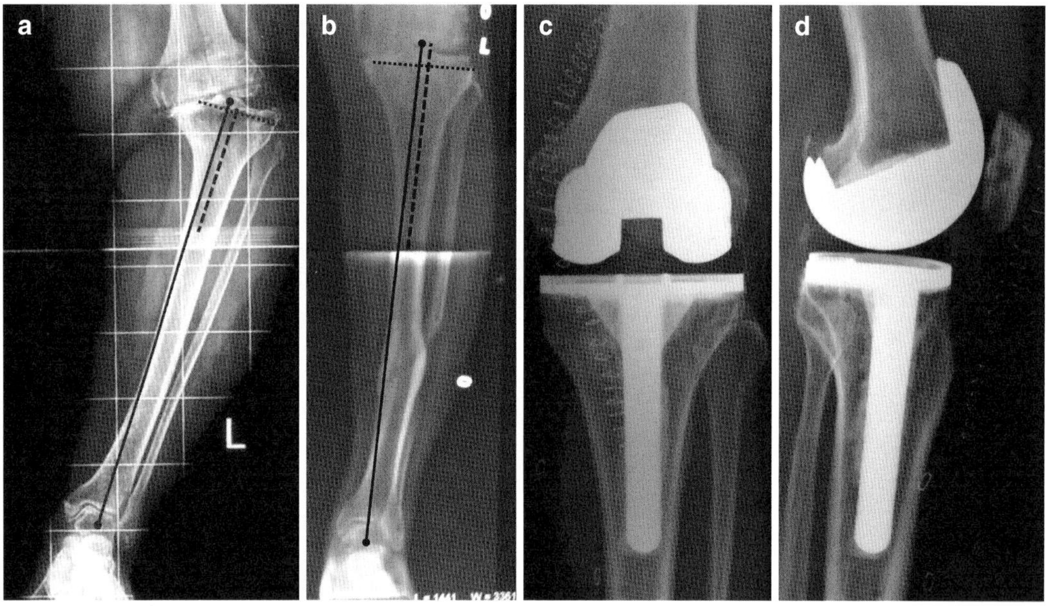

Fig. 8.12 Positioning the tibial tray in the presence of tibial extra-articular deformity. (**a**) Lateral offset of the proximal tibial medullary axis (*dashed line*) with respect to the tibial mechanical axis (*solid line*) and the tibial cut (*dotted line*) in the presence of tibia vara. (**b**) Preoperative standing, full-length tibia radiograph showing lateral offset of the proximal tibial medullary axis (*dashed line*) with respect to the tibial mechanical axis (*solid line*) and the tibial cut (*dotted line*) in the presence of a malunited fracture of the distal ½ of the tibial shaft. (**c**) Postoperative anteroposterior knee radiograph of the same patient (b) showing central position of the long tibial stem within the medullary canal. The tibial component was implanted after lateralisation in line with the proximal tibial medullary axis. (**d**) Postoperative lateral knee radiograph of the same patient (b) showing central position of the long tibial stem within the medullary canal even in the sagittal plane. (**e**) Postoperative standing, full-length tibial radiograph of the same patient (b) showing the tibial component in line with the tibial mechanical axis. (**f**) Preoperative standing, full-length tibial radiograph showing lateral offset of the proximal tibial medullary axis (*dashed line*) with respect to the tibial mechanical axis (*solid line*) and the tibial cut (*dotted line*) in the presence of a malunited fracture of the tibial midshaft with a broken nail in situ. (**g**) Postoperative anteroposterior knee radiograph of the same patient (f) showing the all polyethylene tibial component in line with the tibial mechanical axis (*solid line*). (**h**) Preoperative standing, full-length tibia radiograph showing lateral offset of the proximal tibial medullary axis (*dashed line*) with respect to the tibial mechanical axis (*solid line*) and the tibial cut (*dotted line*) in the presence of a malunited fracture of the tibial midshaft. (**i**) Postoperative anteroposterior knee radiograph of the same patient (h) showing the tibial component in line with the tibial mechanical axis (*solid line*). (**j**) Preoperative standing, full-length tibial radiograph showing significant extra-articular deformity due to malunited fracture of the proximal 1/3 of the tibial shaft. The proximal tibial medullary axis (*dashed line*) is angled away with respect to the tibial mechanical axis (*solid line*) and the tibial cut (*dotted line*). (**k**) Postoperative anteroposterior knee radiograph of the same patient (j) showing the all polyethylene tibial component with a short stem in line with the tibial mechanical axis. The tibial component was implanted in line with the mechanical axis of the tibia (*solid line*)

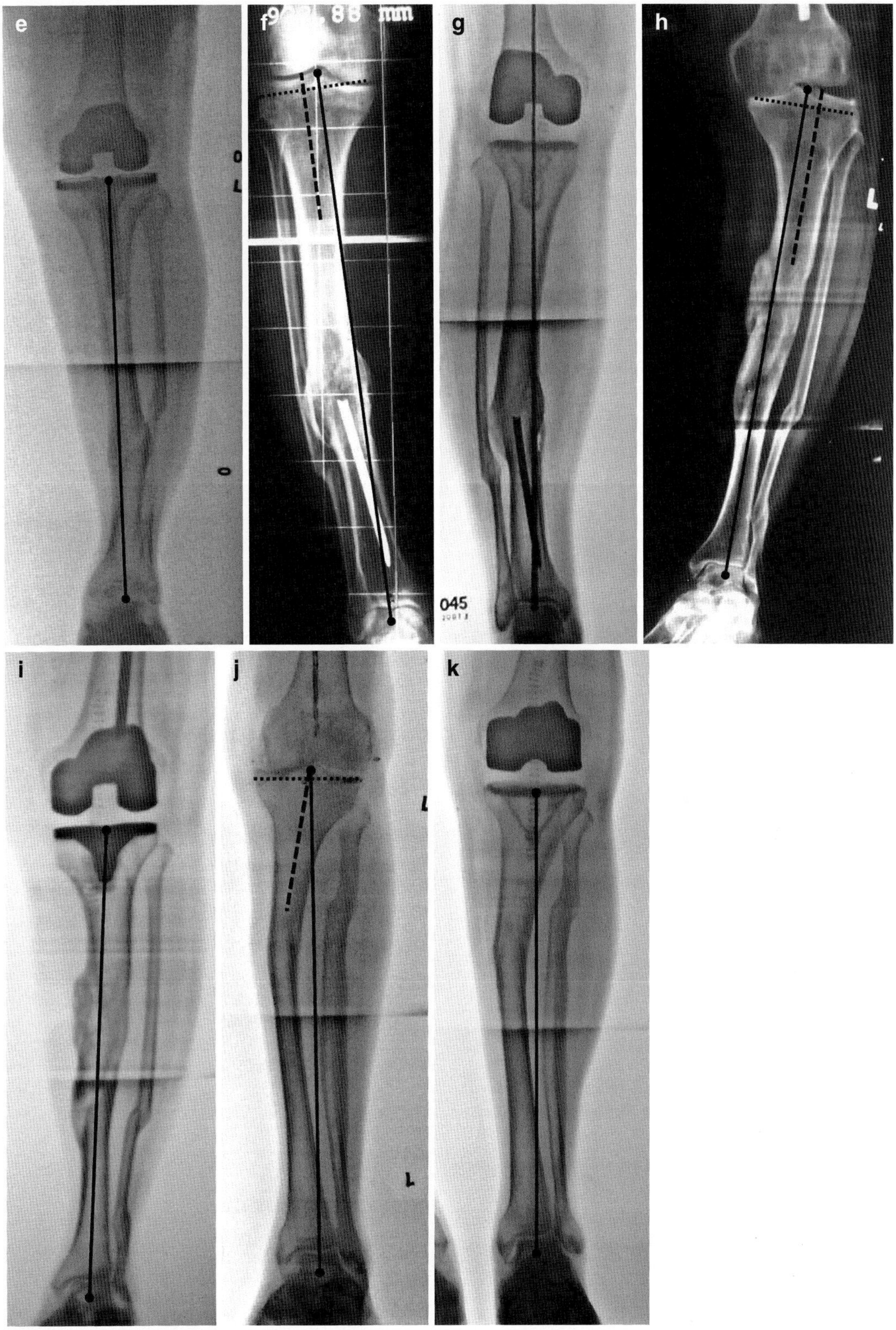

Fig. 8.12 (continued)

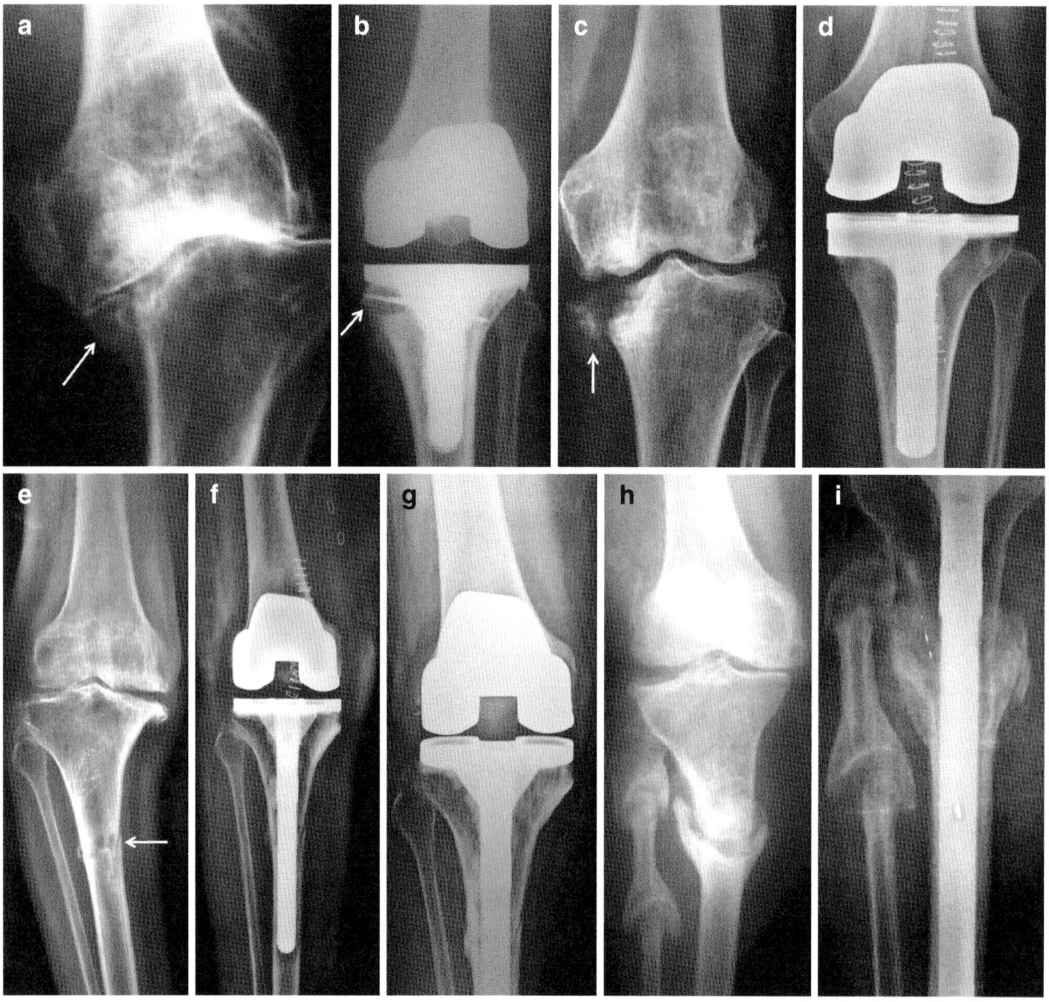

Fig. 8.13 Treatment of tibial stress fractures during TKA. (**a**) Preoperative standing knee radiograph showing an intra-articular ununited tibial stress fracture (*arrow*). (**b**) Postoperative standing knee radiograph of same patient (a) showing the medial tibial bone defect caused by the stress fracture treated with autologous bone graft fixed with Kirschner wires (*arrow*) and stabilised with a tibial stem extender. (**c**) Preoperative standing knee radiograph showing an intra-articular ununited tibial stress fracture with significant bone loss of the medial tibial plateau (*arrow*). (**d**) Postoperative standing knee radiograph of same patient (c) showing the medial tibial bone defect treated with a metal augment and stabilised with a tibial stem extender. (**e**) Preoperative standing knee radiograph showing an extra-articular acute stress fracture (*arrow*) of the proximal tibial shaft. (**f**) Postoperative standing knee radiograph of the same patient (**e**) showing the fracture stabilised with a long tibial stem extender. (**g**) Standing knee radiograph of the same patient (**e**) at 3 months postoperatively showing union at the fracture site. (**h**) Preoperative standing knee radiograph showing an extra-articular ununited stress fracture of the proximal tibial shaft. (**h**) Standing knee radiograph of the same patient (f) at 6 months postoperatively showing union at the fracture site

the proximal tibia due to previous osteotomy may require a corrective osteotomy to achieve optimum limb and component alignment and also soft-tissue balance (Fig. 8.15e–f).

Significant soft-tissue imbalance due to previous HTO primarily depends on whether the knee has been overcorrected (valgus) or undercorrected (varus) and to what extent has the tibial slope altered. Overcorrection by HTO will cause stretching of the medial soft-tissue structures along with the already stretched out lateral soft-tissue structures (due to pre-HTO medial

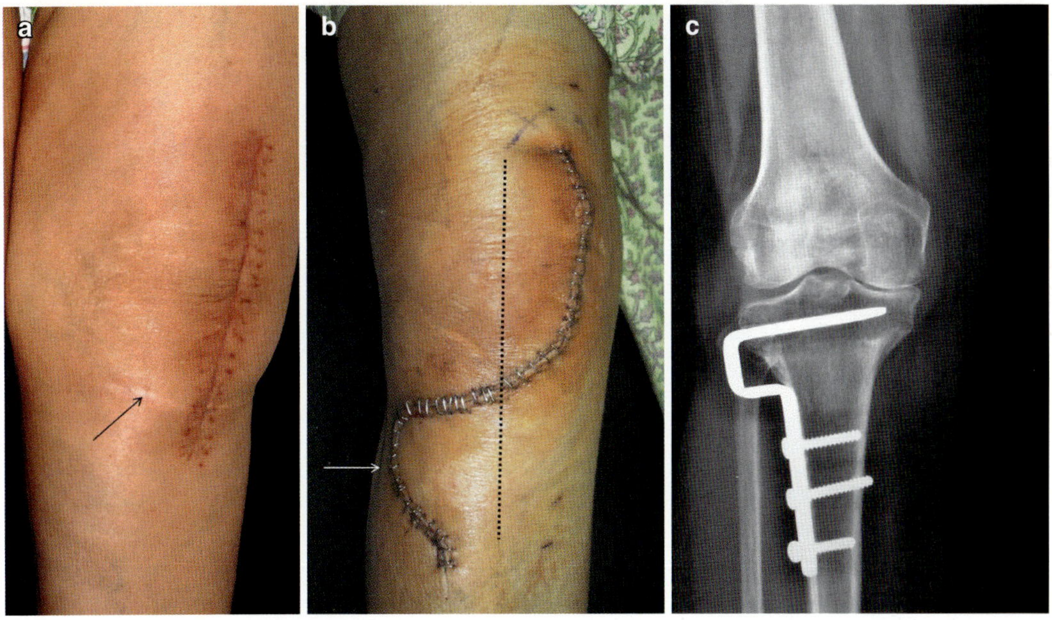

Fig. 8.14 Previous skin incisions encountered during TKA performed in post-high tibial osteotomy (*HTO*) knees. (**a**) Clinical photograph of the knee taken 1 month postoperatively after TKA. A previous horizontal incision (*arrow*) does not interfere with healing of the subsequent vertical incision used for TKA. (**b**) Clinical photograph of another patient taken 2 weeks postoperatively after TKA during suture removal. A curved anterolateral incision (*arrow*) used for a previous HTO poses a challenge for the subsequent vertical, midline TKA incision (*dotted line*). A vertical incision in this case could have jeopardised the vascularity of the flap distally. In this case, we extended the incision proximally and medially in line with the previous incision. (**c**) Preoperative knee radiograph of the same patient in (b) shows a large plate and multiple screws used to fix the HTO. Since the hardware had to be removed before start of TKA, a more extensive approach to include the previous curved anterolateral incision [as seen in (b)] was used

OA). Hence, overcorrected limbs will show significant laxity on both medial and lateral sides, causing increase in the extension gap. Similarly, anterior sloping will cause the knee to go into hyperextension, laxity of posterior soft-tissue structures and a large extension gap. Both these scenarios require the surgeon to minimise resection from not only the proximal tibia but also the distal femur. Hence, a thicker tibial insert or very rarely constrained implant may be required in post-HTO knees during TKA. Furthermore, significant medial tibial bone loss and the resultant tibial cut will cause increase in both extension and flexion gap. Hence, the femoral component may have to be upsized in order to balance the flexion gap with the extension gap.

In all patients treated with intra-articular correction only, routine postoperative rehabilitation is carried out with bedside knee range of motion, and quadriceps strengthening exercises and ambulation with walking frame usually commenced within 6 h after surgery. In patients where a lateral epicondylar or a sliding medial condylar osteotomy has been performed, the patient is allowed full weight-bearing ambulation with a long knee brace. Knee movement is not allowed for 2 weeks after which the patient is advised to remove the brace three to four times a day and perform gentle, active knee flexion and extension. Knee brace is discontinued at 4 weeks and patient allowed full activity. In patients where a corrective osteotomy is performed, knee movements and partial weight-bearing ambulation in long-leg knee brace are commenced the next day postoperatively. If x-rays at 4–6 weeks show satisfactory healing, patients are allowed full weight-bearing ambulation with a stick but are advised to wear the brace. After 3 months, the brace and stick may be discontinued once x-rays show that the osteotomy site has consolidated.

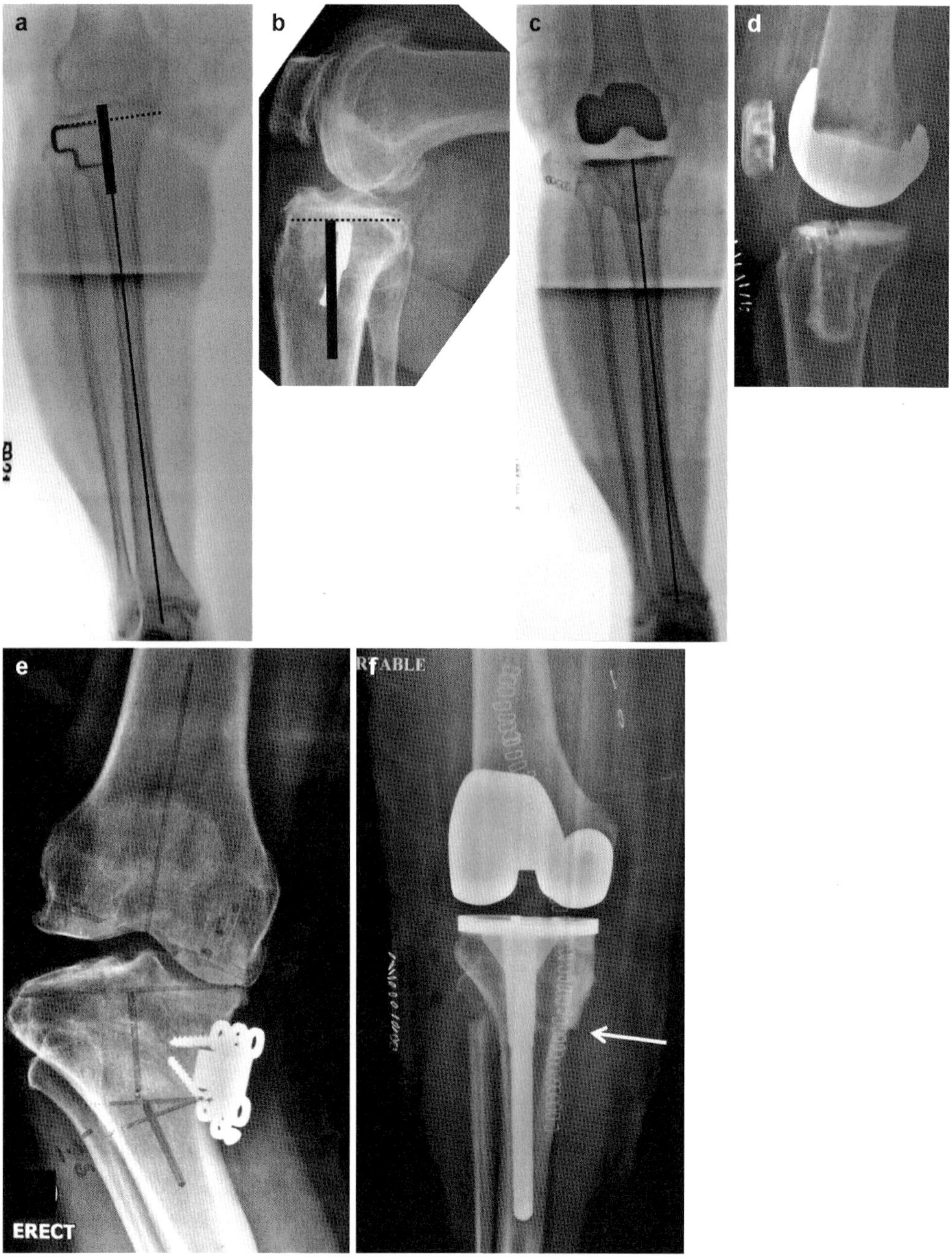

Fig. 8.15 TKA in knees with previous HTO. (**a**) Preoperative standing, full-length tibial radiograph showing a lateral closing wedge HTO fixed with staples. Tibial component if aligned with respect to the tibial mechanical axis (*solid thin line*) will lateralise the tibial stem (*short thick line*), close to the lateral cortex of the tibia. *Dotted line* in (**a**) is tentative position of the tibial tray. (**b**) Preoperative lateral knee radiograph showing tentative position of the tibial tray (*dotted line*) and its stem (*solid thick line*) with respect to the proximal tibial intramedullary axis. (**c**) Postoperative standing, full-length tibial radiograph of same patient (a) showing the tibial component aligned along the tibial mechanical axis (*solid thin line*). Note that the tibial stem is lateral and closer to the lateral cortex of the tibia as expected. (**d**) Postoperative lateral knee radiograph showing final position of the tibial tray and its stem in the sagittal plane. (**e**) Severe extra-articular varus deformity (25° varus) of the proximal tibia with implant in situ. A corrective osteotomy is required here to restore limb alignment considering the severity and proximity of the extra-articular deformity to the knee joint, significant lateral soft-tissue laxity and the deficiency of osteophytes. (**f**) Postoperative standing knee radiograph of same patient (e) showing the final position of the tibial component and stem following a corrective osteotomy (*arrow*)

Computer-Assisted Technique

Navigation systems determine mechanical axis of femur, tibia and the lower limb using specific points (centre of the hip, knee and ankle) acquired during registration. Hence, navigation has the ability to determine the mechanical axis and the position of components irrespective of the presence of any EAD of femur or tibia or hardware in between. In contrast, conventional TKA requires the use of alignment devices (intramedullary for the femur) to determine implant position and limb mechanical alignment. The presence of a distorted femoral canal and/or hardware will require the surgeon to use an extramedullary guide, remove the obstructing hardware or correct the deformity with a corrective osteotomy. Navigation, therefore, is a better option compared to conventional techniques when TKA is performed in the presence of significant EAD especially in the presence of hardware [1, 18].

An osteotomy (lateral epicondylar, SMCO or corrective osteotomy) may have to be performed simultaneously with TKA in cases with severe EADs as previously discussed. Conventional measuring techniques to determine the amount of correction required or the amount by which the medial condyle or lateral epicondyle needs to be shifted can be imprecise and unreliable. Navigation helps to accurately measure the degree of deformity and the amount of gap imbalance and therefore helps the surgeon to accurate quantify the amount of correction required in alignment and gap imbalance. Therefore, navigation can be a more accurate and quantitative method to perform osteotomies during TKA [9, 10, 18]. However, the surgeon must be well versed with the navigation before attempting to perform simultaneous computer-assisted osteotomies during TKA.

References

1. Mullaji A, Shetty GM. Computer-assisted total knee arthroplasty for arthritis with extra-articular deformity. J Arthroplasty. 2009;24:1164–9.
2. Mullaji A, Shetty G. Total knee arthroplasty for arthritic knees with tibiofibular stress fractures classification and treatment guidelines. J Arthroplasty. 2010;25:295–301.
3. Wang JW, Wang CJ. Total knee arthroplasty for arthritis of the knee with extra-articular deformity. J Bone Joint Surg Am. 2002;84:1769–74.
4. Fehring TK, Mason JB, Moskal J, Pollock DC, Mann J, Williams VJ. When computer-assisted knee replacement is the best alternative. Clin Orthop Relat Res. 2006;452:132–6.
5. Chou WY, Ko JY, Wang CJ, Wang FS, Wu RW, Wong T. Navigation-assisted total knee arthroplasty for a knee with malunion of the distal femur. J Arthroplasty. 2008;23:1239.e13–9.
6. Klein GR, Austin MS, Smith EB, Hozack WJ. Total knee arthroplasty using computer-assisted navigation in patients with deformities of the femur and tibia. J Arthroplasty. 2006;21:284–8.
7. Bottros J, Klika AK, Lee HH, Polousky J, Barsoum WK. The use of navigation in total knee arthroplasty for patients with extra-articular deformity. J Arthroplasty. 2008;23:74–8.
8. Kim KI, Ramteke AA, Bae DK. Navigation-assisted minimal invasive total knee arthroplasty in patients with extra-articular femoral deformity. J Arthroplasty. 2009;25:658.e17–22.
9. Mullaji AB, Shetty GM. Lateral epicondylar osteotomy using computer navigation in total knee arthroplasty for rigid valgus deformities. J Arthroplasty. 2010;25:166–9.
10. Mullaji AB, Shetty GM. Surgical technique: computer-assisted sliding medial condylar osteotomy to achieve gap balance in varus knees during TKA. Clin Orthop Relat Res. 2013;471:1484–91.
11. Mullaji AB, Marawar SV, Mittal V. A comparison of coronal plane axial femoral relationships in Asian patients with varus osteoarthritic knees and healthy knees. J Arthroplasty. 2009;24:861–7.
12. Bonnin M, Zayni R. Total knee arthroplasty after failed high tibial osteotomy. In: Bonnin M, Amendola NA, Bellemans J, MacDonald SJ, Menetrey J, editors. The knee joint. Paris: Springer; 2012. p. 923–32.
13. Madan S, Ranjith RK, Fiddian NJ. Total knee replacement following high tibial osteotomy. Bull Hosp Jt Dis. 2002–2003;61:5–10.
14. Mullaji AB, Shetty GM, Kanna R, Vadapalli RC. The influence of preoperative deformity on valgus correction angle: an analysis of 503 total knee arthroplasties. J Arthroplasty. 2013;28:20–7.

15. Mullaji A, Kanna R, Marawar S, Kohli A, Sharma A. Comparison of limb and component alignment using computer-assisted navigation versus image intensifier-guided conventional total knee arthroplasty: a prospective, randomized, single-surgeon study of 467 knees. J Arthroplasty. 2007;22:953–9.
16. Mullaji AB, Padmanabhan V, Jindal G. Total knee arthroplasty for profound varus deformity: technique and radiological results in 173 knees with varus of more than 20 degrees. J Arthroplasty. 2005;20:550–61.
17. Mullaji AB, Shetty GM. Correction of varus deformity during TKA with reduction osteotomy. Clin Orthop Relat Res. 2014;472:126–32.
18. Mason JB, Fehring TK. Management of extra-articular deformity in total knee arthroplasty with navigation. In: Scott WN, editor. Insall & scott surgery of the knee. Philadelphia: Elsevier Churchill Livingstone; 2012. p. 1234.

9 The Stiff Knee

Introduction

A stiff knee is defined as having a range of motion of less than 50° [1]. The most common cause of stiffness in an arthritic knee is osteoarthritis and rheumatoid arthritis [2–6]. Less common causes include previous trauma, surgery, infection, ankylosing spondylitis, psoriatic arthritis and haemophilic arthropathy [2–6].

Approaching a stiff knee for TKA is not only difficult but is fraught with risks. This is one situation where a tibial tubercle osteotomy or a quadriceps snip may be required to achieve adequate exposure [7]. Furthermore, stiffness of soft tissues and the associated osteoporosis put these knees at high risk for inadvertent intraoperative fractures or soft-tissue avulsions [3, 4]. Apart from the difficulty in approaching the knee during TKA, stiff knees usually have significant changes in the intra- and periarticular soft tissues which make soft-tissue release and balancing more challenging. In addition to excessive fibrous tissue within the joint, important soft-tissue structures such as the quadriceps, cruciates and collateral ligaments and the joint capsule may be scarred and contracted. Hence, the integrity and competence of these important soft-tissue stabilisers of the knee is unclear and often difficult to assess.

Although technically demanding, TKA in stiff knees has been reported to significantly improve knee range of motion and function [2–4, 8–10]. However, meticulous surgical technique and aggressive postoperative rehabilitation is the key to improve overall function after TKA in stiff knees. In this chapter, the authors describe their approach to treating stiff arthritic knees with TKA.

Pathoanatomy

Stiffness in arthritic knees undergoing TKA is mainly a consequence of severe soft-tissue adhesions within and around the joint. This is more pronounced in stiffness caused due to previous trauma, surgery or infection. In cases with osteoarthritis and rheumatoid arthritis, large multiple osteophytes and adaptive bone changes may cause mechanical blocks to knee movement, further aggravating the stiffness.

Adhesions tethering the quadriceps muscle in the suprapatellar area along with severe patellofemoral arthritis (Fig. 9.1) can be a major cause of limited flexion. Contraction of the posterior capsule along with large osteophytes posteriorly can block extension (Fig. 9.1). Fibrous tissue in the lateral and medial gutters, posterior compartment and the suprapatellar pouch and around soft-tissue structures such as cruciates, collaterals, quadriceps and flexor tendons can severely restrict joint range of motion.

A thorough examination of the knee under anaesthesia will give clues about the actual type of deformity in the coronal plane (varus or valgus) and the amount of medio-lateral laxity present

A.B. Mullaji, G.M. Shetty, *Deformity Correction in Total Knee Arthroplasty*,
DOI 10.1007/978-1-4939-0566-9_9,

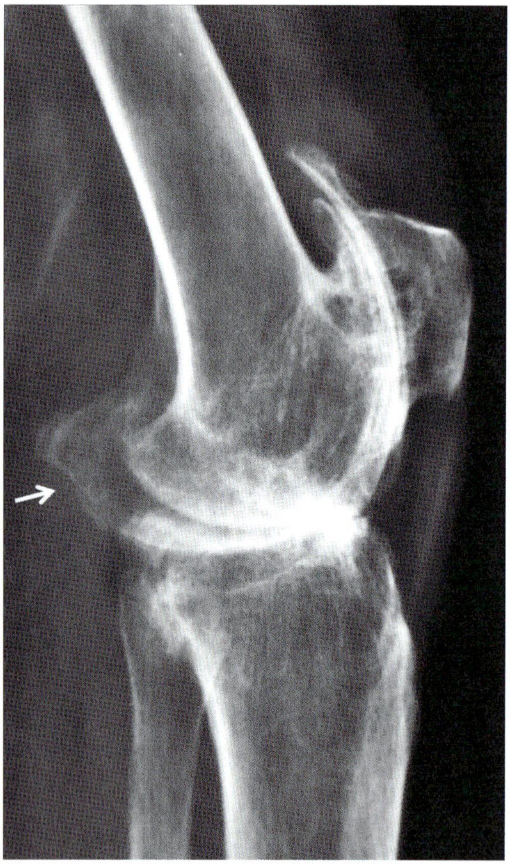

Fig. 9.1 Preoperative lateral knee radiograph showing severe patellofemoral arthritis which will restrict knee flexion and large posterior femoral osteophyte (*arrow*) which will restrict knee extension

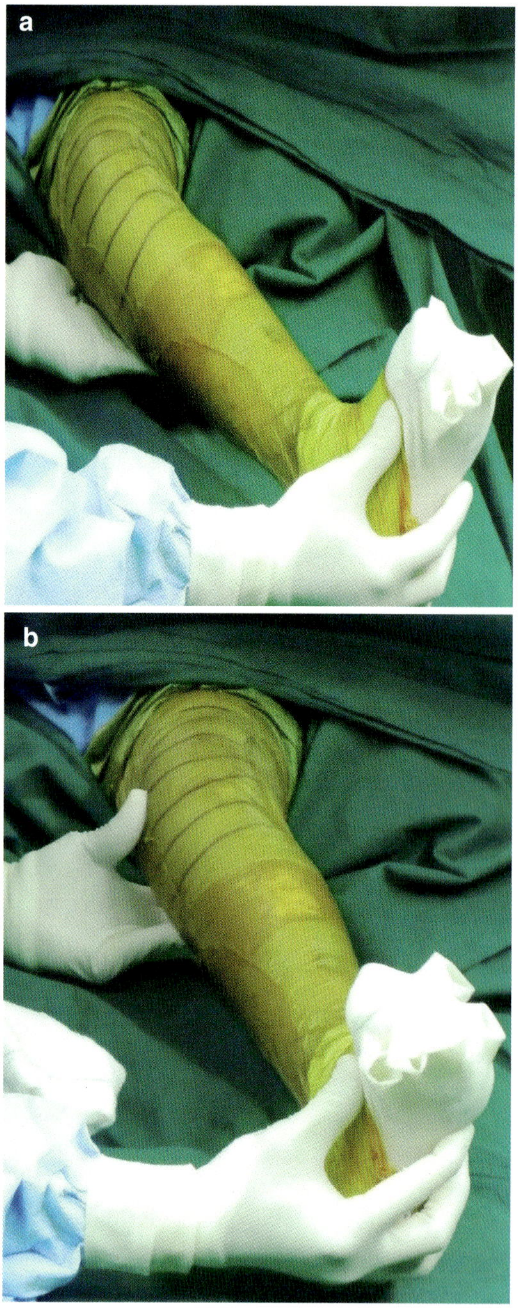

Fig. 9.2 Examination of the knee under anaesthesia to determine the type of coronal deformity and severity of knee stiffness. (**a**) Medial laxity with a valgus stress at the knee joint. (**b**) Lateral laxity with a varus stress at the knee joint. (**c**) Maximum knee flexion. (**d**) Maximum knee extension

(Fig. 9.2). It will also enable the surgeon to assess the actual knee ROM which might be severely restricted if examined without anaesthesia due to pain and reactive (muscular) spasm. A proper assessment of medio-lateral soft-tissue imbalance can only be possible once the knee has been exposed and the range of motion improves with excision of fibrous tissue, cruciates and osteophytes. The key is to proceed with caution and patience and release all the fibrous tissue and tethered soft-tissue structures and excise all the osteophytes. In most cases, this will correct the flexion and extension deformity to a large extent, and the surgeon will achieve adequate exposure of the joint to proceed with the actual TKA procedure.

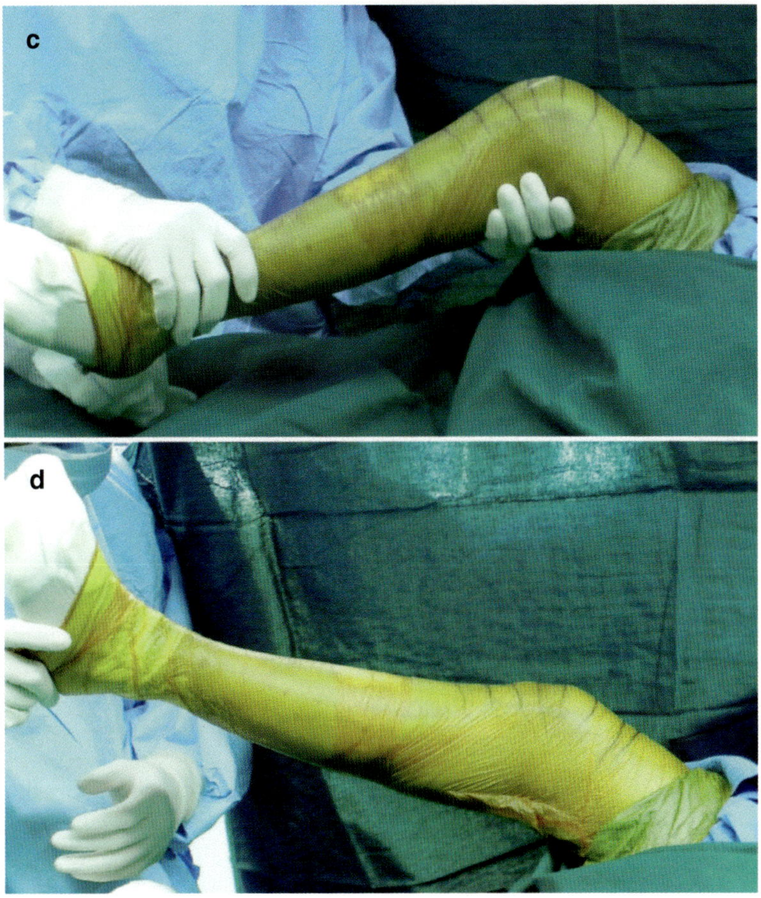

Fig. 9.2 (continued)

Patients with a stiff knee need to be counselled in detail about their expectations and the likely outcome. They must be told that they may not achieve as much flexion as a person without long-standing stiffness and must not compare their progress with other patients undergoing routine TKA! Also it must be emphasised to them that they will need to undergo extensive physiotherapy to maintain and augment the range obtained at surgery.

Surgical Technique

Adequate exposure of the joint is initially restricted due to immobility of the extensor apparatus. After a medial parapatellar arthrotomy, exposure is extended in the deeper planes with the knee in extension (Fig. 9.3). All the parapatellar and anteromedial femoral osteophytes are excised. A thorough synovectomy is performed. The infrapatellar fat pad, medial patellofemoral ligament, fibrous tissue in the suprapatellar pouch (or any fibrous bands tethering the quadriceps muscle) and medial gutter are excised, and the tibial attachment of anteromedial capsule is released using electrocautery. A block pin is inserted into the patellar tendon attachment on the tibial tuberosity to prevent any inadvertent avulsion while the knee is flexed.

The aim should not be to achieve eversion but to obtain sufficient lateral subluxation of the patella. A preliminary release of the lateral retinaculum may be required to achieve sufficient mobility of the patella. With the patella laterally displaced and held in place using a Hohmann's

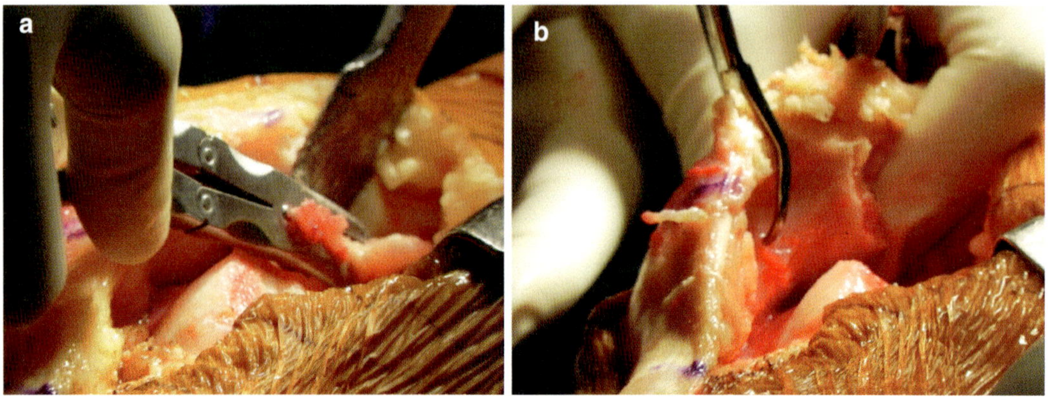

Fig. 9.3 Intraoperative photographs showing approaches for the stiff knee in extension. (**a**) The parapatellar and anteromedial femoral osteophytes are removed using a rongeur and osteotome. (**b**) The patella is gently lifted using a towel clip to reach the lateral aspect for a retinacular release

retractor applied on the lateral side of the tibia, the knee is then gently flexed as much as possible. Intercondylar notch osteophytes are now removed using a narrow osteotome, and both cruciates and the medial meniscus are excised. Osteophytes on the lateral aspect of the femoral condyle and the medial aspect of the tibial plateau are now excised. A preliminary medial soft-tissue release (deep medial collateral ligament, posteromedial capsule and semimembranosus) is now done using electrocautery to achieve anterior dislocation of the tibia. The lateral meniscus is excised after the tibia has been displaced forwards. Rarely, large posterior osteophytes may act as a mechanical block and prevent anterior displacement of the tibia (Fig. 9.4). In such cases, they need to be detached using a thin, narrow osteotome inserted in the joint gap. The remainder of these osteophytes are removed after the tibial cut has been performed for better access. All these steps will further improve knee flexion and expose the tibial plateau for bone cut. A posterior capsular release may be required for residual flexion deformity present despite excision of osteophytes; this is done at its attachment to the posterior femoral condyles. The TKA is then performed in a routine manner in terms of deformity correction and ligament/gap balance (Fig. 9.5).

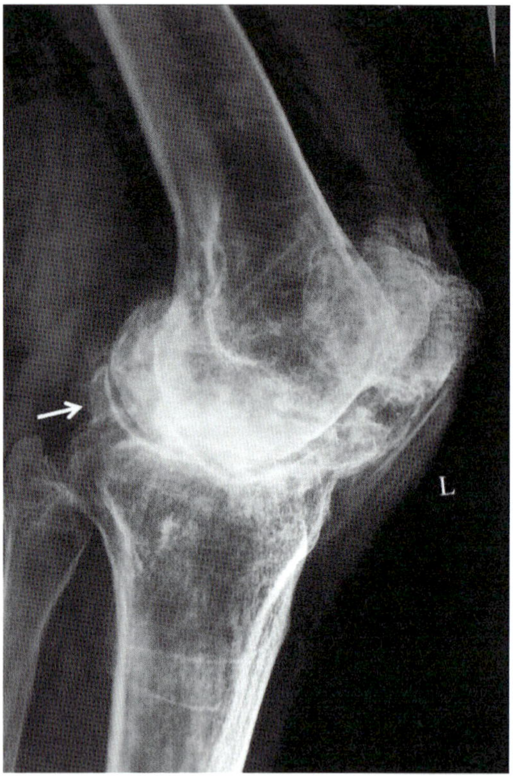

Fig. 9.4 Preoperative lateral knee radiograph showing a large posterior tibial osteophyte (*arrow*) which acts as a mechanical block and prevents anterior dislocation of the tibia

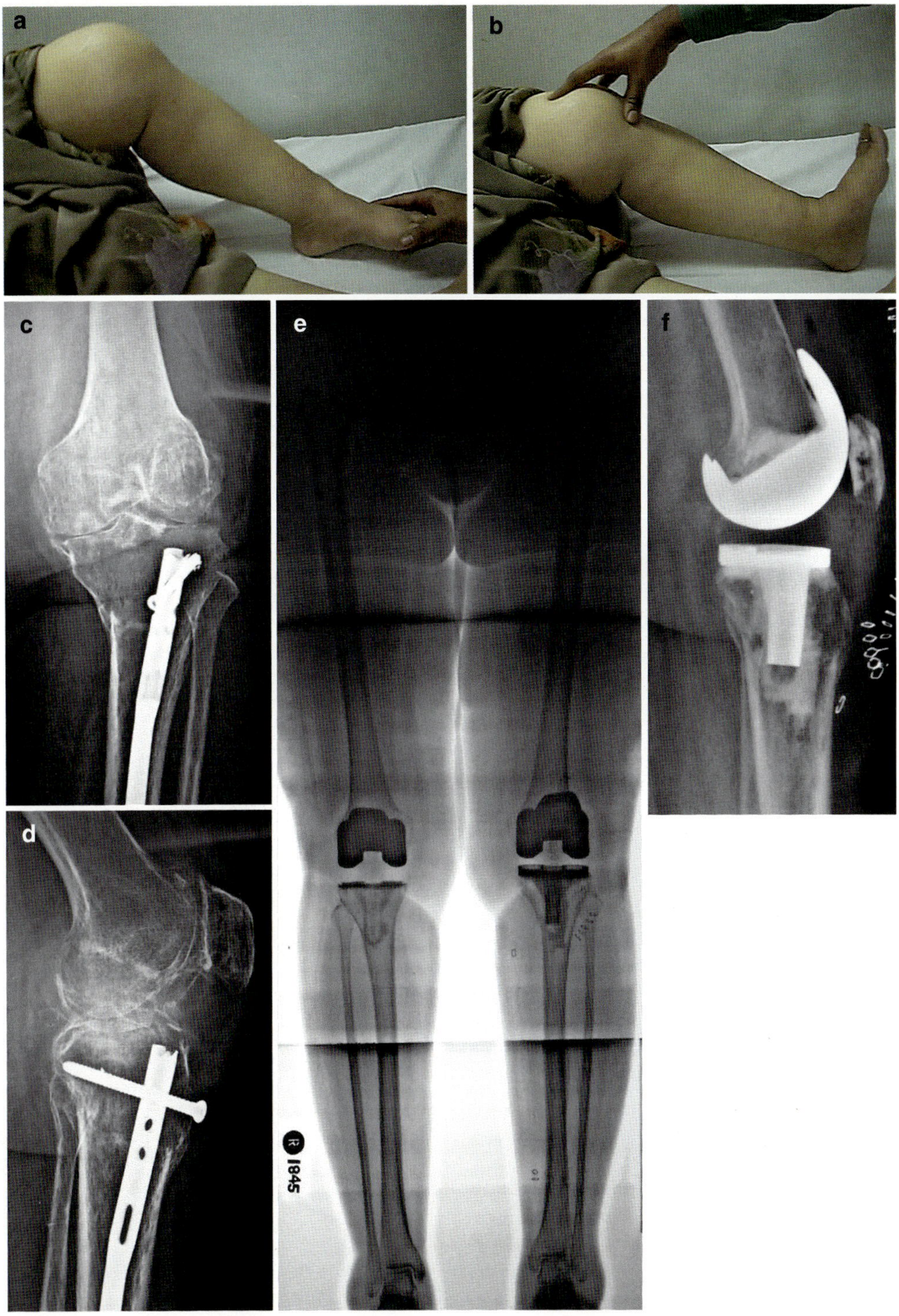

Fig. 9.5 Postsurgical stiff arthritic knee treated with a cruciate-substituting (CS) design. (**a**) Preoperative clinical photograph showing maximum knee flexion. (**b**) Preoperative clinical photograph showing maximum knee extension. (**c**) Preoperative anteroposterior standing knee radiograph of the same patient (a, b) showing an intramedullary tibial nail in situ. (**d**) Preoperative lateral knee radiograph of the same patient. (**e**) Postoperative full-length hip-to-ankle radiograph of the same patient (c) showing complete restoration of limb mechanical axis with a cruciate-substituting knee implant. Note that the tibial nail had to be removed before TKA to facilitate implantation of the tibial component. (**f**) Postoperative lateral knee radiograph of the same patient (c)

The authors occasionally perform a quadriceps snip but never a V-Y plasty or turndown to achieve exposure. Very rarely, a tibial tubercle osteotomy (TTO) may have to be performed to achieve adequate exposure. However, the authors use a more conservative modification of the conventional TTO technique which involves detaching the patellar tendon from the tibial tubercle with a thin layer of bone using a sharp osteotome (refer to Chap. 11), leaving the extensor mechanism intact distally and laterally. The osteotomised bone fragment detached with the tendon heals when the capsulotomy is repaired without the need for fixation in this technique.

A quadricepsplasty is a useful technique to achieve greater flexion in these stiff knees. This is initiated by isolating 3–5 cm length of the deeper layer of the vastus intermedius tendon from the rest of the quadriceps tendon insertion into the upper pole of the patella. A length of 2 cm or so of the intermedius tendon is excised. The knee is gently manipulated to check the improvement in flexion. If more range is desired, pie crusting of the rectus tendon is performed using an 11 number stab knife to make multiple transverse nicks in the tendon in a staggered fashion. The knee is then manipulated again so that there is lengthening of the tendon and further flexion achieved.

Postoperatively, aggressive physiotherapy is recommended to maintain and improve on the range of motion gained after TKA. A 90/90 anterior splint from the proximal thigh to the ankle is applied in the operation theatre before the patient is shifted. This is removed along with the drain the next day morning, and the patient is put on continuous passive motion (CPM) machine for the next 48 h. A muscle relaxant is given orally to the patient along with analgesic/anti-inflammatory medications to prevent muscle spasms and pain while the patient is on CPM. Quadriceps strengthening exercises along with electric stimulation and gravity-assisted active knee flexion and extension exercises and full weight-bearing walking with support are started after 48 h. Working closely with a physiotherapist and frequent monitoring of their progress are essential to obtain optimal function in these difficult cases. Subsequently, stationary bicycling and swimming are encouraged.

References

1. Aglietti P, Windsor RE, Buzzi R, Insall JN. Arthroplasty for the stiff or ankylosed knee. J Arthroplasty. 1989;4:1–5.
2. Rajgopal A, Ahuja N, Dolai B. Total knee arthroplasty in stiff and ankylosed knees. J Arthroplasty. 2005;20:585–90.
3. Bhan S, Malhotra R, Kiran EK. Comparison of total knee arthroplasty in stiff and ankylosed knees. Clin Orthop Relat Res. 2006;451:87–95.
4. Massin P, Lautridou C, Cappelli M, Petit A, Odri G, Ducellier F, Sabatier C, Hulet C, Canciani JP, Letenneur J, Burdin P, Société d'Orthopédie de l'Ouest. Total knee arthroplasty with limitations of flexion. Orthop Traumatol Surg Res. 2009;95(4 Suppl 1):S1–6.
5. Su EP, Su SL, Della Valle AG. The stiff knee – exposure and management. Tech Orthop. 2011;26:105–10.
6. Argenson JN, Vinel H, Aubaniac JM. Total knee arthroplasty for the stiff knee. In: Bonnin M, Chambat P, editors. Osteoarthritis of the knee – surgical treatment. Paris: Springer; 2008. p. 315–21.
7. Barrack R. Surgical exposure of the stiff knee. Acta Orthop Scand. 2000;71:85–9.
8. Bae DK, Yoon KH, Kim HS, Song SJ. Total knee arthroplasty in stiff knees after previous infection. J Bone Joint Surg Br. 2005;87:333–6.
9. Fosco M, Filanti M, Amendola L, Savarino LM, Tigani D. Total knee arthroplasty in stiff knee compared with flexible knees. Musculoskelet Surg. 2011;95:7–12.
10. Hsu CH, Lin PC, Chen WS, Wang JW. Total knee arthroplasty in patients with stiff knees. J Arthroplasty. 2012;27:286–92.

The Unstable Knee

10

Introduction

Excessive soft-tissue laxity is frequently encountered in severely deformed arthritic knees undergoing TKA [1]. It is usually uni- or biplanar where the lateral side (in varus deformity) or medial side (in valgus deformity) shows excessive laxity with or without an associated posterior laxity (in hyperextension deformity) [2]. However, rarely, an arthritic knee undergoing TKA may also show multiplanar or global laxity where there is significant medial, lateral and posterior ligamentous insufficiency along with significant bone loss. Although extremely rare in osteoarthritis or rheumatoid arthritis, severe or global knee instability may be secondary to a neuromuscular disorder (such as post-poliomyelitis, spinal neuropathy) or due to post-traumatic global ligamentous insufficiency [2–7].

Lack of competent and functional collateral ligaments makes it extremely difficult for the surgeon to achieve optimum soft-tissue balance in an unstable knee using conventional cruciate-substituting implants. This gets even more challenging when the knee has an associated hyperextension due to lax and stretched out posterior soft-tissue structures. Hence, an unstable knee is one of the rare occasions where a constrained or hinged prosthesis may be required during primary TKA. This chapter outlines the management of instability during primary TKA.

Pathoanatomy

Severe arthritic knee deformities are associated with significant tibio-femoral bone erosions and adaptive changes in the periarticular ligaments and soft tissues. In varus deformities, bony erosion of the medial tibia and femur, periarticular inflammation and osteophytes cause gradually relative shortening and stiffness of the medial soft-tissue structures [2]. The patient subsequently walks with a varus moment at the knee causing gradual adaptive elongation of the lateral soft-tissue structures [2]. Hence, severe varus deformities typically present with medial soft-tissue contracture and excessive laxity on the lateral side. Similarly, in valgus knees, the lateral soft-tissue structures show contracture and there is laxity on the medial side. This scenario may be compounded by additional laxity or contracture of posterior soft-tissue structures if there is an associated hyperextension or flexion deformity. This complex situation results in medio-lateral as well as flexion-extension gap asymmetry.

Although most arthritic knees undergoing TKA can be dealt with using standard cuts, graduated soft-tissue release and a cruciate-substituting knee design, knees with significant laxity or instability need to be tackled differently.

Based on the authors' experience, instability encountered in arthritic knees undergoing TKA can be classified into three types (Table 10.1): Type 1, severe coronal plane (medial or lateral) laxity; Type 2, severe coronal (medial or lateral)

A.B. Mullaji, G.M. Shetty, *Deformity Correction in Total Knee Arthroplasty*,
DOI 10.1007/978-1-4939-0566-9_10,

Table 10.1 Classification of instability

Type 1:	Severe coronal plane (medial or lateral) laxity
Type 2:	Severe coronal (medial or lateral) and sagittal (posterior) plane laxity
Type 3:	Global (medial, lateral and posterior) laxity

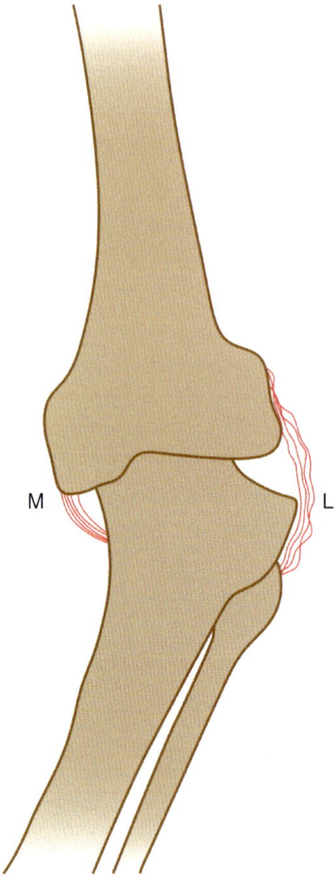

Fig. 10.1 Type 1 instability. The lateral side (*L*) in varus knees or the medial side (*M*) in valgus knees shows excessive laxity

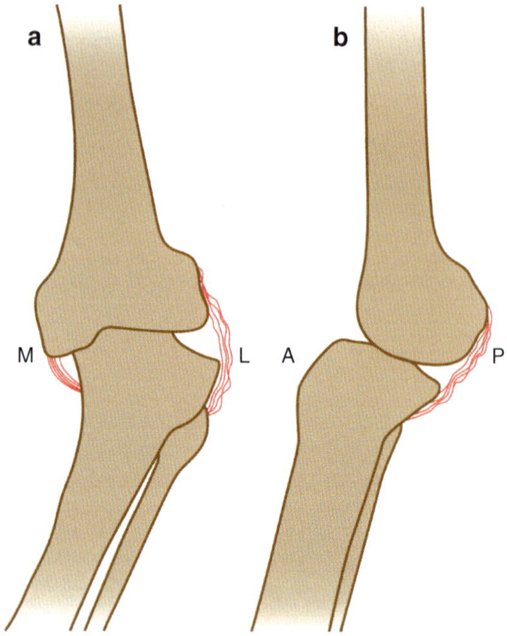

Fig. 10.2 Type 2 instability. The lateral side (*L*) in varus knees or the medial side (*M*) in valgus knees (**a**) and the posterior aspect (*P*) of the knee (**b**) show excessive laxity

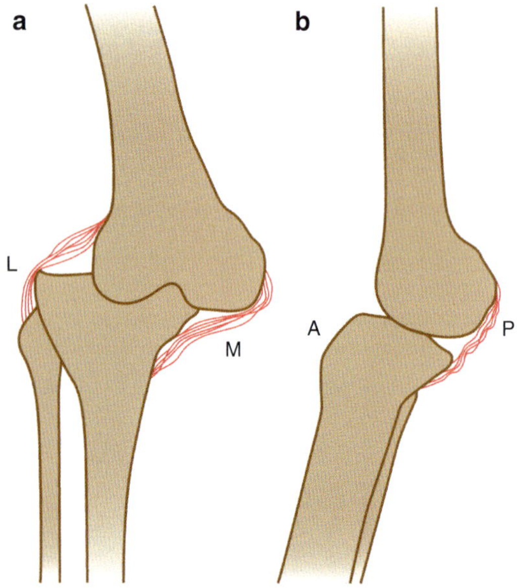

Fig. 10.3 Type 3 instability. The lateral (*L*), medial (*M*) (**a**) and posterior (*P*) aspect (**b**) of the knee show excessive laxity

and sagittal plane (posterior) laxity; and Type 3, global (medial, lateral and posterior) laxity. In Type 1 instability, the lateral (in varus deformity) or medial (in valgus deformity) soft-tissue structures may show significant laxity and pose a challenge in equalising the medio-lateral gap balance (Fig. 10.1). In Type 2 instability, in addition to the lax lateral or medial soft-tissue structures, the posterior structures may be attenuated due an associated hyperextension deformity (Fig. 10.2). In Type 3 instability, three sides of the knee (medial, lateral and posterior) shows significant laxity and the patient may present with a subluxated or a dislocated knee joint (Fig. 10.3).

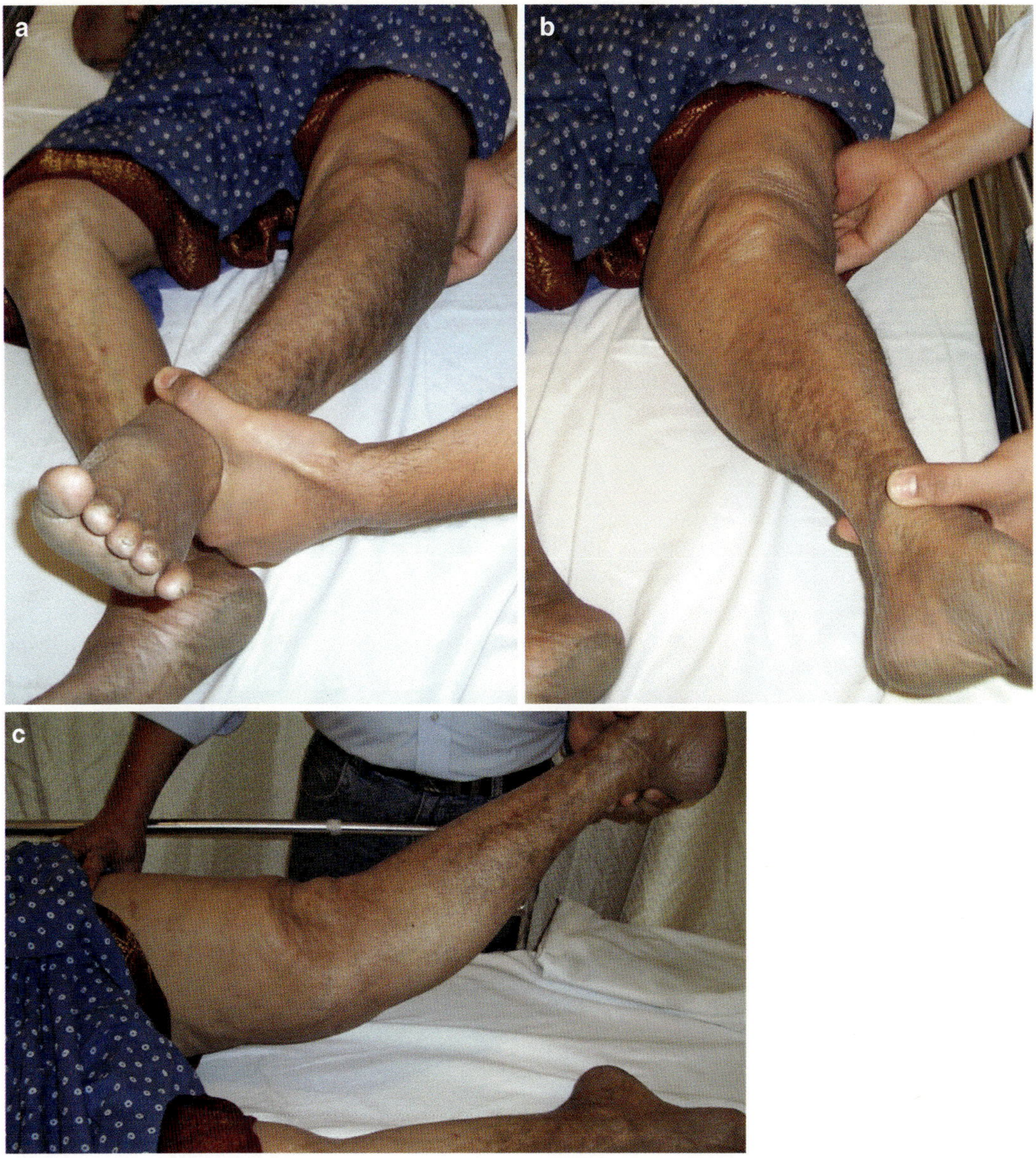

Fig. 10.4 Clinical photographs of a patient showing global or Type 3 instability. (**a**) Excessive laxity on the lateral side on applying a varus stress at the knee. (**b**) Excessive laxity on the medial side on applying a valgus stress at the knee. (**c**) Excessive laxity posteriorly resulting in a hyperextension deformity at the knee

Global laxity as seen in Type 3 instability, although rare, is usually associated with an underlying neuropathic component (Fig. 10.4). A common cause for it is spinal degeneration and the resulting neuropathy involving both lower limbs. Furthermore, many of these patients have not been walking due to severe arthritic pain and knee instability, and the resultant muscular atrophy especially of the knee extensors accentuates posterior instability. Hence, such patients with Type 3 instability who undergo TKA will require prolonged postoperative physiotherapy to improve muscle strength around the knee joint and treatment of the underlying neuropathy.

Surgical Technique

In view of excessive laxity and bony erosion commonly associated with unstable knees, the tibial and the distal femoral cuts need to be conservative (typically less than 8 mm). However, in Type 1 instability where the patient has an associated fixed flexion deformity, the tibial cut needs to be adequate (8–10 mm) since the extension gap may be smaller when compared to the flexion gap. Surgical technique may have to be modified based on the type of instability present.

Type 1 Instability

For varus knees, a graduated stepwise medial soft-tissue release is performed in order to correct the varus deformity. However, typically, although the mechanical axis may get fully restored to 180°, the lateral side will still show excessive laxity vis-à-vis the medial side. This can be confirmed by applying a varus stress at the knee with the knee in full extension. A reduction osteotomy by downsizing the tibia tray (compatible with the femur size) at this point will help further reduce this medio-lateral discrepancy in the extension gap (Fig. 10.5). In view of the substantial soft-tissue release done, the flexion gap may be much larger than the extension gap which may require upsizing of the femur to achieve flexion-extension balance. This may sometimes have to be combined with a constrained design to account for the large flexion gap (Fig. 10.6). Rarely, a medial condylar or lateral epicondylar osteotomy may be required if the medial or lateral gap is tighter despite maximum soft-tissue release in varus or valgus knees, respectively (Fig. 10.7).

Type 2 Instability

On account of the posterior laxity encountered in Type 2 instability, soft-tissue release should be strictly avoided posteriorly, and the tibial and distal femur bone cuts must be conservative. Although the technique to achieve medio-lateral balance in extension is similar to Type 1, due to

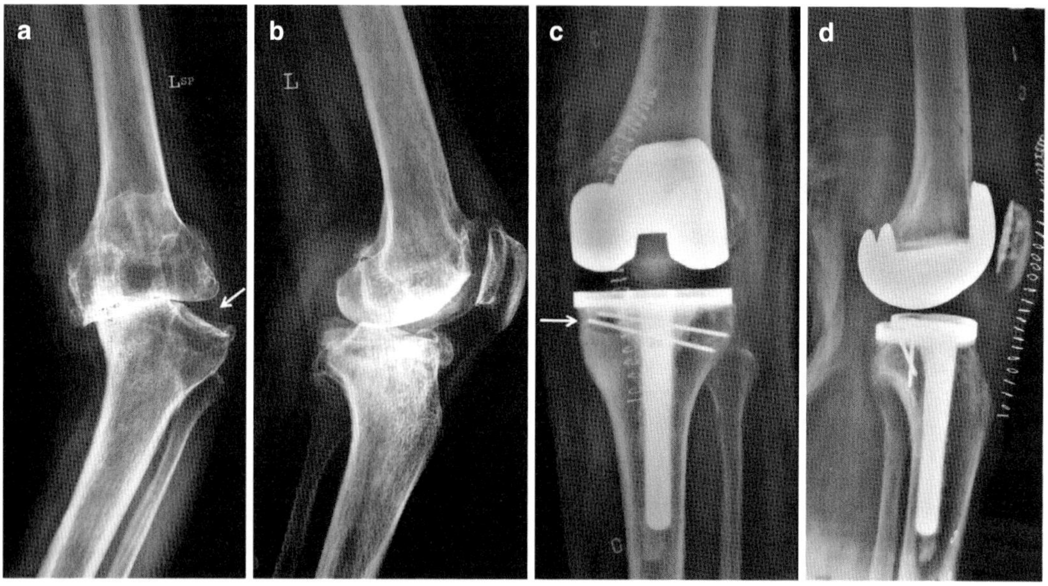

Fig. 10.5 Type 1 instability in a varus arthritic knee treated with a cruciate-substituting (*CS*) design. (**a**) Preoperative anteroposterior standing knee radiograph showing excessive opening of the lateral joint space (*arrow*) implying excessive soft-tissue laxity on the lateral side. (**b**) Preoperative lateral knee radiograph showing mild flexion deformity. (**c**) Postoperative anteroposterior standing knee radiograph showing the same patient (a) treated with a simple CS design. Note that medial tibial bone defect has been treated with an autologous bone graft fixed with Kirschner wires (*arrow*) and supplemented with a long tibial stem. (**d**) Postoperative lateral knee radiograph of the same patient (c)

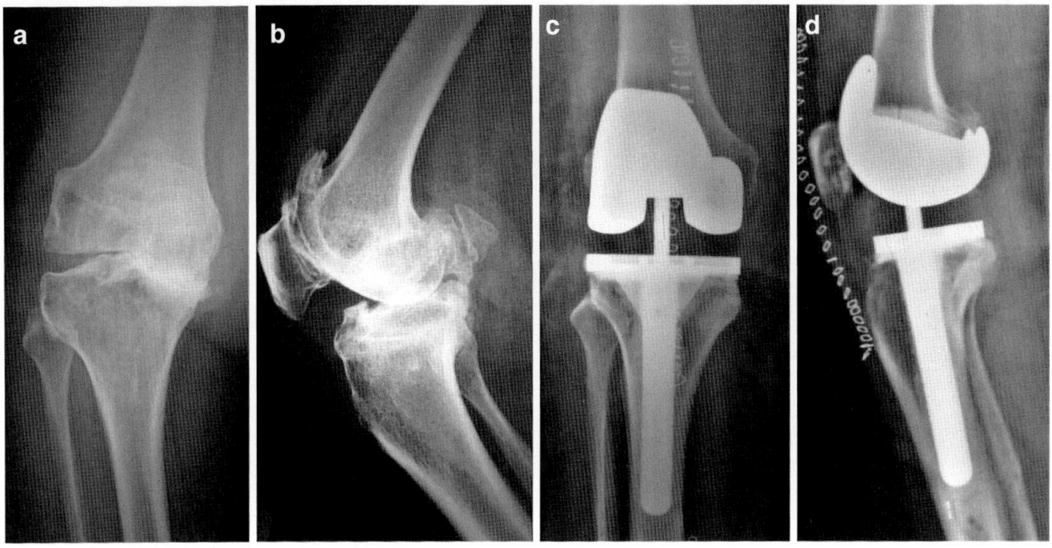

Fig. 10.6 Type 1 instability in a varus arthritic knee treated with a constrained design. (**a**) Preoperative anteroposterior standing knee radiograph showing excessive opening of the lateral joint space implying excessive soft-tissue laxity on the lateral side. (**b**) Preoperative lateral knee radiograph showing flexion deformity. (**c**) Postoperative anteroposterior standing knee radiograph showing the same patient (a) treated with a constrained design. (**d**) Postoperative lateral knee radiograph of the same patient (c)

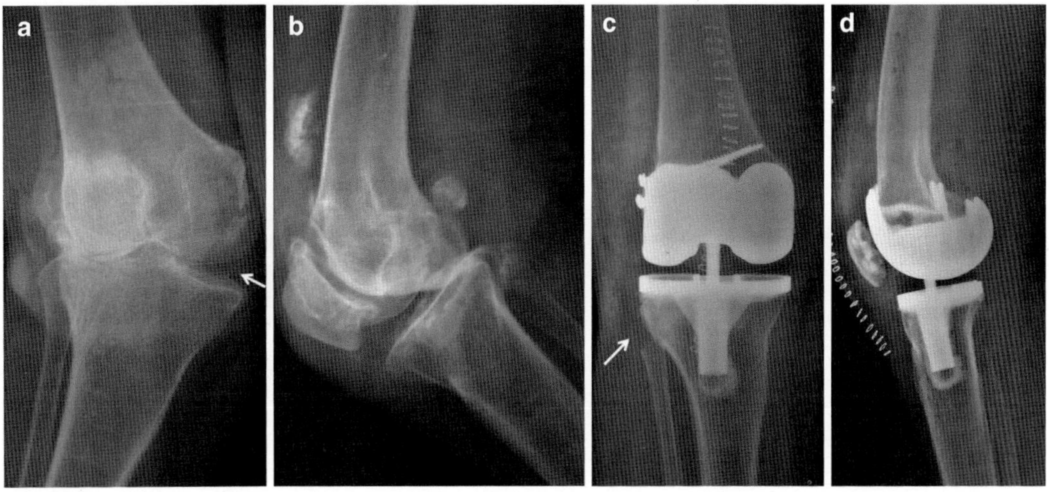

Fig. 10.7 Type 1 instability in a valgus arthritic knee treated with a lateral epicondylar osteotomy and constrained design. (**a**) Preoperative anteroposterior standing knee radiograph showing excessive opening of the medial joint space (*arrow*) implying excessive soft-tissue laxity on the medial side. (**b**) Preoperative lateral knee radiograph showing mild flexion deformity. (**c**) Postoperative anteroposterior standing knee radiograph showing the same patient (a) treated with a constrained design. Note that a lateral epicondylar osteotomy along with subperiosteal excision of the fibular head (*arrow*) was required in order to equalise the rigid lateral gap with the lax medial gap. The resultant large flexion gap necessitated the use of a constrained design. (**d**) Postoperative lateral knee radiograph of the same patient (c)

associated hyperextension, the extension gap is expected to be large [8]. Hence, the femoral component may have to be downsized to match the large extension gap to the smaller flexion gap. However, owing to substantial soft-tissue release to correct the varus/valgus deformity, the flexion gap may also become significant in some knees. Hence, a constrained design is more likely to be

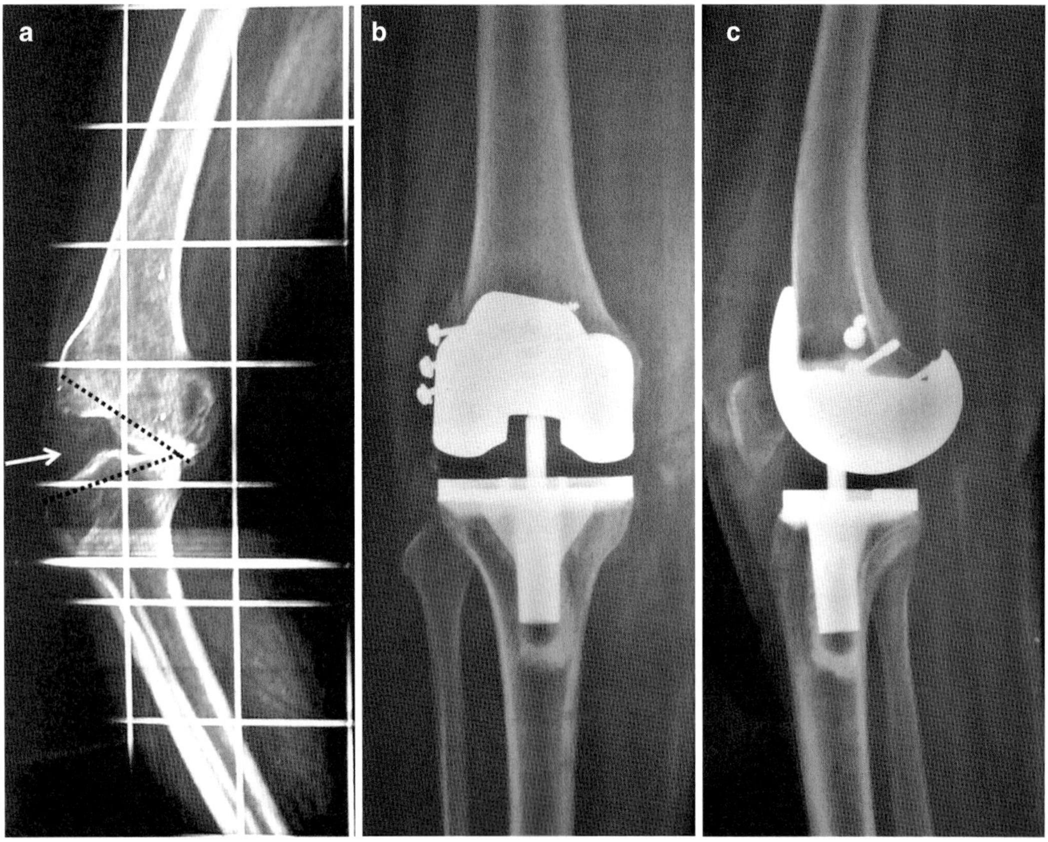

Fig. 10.8 Type 2 instability (post-poliomyelitis) in a varus arthritic knee treated with proximalisation of the lateral epicondyle and a constrained design. (**a**) Preoperative anteroposterior standing knee radiograph showing excessive opening of the lateral joint space (*arrow*) and a large joint divergence angle (*dashed line*). The patient had post-poliomyelitis residual paralysis of the right lower limb and a combination of varus and hyperextension knee deformity on the right side. (**b**) Postoperative anteroposterior standing knee radiograph showing the same patient (a) treated with a constrained design. Owing to the enormous discrepancy between the lateral and medial side, the lateral collateral ligament was shortened using a lateral epicondylar osteotomy where the lateral epicondyle was proximalised and fixed with cancellous crews. (**c**) Postoperative lateral knee radiograph of the same patient (b)

used here than in Type 1 instability. Rarely, the lateral collateral ligament (LCL) may show enormous elongation (such as in post-poliomyelitis limbs) in varus knees where a lateral epicondylar osteotomy with *proximalisation* of the LCL attachment (to effectively shorten the LCL) is warranted (Fig. 10.8). This procedure is especially preferred in young patients where a hinge knee design is best avoided. Significant bone loss which is frequently encountered in such cases needs to be addressed using autologous bone grafts supplemented with a long tibial stem (Fig. 10.9).

Type 3 Instability

Incompetent collateral ligaments along with an attenuated posterior capsule pose a complex challenge to the surgeon in terms of ligament balance during TKA. Such knees also show significant joint subluxation and bone loss (Fig. 10.10). Although optimal ligament balance may be elusive in such cases, the surgeon must follow the basic principles of conservative tibial and distal femoral bone cuts and minimal soft-tissue release in these cases. Owing to large extension and flexion gaps, a simple CS or constrained prosthesis

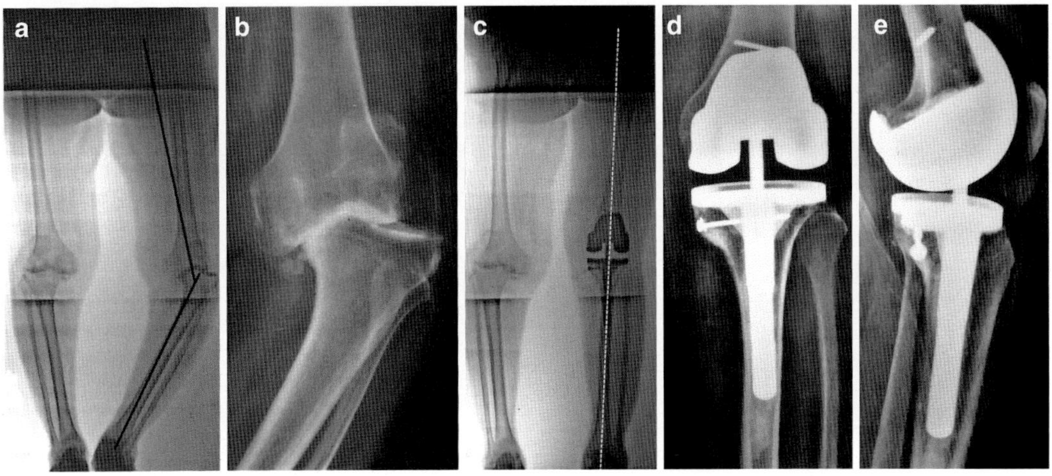

Fig. 10.9 Type 2 instability in a varus arthritic knee treated with a constrained design. (**a**) Preoperative standing, full-length hip-to-ankle radiograph showing profound varus deformity of approximately 40° on the left side. (**b**) Preoperative anteroposterior standing knee radiograph of the same patient (a) showing joint subluxation and significant medial tibial bone loss. (**c**) Postoperative standing, full-length hip-to-ankle radiograph showing complete restoration of limb alignment (*dotted line*) after TKA with constrained prosthesis. (**d**) Postoperative anteroposterior standing knee radiograph of the same patient (c) showing TKA done with a constrained design and the medial tibial bone loss treated with autologous bone graft fixed with screw. (**e**) Postoperative lateral knee radiograph of the same patient (d)

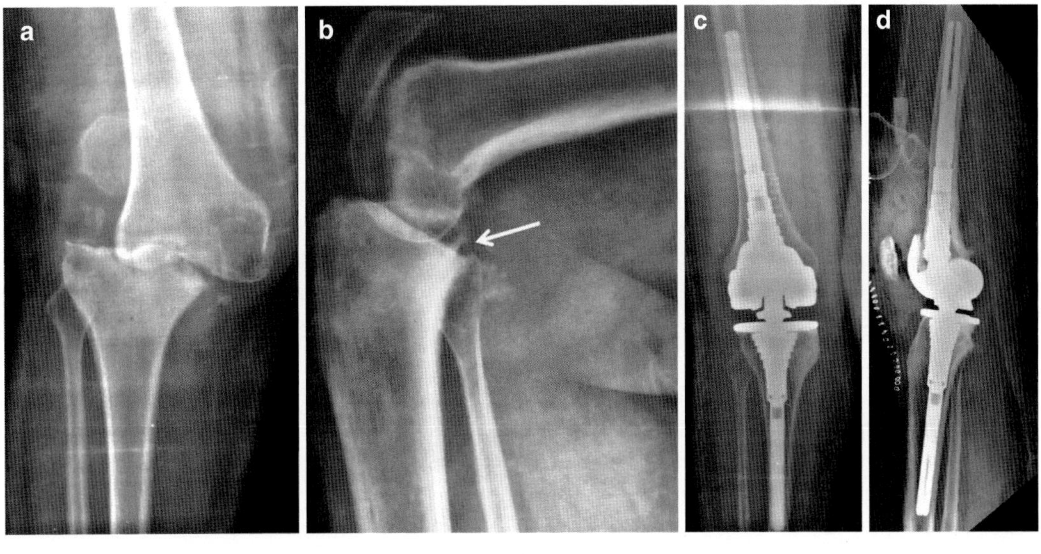

Fig. 10.10 Type 3 instability treated with a hinge knee. (**a**) Preoperative anteroposterior standing knee radiograph significant joint subluxation and significant medial tibial bone loss. (**b**) Preoperative lateral knee radiograph showing severe posterior tibial bone loss and a large slope (*arrow*). (**c**) Postoperative anteroposterior standing knee radiograph showing the same patient (a) treated with a hinge knee. (**d**) Postoperative lateral knee radiograph of the same patient (c)

(such as TC3 or VVC) may not be sufficient to provide stability, and most of these knees may require a hinged prosthesis which requires more solid fixation in the femur and tibia to withstand the additional stresses on the implant/cement/bone interface [3]. A rotating hinge is preferable to reduce the forces on the fixation, and tibial and femoral sleeves and/or stems are essential [3].

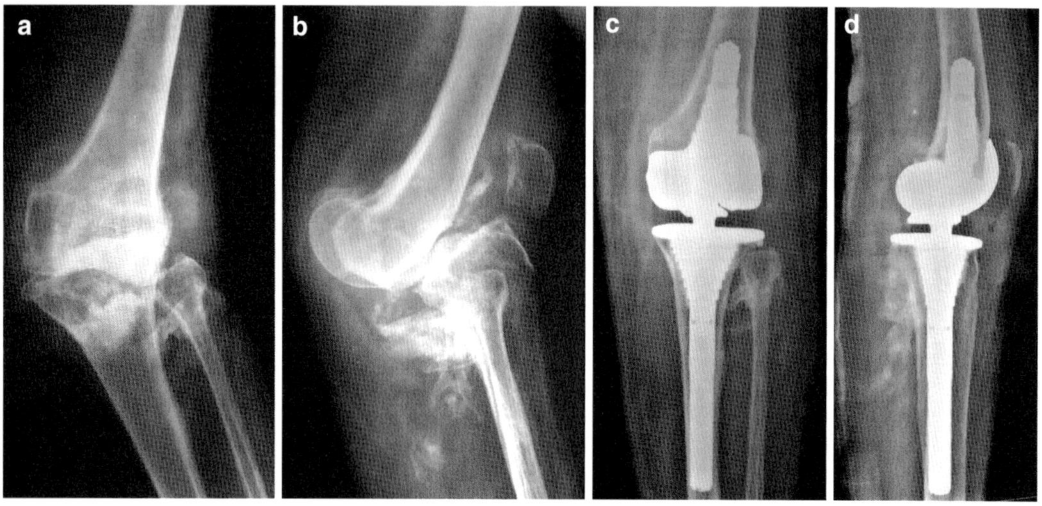

Fig. 10.11 Type 3 instability treated with a hinge knee (same patient from Fig. 10.4). This patient had severe sensorimotor neuropathy of both lower limbs due to lumbar spine degeneration. (**a**) Preoperative anteroposterior standing knee radiograph. (**b**) Preoperative lateral knee radiograph showing complete dislocation of the knee joint with the anterior cortex of the distal femur resting on the tibial spine. (**c**) Postoperative anteroposterior standing knee radiograph showing the same patient (a) treated with a hinge knee. Note that a femoral stem could not be used in this patient owing to a narrow and bowed distal femoral canal. (**d**) Postoperative lateral knee radiograph of the same patient (c). Note the excessive anteroposterior curvature of the distal femur

However, the surgeon must be cautious and vigilant while preparing the tibia and femur for sleeves and stems. The distal femur is typically osteoporotic in the elderly and may be narrow which puts it at high risk for fracture while impacting with trial sleeves. The surgeon may have to perform prophylactic wire cerclage before preparing the distal femur for sleeves to prevent this complication. Furthermore, the distal femoral and tibial canal may be too narrow or bowed in the coronal or sagittal plane to accommodate a long intramedullary stem. The surgeon needs to take care while reaming the canal to prevent any inadvertent cortical penetration, and very rarely the prosthesis may have to be implanted without the stem (and only sleeve) if the canal is too narrow or bowed on the femoral side (Fig. 10.11).

Postoperative rehabilitation is routine for TKAs performed for Type 1 or Type 2 instability. However, in cases where an epicondylar/condylar osteotomy has been performed, the patient is allowed full weight-bearing ambulation with a long knee brace on the first postoperative day. Knee movement is not allowed for 2 weeks after which the patient is advised to remove the brace three to four times a day and perform gentle, active knee flexion and extension. Knee brace is discontinued at 4 weeks and patient allowed full activity. A long knee brace is also advised while walking in patients with preoperative Type 2 instability with long-standing hyperextension deformity for 1 month to prevent recurrence of recurvatum; they are also advised to use a pillow under the knee while sleeping for 2–4 weeks. In Type 3 instability, although most patients show satisfactory early functional recovery, the authors advice the use of a long knee brace and walker during ambulation till the patient regains sufficient muscle strength (knee and hip muscles) and risk of fall is minimised (Fig. 10.12).

In patients where the contralateral knee is unaffected or less severely deformed, we warn the patients before surgery that there may be some leg-length discrepancy between the two legs which may require a shoe lift on the unoperated side. This is unlikely however when both knees are affected to a nearly equal extent in terms of angular deformity and ligament elongation.

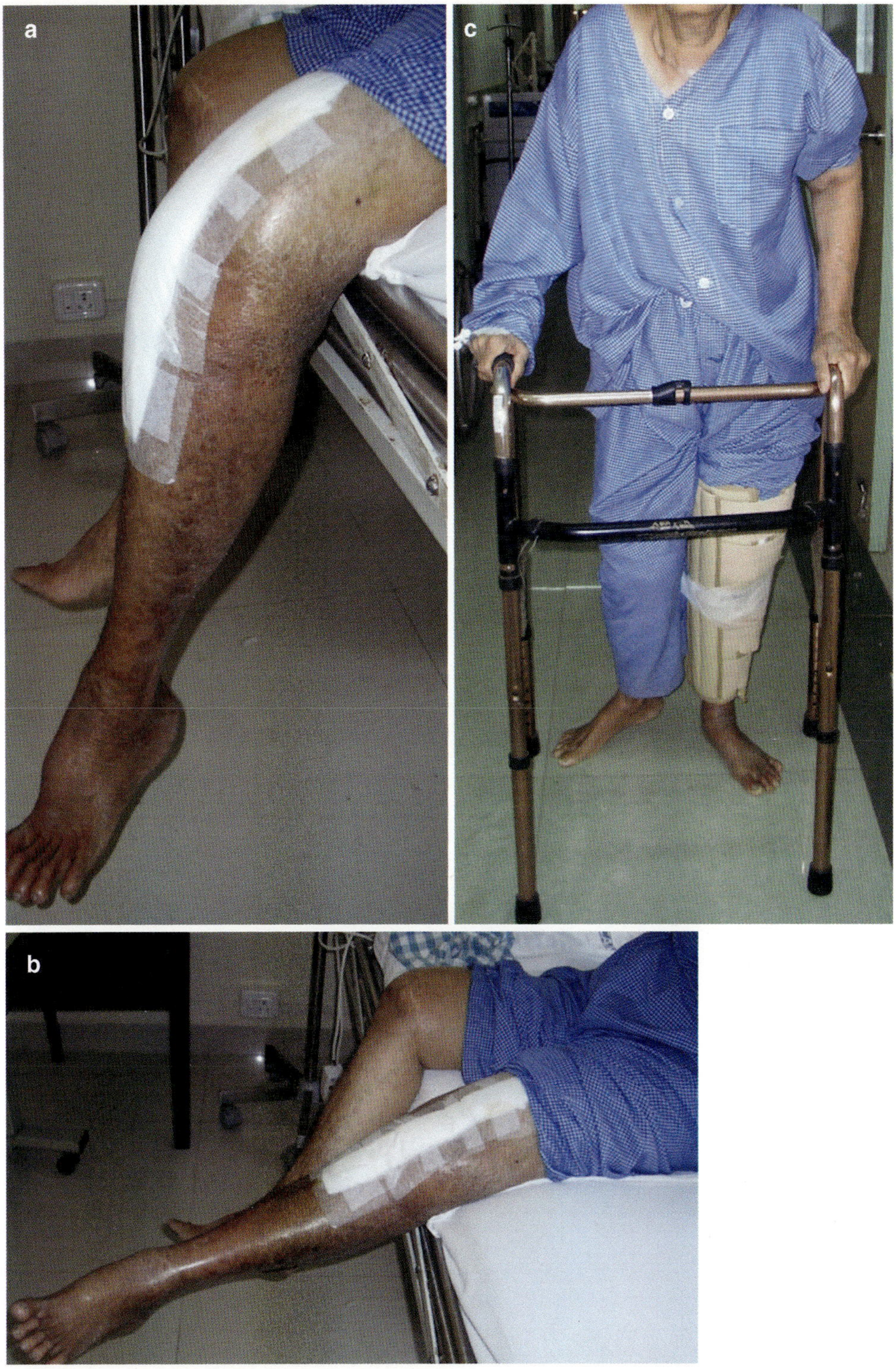

Fig. 10.12 Clinical photographs showing functional recovery (at 72 h postoperatively) in a patient with Type 3 instability where a hinge knee was used (same patient from Figs. 10.4 and 10.11). (**a**) Gravity-assisted active knee flexion. (**b**) Active knee extension in the sitting position. (**c**) Full weight-bearing ambulation with a walker. Note that a long knee brace has been applied on the operated side while walking

References

1. Mullaji AB, Shetty GM, Lingaraju AP, Bhayde S. Which factors increase risk of malalignment of the hip-knee-ankle axis in TKA? Clin Orthop Relat Res. 2013;471:134–41.
2. Vail TP, Lang JE, Van Sikes C. Surgical techniques and instrumentation in total knee arthroplasty. In: Scott WN, editor. Insall & Scott surgery of the knee. Philadelphia: Elsevier/Churchill Livingstone; 2012. p. 1075–86.
3. Morgan H, Battista V, Leopold SS. Constraint in primary total knee arthroplasty. J Am Acad Orthop Surg. 2005;13:515–24.
4. Tigani D, Fosco M, Amendola L, Boriani L. Total knee arthroplasty in patients with poliomyelitis. Knee. 2009;16:501–6.
5. Jordan L, Kligman M, Sculco TP. Total knee arthroplasty in patients with poliomyelitis. J Arthroplasty. 2007;22:543–8.
6. Hernández-Vaquero D, Sandoval-García MA. Hinged total knee arthroplasty in the presence of ligamentous deficiency. Clin Orthop Relat Res. 2010;468:1248–53.
7. Springer BD, Hanssen AD, Sim FH, Lewallen DG. The kinematic rotating hinge prosthesis for complex knee arthroplasty. Clin Orthop Relat Res. 2001;392:283–91.
8. Mullaji A, Lingaraju AP, Shetty GM. Computer-assisted total knee replacement in patients with arthritis and a recurvatum deformity. J Bone Joint Surg Br. 2012;94:642–7.

11 Osteotomies in Total Knee Arthroplasty

Introduction

Bone cuts and soft-tissue releases are the principal steps in TKA. However, some knees undergoing TKA may require an additional procedure in the form of an osteotomy. An osteotomy in primary TKA is usually indicated in rigid or severe deformities to facilitate soft-tissue balance and deformity correction, to concomitantly correct an extra-articular deformity or rarely to facilitate exposure of the joint. Frequently, in varus arthritic knees undergoing TKA, the medial and posteromedial side of the tibial plateau shows adaptive changes resulting in the formation of a prominent bony flare in this area (Fig. 11.1a). This causes local tenting of the medial soft-tissue structures and contributes to knee deformity and mediolateral soft-tissue imbalance (Fig. 11.1b). A reduction osteotomy involves excision of this medial bony flare to decompress the medial soft-tissue structures [1, 2]. Rarely, despite extensive soft-tissue release and a reduction osteotomy, a knee deformity may be too rigid and/or the medio-lateral soft-tissue imbalance too severe to correct. In such cases a sliding medial condylar osteotomy (SMCO) in a varus knee [3] or a lateral epicondylar osteotomy (LEO) in a valgus knee [4] may be required to achieve optimum limb alignment and soft-tissue balance.

In cases with severe extra-articular deformities, a corrective osteotomy may be required simultaneously with the TKA in order to facilitate restoration of limb alignment [5–7]. However, in severe tibial extra-articular deformities where a medial closing wedge corrective osteotomy is required, the intact fibula at the apex may not allow complete closure at the osteotomy site, and therefore a segmental fibular osteotomy will have to be performed [6]. Sometimes in a stiff knee, excessive soft-tissue contractures and severe arthritis of the patellofemoral joint may result in poor exposure through the routine arthrotomy approach. A tibial tubercular osteotomy in such cases will facilitate adequate exposure of the joint for TKA. Hence, the main indications of an osteotomy in primary TKA are (a) correction of limb malalignment in knee arthritis due to an associated extra-articular deformity, (b) soft-tissue balance in severe and/or rigid knee deformities and (c) surgical exposure in a stiff or ankylosed knee joint. Each osteotomy as discussed above has a specific role to play during TKA (Fig. 11.2). This chapter aims to outline the indications and technique of various osteotomies used in primary TKA.

Types of Osteotomies and Technique

Reduction Osteotomy of the Tibia

Principle: A reduction osteotomy involves excision of the posteromedial bony flare on the tibial plateau to decompress medial soft-tissue structures in a varus arthritic knee undergoing TKA (Fig. 11.1). This osteotomy works similar to the excision of osteophytes where they cause tenting

A.B. Mullaji, G.M. Shetty, *Deformity Correction in Total Knee Arthroplasty*,
DOI 10.1007/978-1-4939-0566-9_11, © Springer Science+Business Media New York 2014

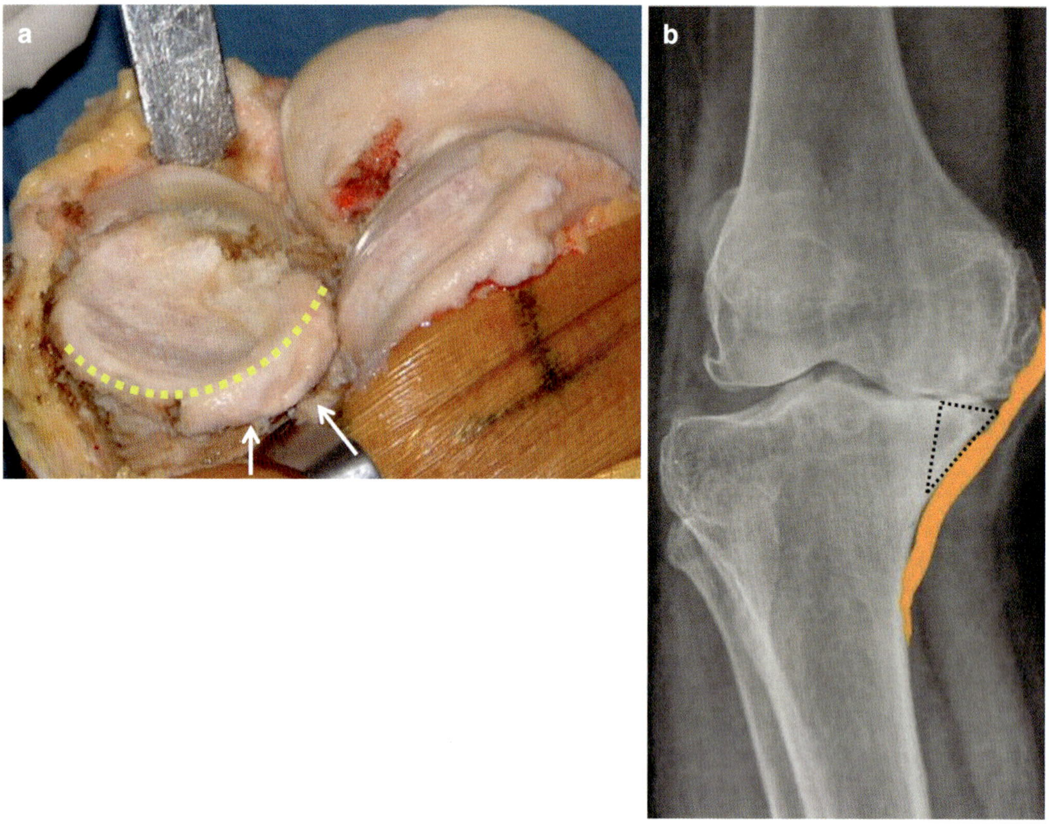

Fig. 11.1 Medial and posteromedial bony changes of the tibial plateau in varus arthritic knees. (**a**) Intraoperative photograph showing posteromedial bony flare (*dotted line*) of the tibial plateau (*arrows*). (**b**) Preoperative knee standing radiograph showing the bony flare (*triangle*) which causes tenting of the medial soft-tissue structures in varus arthritic knee

Fig. 11.2 Step-by-step technique of reduction osteotomy performed to achieve deformity correction and/or medio-lateral soft-tissue balance in varus arthritic knees undergoing TKA. (**a**, **b**) Step 1 – Intraoperative recording of varus deformity of 17.5° (**a**) and maximum correctibility up to 6.5° varus (**b**) on applying a valgus stress at the knee. (**c**) Step 2 – Posteromedial soft-tissue release (deep medial collateral ligament, posteromedial capsule and semimembranosus) to achieve deformity correction and medio-lateral soft-tissue balance. (**d**) Step 3 – Intraoperative recording of final correction achieved after posteromedial release shows a residual varus deformity of 2.5° on applying a valgus stress at the knee. Based on the "2-mm excision for 1° degree correction" principle, a reduction osteotomy of 5 mm is required in this case to achieve full correction (or neutral alignment). (**e**, **f**) Step 4 – Using the tibial tray of appropriate size as reference, the required amount of osteotomy is marked on the tibial cut surface (distance AB) along the margin of the tibial tray as seen in the axial (**e**) and frontal (**f**) views. (**g**, **h**) Step 5 – Reduction osteotomy performed along the *marked line* using an osteotome as seen intraoperatively (**g**) and on a schematic diagram (**h**)

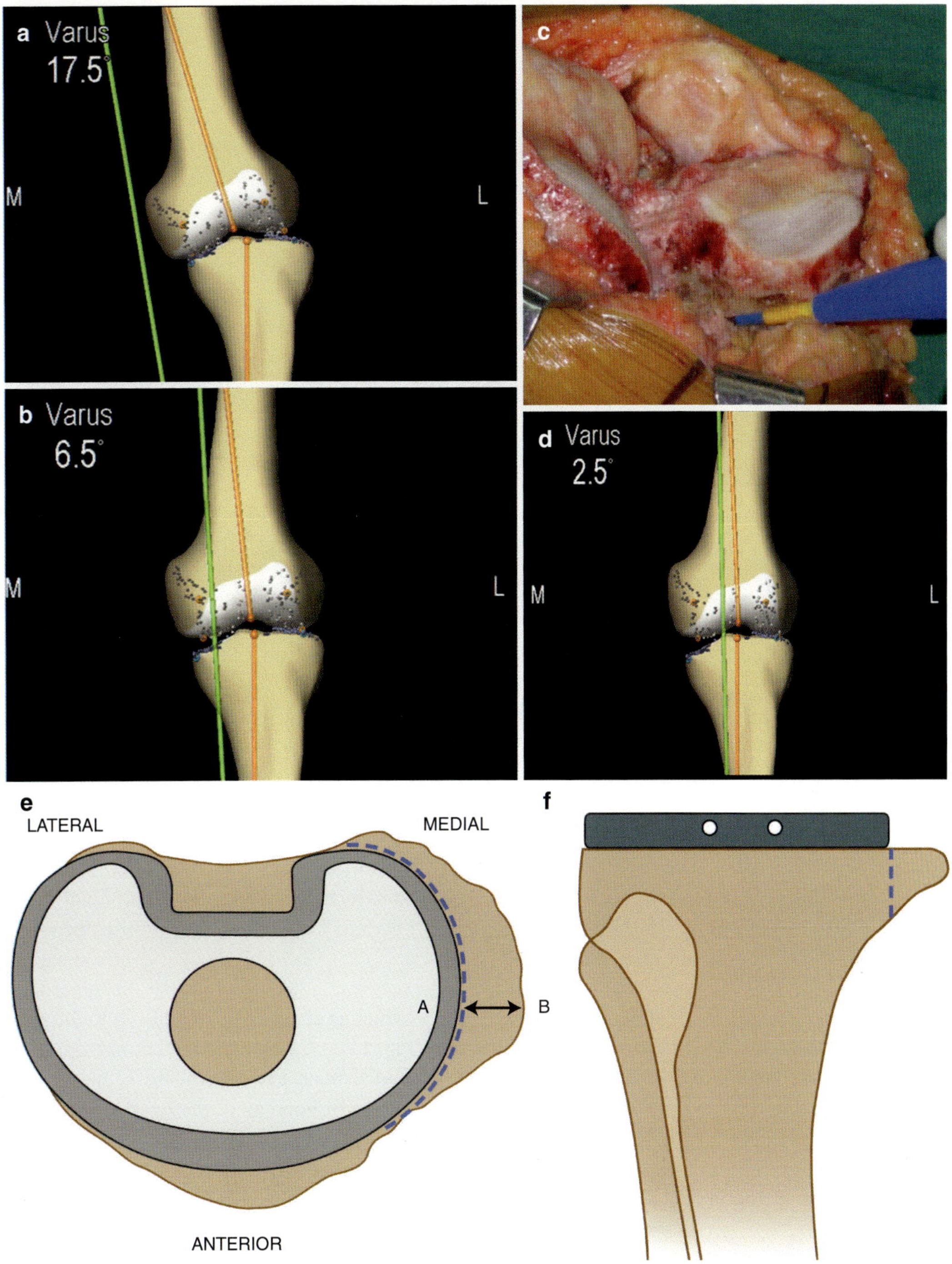
a Varus
17.5°
M
L
b Varus
6.5°
M
L
c
d Varus
2.5°
M
L
e
LATERAL
MEDIAL
A
B
ANTERIOR
f

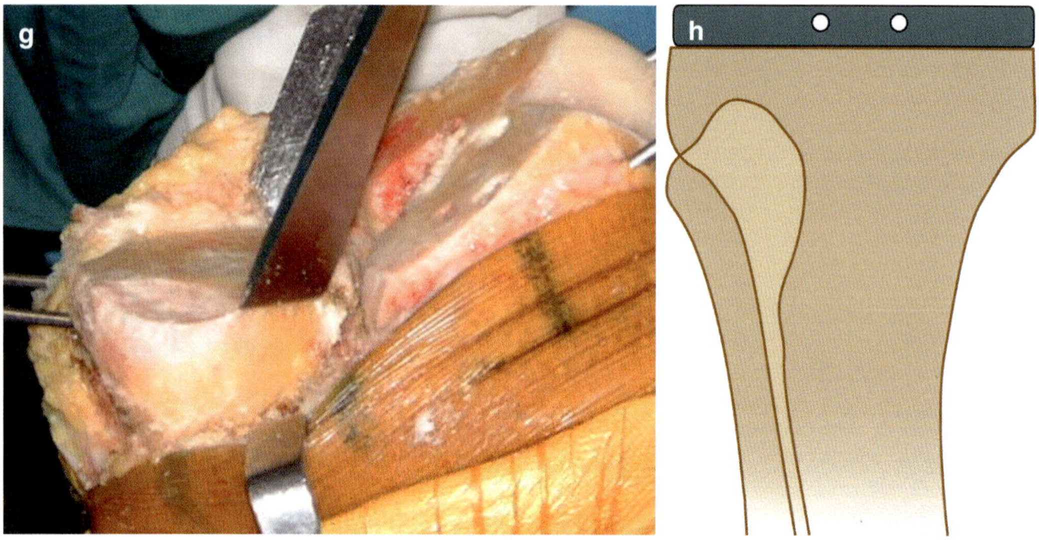

Fig. 11.2 (continued)

and a bowstring effect on the adjoining medial soft-tissue structure (Fig. 11.1). Reduction osteotomy allows correction of deformity and medio-lateral soft-tissue balance without having to resort to excessive soft-tissue release and acts as a soft-tissue sparing step.

Indications: These include residual varus deformity of >2° (when measured using computer navigation) or medio-lateral soft-tissue imbalance (excessive medial tightness or excessive lateral laxity) despite sufficient medial soft-tissue release (deep MCL, posteromedial capsule and semimembranosus) in a varus arthritic knee undergoing TKA.

Technique: Reduction osteotomy can achieve deformity correction in a predictable manner using the "2-mm excision for 1° degree correction" formula especially in knees with <15° preoperative varus deformity [1]. However, this formula may not be as predictable in knees with >15° preoperative varus deformity due to associated severe medial soft-tissue contracture or lateral soft-tissue laxity and/or an associated extra-articular deformity [1]. A step-by-step technique for this osteotomy is illustrated in Fig. 11.2.

Precautions: Since reduction osteotomy can achieve deformity correction in a predictable manner (1° correction for every 2 mm of excision) especially in arthritic knees with <15° preoperative varus deformity, the surgeon should be careful not to perform it in limbs where the varus deformity is <5° or where the deformity is fully correctible as it may lead to excessive slackening of soft tissue medially and overcorrection [1]. Furthermore, the surgeon needs to take care that only the medial bony flare is excised (as previously measured in relation to the residual varus deformity and keeping the tibial tray as the reference) and the osteotomy should not be too medial and excessive as this may detach the superficial MCL which is attached 6–7 cm distal to the joint line (Fig. 11.3). In case the patient has a significant medial bone loss which has been built up with cement or bone graft, the fixation should be supplemented with a long tibial stem (Fig. 11.4).

Postoperative Care: Postoperative physiotherapy is similar to that of a routinely performed TKA and no postoperative bracing is required.

Sliding Medial Condylar Osteotomy (SMCO)

Principle: A sliding medial condylar osteotomy involves detachment of a bony segment medially from the medial femoral condyle with the medial

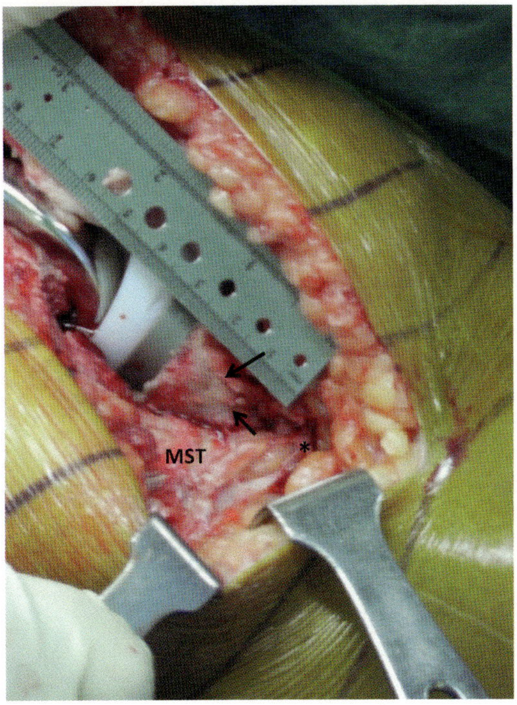

Fig. 11.3 Intraoperative photograph showing relation of the reduction osteotomy (*arrows*) to the medial soft-tissue sleeve (*MST*). Note that the attachment of the superficial MCL (*asterisk*) is distal to the distal border of the reduction osteotomy (*arrows*)

collateral ligament (MCL) attached to it. This allows distal displacement and fixation of the femoral attachment of the MCL (while preserving its attachment to bone) to increase the medial gap vis-à-vis the lateral gap in varus arthritic knees during TKA. Subperiosteal stripping of tibial attachment of MCL or its detachment from the femoral side with a wafer of bone is an imprecise technique and carries the risk of overrelease and medio-lateral instability [8], whereas SMCO is precise and quantitative and allows repositioning the MCL more accurately.

Indications: These include rigid, recalcitrant varus deformities not amenable to full correction of limb alignment and/or medio-lateral imbalance despite extensive medial soft-tissue release (except superficial MCL and pes anserinus) and a reduction osteotomy during TKA.

Technique: A step-by-step technique for this osteotomy is illustrated in Fig. 11.5.

Precautions: This osteotomy is best avoided in knees where the distal femur is small in size and where performing a SMCO carries the risk of intraoperative fracture of the medial femoral condyle. The condylar bone block with the attached

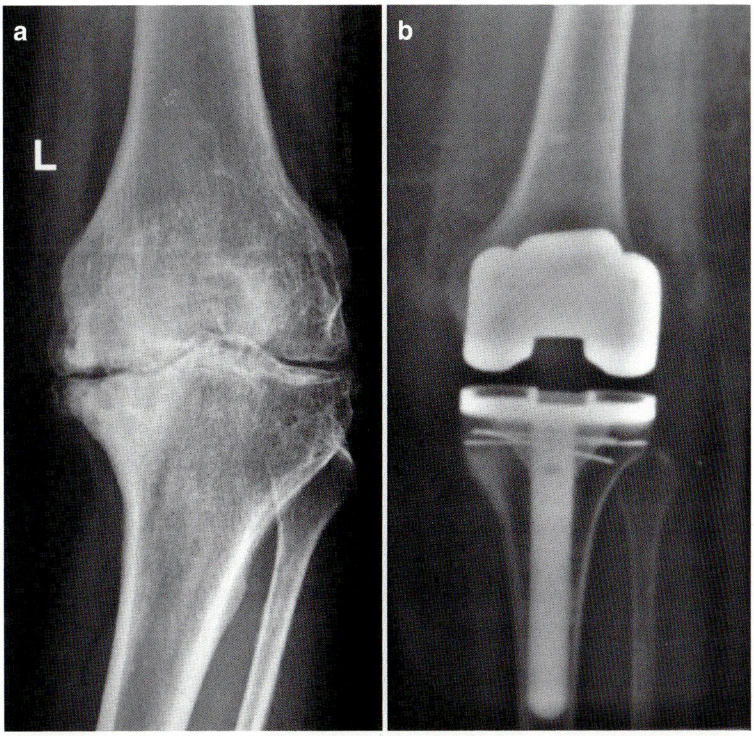

Fig. 11.4 Pre- and postoperative standing knee radiograph of a case with varus arthritis in which reduction osteotomy has been performed as part of TKA. (**a**) Preoperative radiograph showing prominent medial tibial bony flare with medial tibial bone loss. (**b**) Postoperative radiograph of the same patient showing final alignment after TKA with a reduction osteotomy. The medial bone loss has been built up using bone autograft fixed with Kirschner wires and supplemented with a long tibial stem

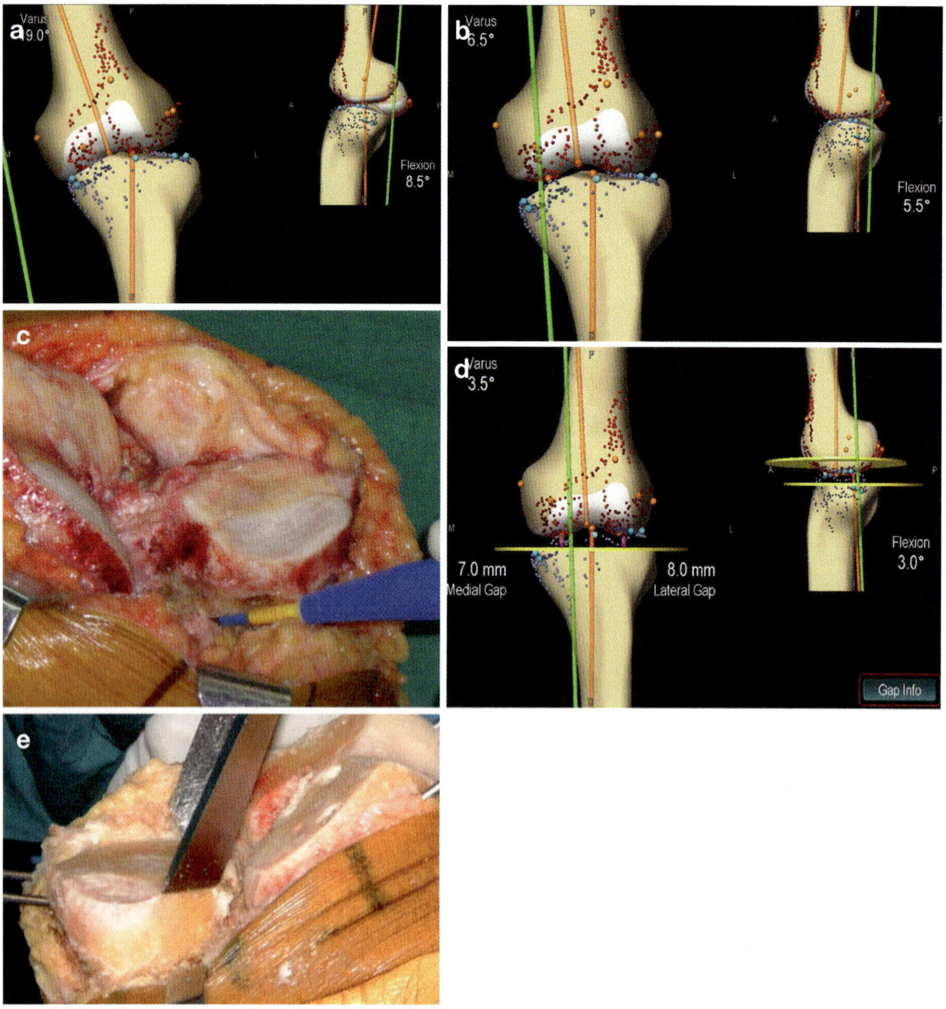

Fig. 11.5 Step-by-step technique of sliding medial condylar osteotomy (SMCO) performed to achieve deformity correction and/or medio-lateral soft-tissue balance in varus arthritic knees undergoing TKA. (**a**, **b**) Step 1 – Intraoperative recording of varus deformity of 17.5° (**a**) and maximum correctibility up to 6.5° varus (**b**) on applying a valgus stress at the knee. (**c**) Step 2 – Posteromedial soft-tissue release (deep medial collateral ligament, posteromedial capsule and semimembranosus) to achieve deformity correction and medio-lateral soft-tissue balance. (**d**) Step 3 – Intraoperative recording shows a residual varus deformity of 3.5° on applying valgus stress at the knee despite posteromedial soft-tissue release. A reduction osteotomy will have to be performed to correct this residual deformity. (**e**) Step 4 – Reduction osteotomy done to correct the residual varus deformity based on the "2-mm excision for 1° degree correction" principle. (**f**, **g**) Step 5 – Intraoperative recording shows complete correction of deformity after reduction osteotomy (**f**): however, on maximum varus stress to the knee the same knee shows excessive lateral soft-tissue laxity (*arrow*) vis-à-vis the medial side (**g**). A SMCO is now required to achieve medio-lateral soft-tissue balance. (**h**) Step 6 – The difference between the medial and lateral gap in knee extension (distance CD–AB) is measured to determine the amount by which the medial condylar block needs to be shifted distally. This distance can be determined using either navigation or a measuring scale. (**i**, **j**) Step 7 – Plane of the osteotomy cut is marked on the medial femoral condyle. The cut starts 5 mm lateral to the medial edge of the bony medial condyle (*red line*) and continues obliquely in the superomedial direction to exit distal to the adductor tubercle (*asterisk*). The osteotomy is performed using a reciprocating saw. (**j**, **k**) Step 8 – The amount by which the medial condylar block needs to be shifted distally is marked on the block using a measuring scale and electrocautery. (**l**) Step 9 – The condylar block is now controlled using sutures (Vicryl no. 1) passed through its soft-tissue attachment. *Dotted line* signifies amount of bone marked on the condylar block which will be excised. (**m**) Step 10 – The amount of bone previously marked on the condylar block is now excised using a bone cutter. (**n**) Step 11 – The condylar block is now gently shifted distally and repositioned in place using the attached sutures. The medio-lateral balance and alignment are then checked with trial implants in full extension and the knee in 90° flexion with the condylar block in its new position. (**o**) Step 12 – After cementing of the final implant, the condylar block is fixed in position using two to three cancellous screws with the knee in 45° flexion

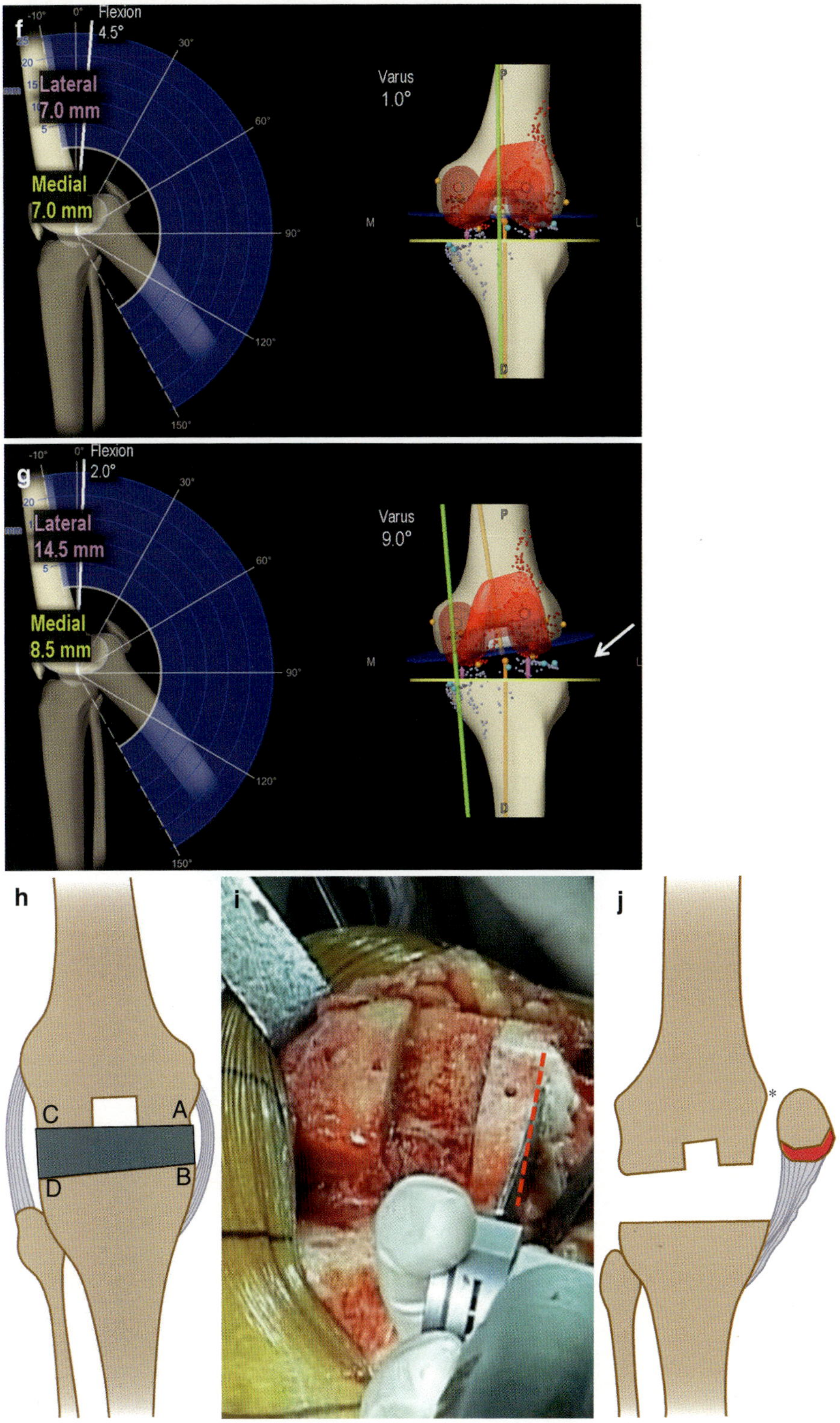

Fig. 11.5 (continued)

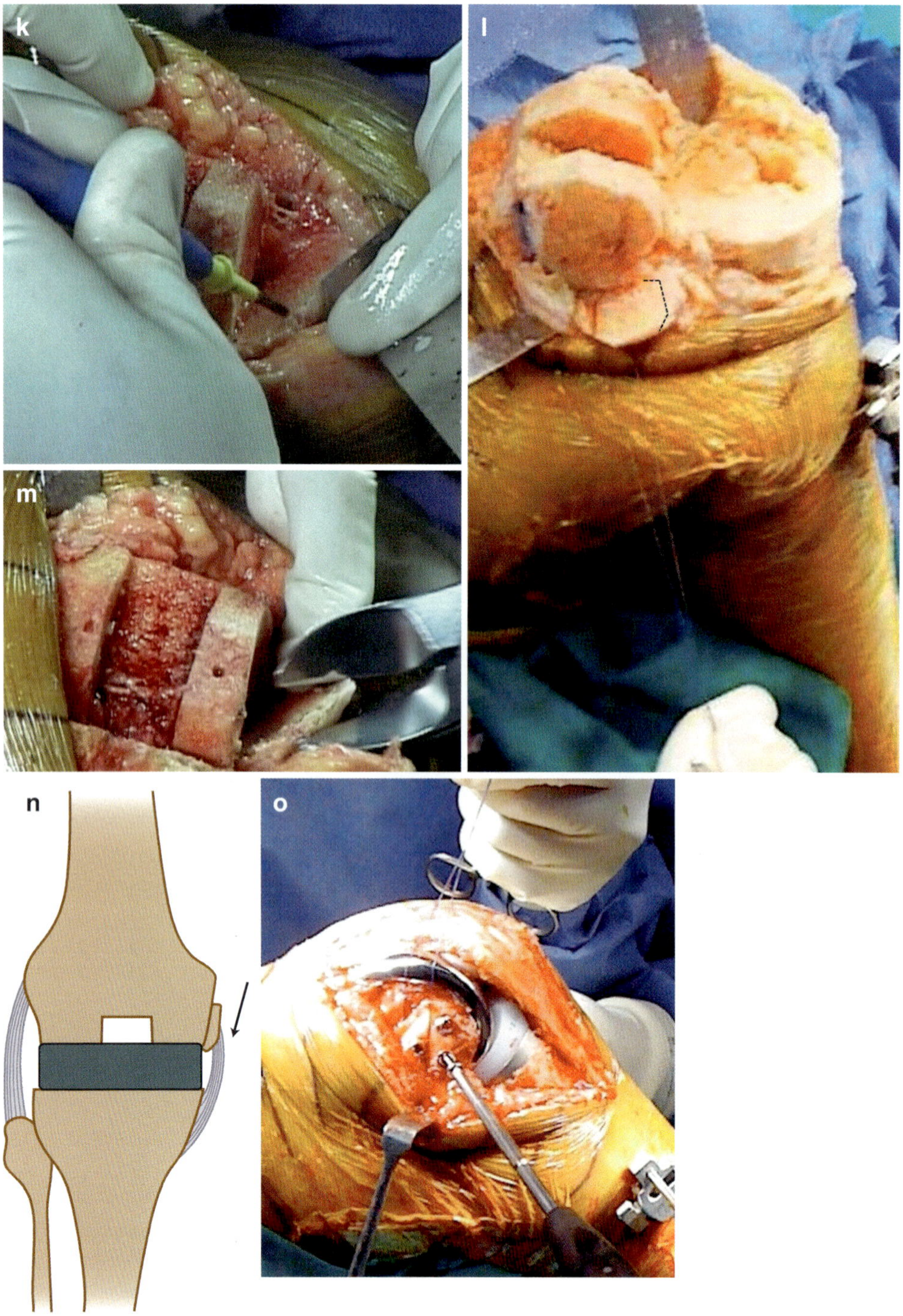

Fig. 11.5 (continued)

MCL must be handled with care once it has been osteotomised from the femoral condyle, with sutures passed through its soft-tissue attachment. The condylar block must be controlled with the attached sutures at all times (especially during knee flexion or extension) as otherwise it may fracture if directly handled using instruments or if it gets entrapped during knee movement. The condylar block should be fixed with the knee in 45° flexion to gain sufficient access to insert the screws and to avoid excessive traction of the block and distraction at the osteotomy fixation site. Although the condylar block is fixed with two to three 4-mm cancellous screws, underdrilling with a 2-mm drill bit is advisable in osteoporotic patients to achieve better purchase of screws.

Postoperative Care: In cases where a SMCO has been performed, the patient is allowed full weight-bearing ambulation with a long knee brace on the first postoperative day. Knee movement is not allowed for 2 weeks after which the patient is advised to remove the brace three to four times a day and perform gentle, active knee flexion and extension. Knee brace is discontinued at 4 weeks and patient allowed full activity. An anteroposterior standing and lateral knee radiograph is performed at 6 weeks to confirm union at the osteotomy site.

Lateral Epicondylar Osteotomy (LEO)

Principle: A lateral epicondylar osteotomy involves detachment of the lateral epicondyle with the lateral collateral ligament (LCL) and popliteus tendon attached to it. This allows distal displacement and fixation of the LCL and popliteus tendon (while preserving its attachment to bone) to increase the lateral gap vis-à-vis the medial gap in valgus arthritic knees during TKA.

Indications: These include rigid, recalcitrant valgus deformities not amenable to full correction of limb alignment and/or medio-lateral balance despite extensive lateral soft-tissue release (including iliotibial band, posterolateral capsule and popliteofibular ligament) during TKA.

Technique: A step-by-step technique for this osteotomy is illustrated in Fig. 11.6.

Precautions: Similar to SMCO, this osteotomy is best avoided in knees where the distal femur is small in size to prevent intraoperative fracture of the lateral femoral condyle. The epicondylar bone block with the attached LCL and popliteus tendon must be handled using sutures passed through its soft-tissue attachment. The block should be fixed with the knee in 45° flexion similar to SMCO, and underdrilling with a 2 mm drill bit is advisable in osteoporotic patients.

Postoperative Care: Similar to SMCO, the patient where a LEO has been performed is allowed full weight-bearing ambulation with a long knee brace on the first postoperative day. Knee movement is not allowed for 2 weeks after which the patient is advised to remove the brace three to four times a day and perform gentle, active knee flexion and extension. Knee brace is discontinued at 4 weeks and patient allowed full activity. An anteroposterior standing and lateral knee radiograph is performed at 6 weeks to confirm union at the osteotomy site.

Corrective Osteotomy

Principle: Corrective osteotomy is performed (usually a closing wedge) at the apex of an extra-articular deformity (EAD) which compounds an already severe intra-articular deformity in arthritic knees undergoing TKA. This allows for restoration of the limb mechanical axis to neutral alignment which may not be possible with intra-articular bony resections and releases alone during TKA.

Indications: Corrective osteotomy may be indicated when bone resections of the distal femur or proximal tibia compromise the collateral attachments or create a large asymmetric soft-tissue gap that may be difficult to balance. Furthermore, corrective osteotomy for EADs is indicated if the EAD is 20° or more in the femur and 30° or more in the tibia in the coronal plane and is close to the knee joint in order to restore limb mechanical axis [5, 7, 9].

Technique: In the femur, an intramedullary femoral guide rod is unsuitable due to distorted medullary canal and/or old hardware and in cases where a corrective osteotomy has been performed and fixed with an intramedullary nail and/or plate and screws and TKA is to be performed subsequently. Hence, computer navigation for TKA is ideal for such situations as it bypasses any distortion of the femoral canal or hardware. Achieving

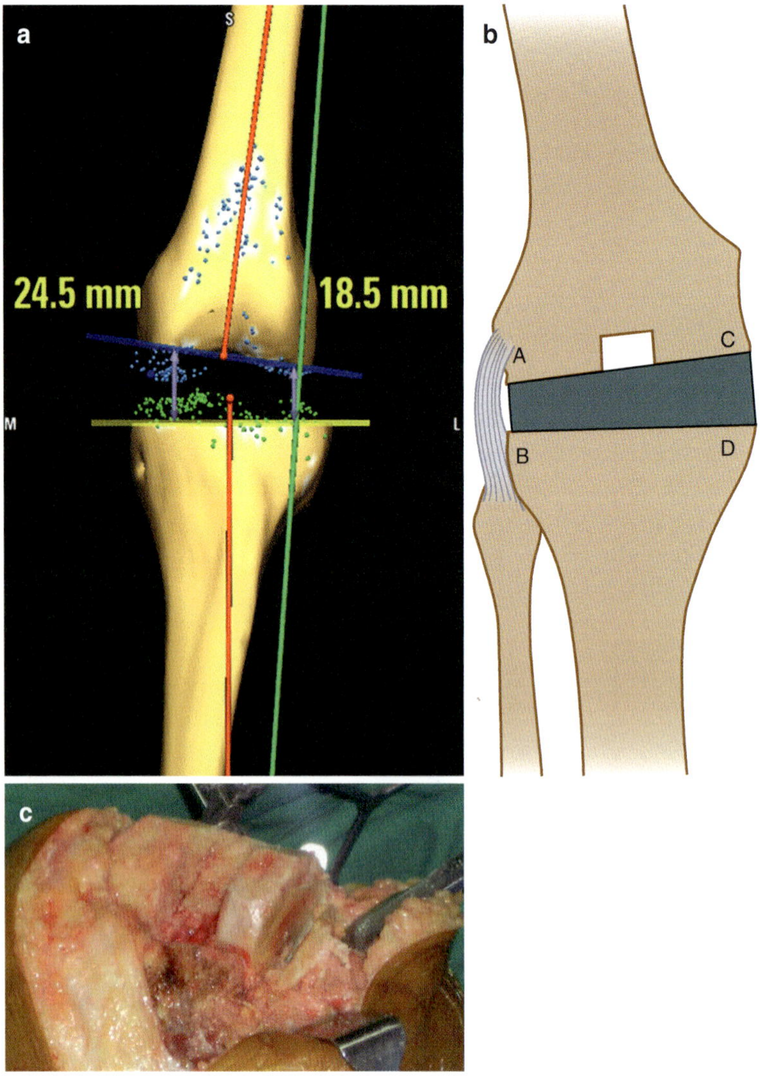

Fig. 11.6 Step-by-step technique of lateral epicondylar osteotomy (LEO) performed to achieve deformity correction and/or medio-lateral soft-tissue balance in valgus arthritic knees undergoing TKA. (**a**) Step 1 – Intraoperative recording of valgus deformity of 8° on applying a varus stress at the knee and a medio-lateral gap mismatch of 6 mm (lateral gap tighter than the medial) despite lateral soft-tissue release (posterolateral capsule, iliotibial band, and popliteofibular ligament). A LEO needs to be performed here to achieve deformity correction and medio-lateral soft-tissue balance. (**b**) Step 2 – The difference between the medial and lateral gap in knee extension (distance *CD–AB*) is measured to determine the amount by which the lateral epicondylar block needs to be shifted distally. This distance can be determined using either navigation or a measuring scale. (**c**) Step 3 – Plane of the osteotomy cut is marked on the lateral femoral condyle. The cut starts 2 mm medial to the lateral edge of the bony lateral condyle and continues obliquely in the superolateral direction. The osteotomy is performed using a reciprocating saw. (**d**) Step 4 – The amount by which the lateral epicondylar block needs to be shifted distally is marked on the block using a measuring scale and electrocautery. The block is then controlled using sutures (Vicryl no. 1) passed through its soft-tissue attachment, and the amount of bone previously marked on the condylar block is now excised using a bone cutter. (**e**) Step 5 – The epicondylar block is now gently shifted distally and repositioned in place using the attached sutures. The medio-lateral balance and alignment are then checked with trial implants in full extension and the knee in 90° flexion with the epicondylar block in its new position. (**f**) Step 6 – After cementing of the final implant, the condylar block is fixed in position using two to three cancellous screws with the knee in 45° flexion

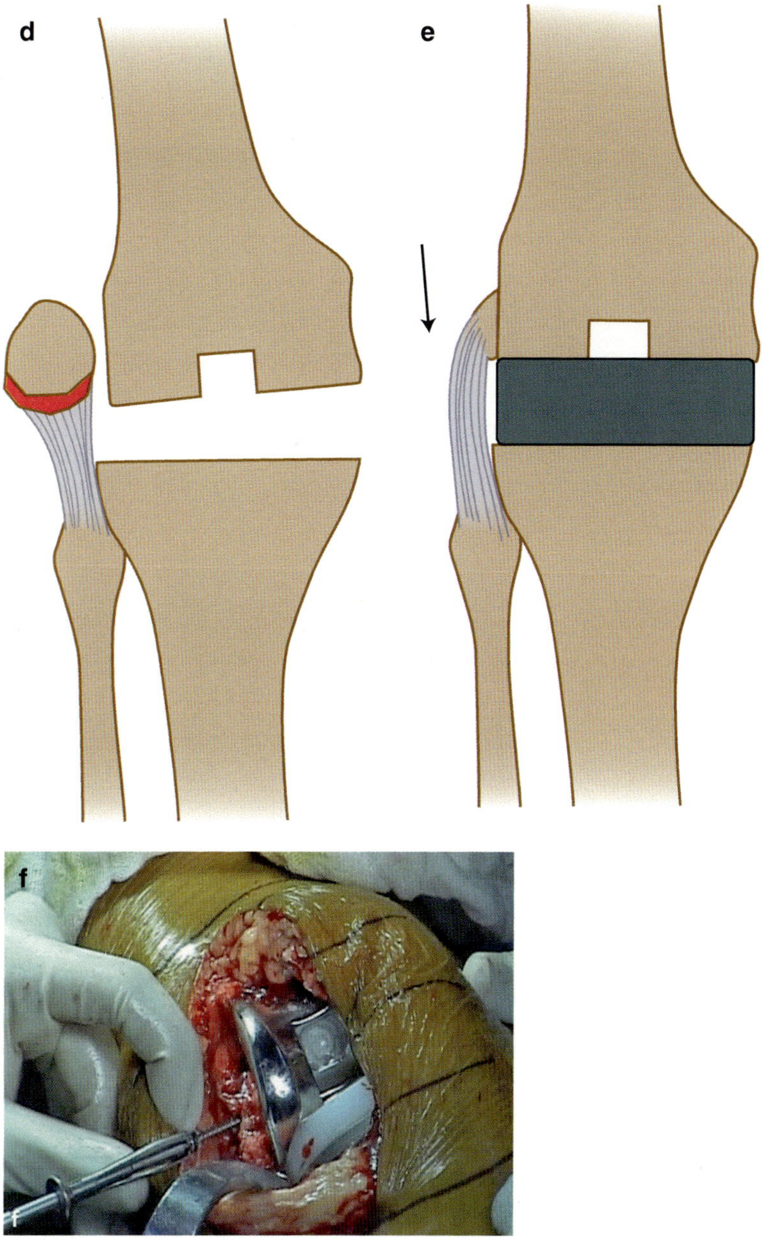

Fig. 11.6 (continued)

stable fixation of the osteotomy performed in the distal third of the femur is challenging due to the distal flaring of the endosteal canal. The authors have used femoral stems, sleeves with stems and retrograde intramedullary locked nails supplemented by a derotation plate to stabilise the osteotomy. A step-by-step technique for corrective osteotomy in the femur is illustrated in Fig. 11.7.

In the tibia, after adequate soft-tissue release and the distal femoral cut, the tibial cut is performed at an angle equal to the residual deformity remaining after soft-tissue release to achieve rectangular

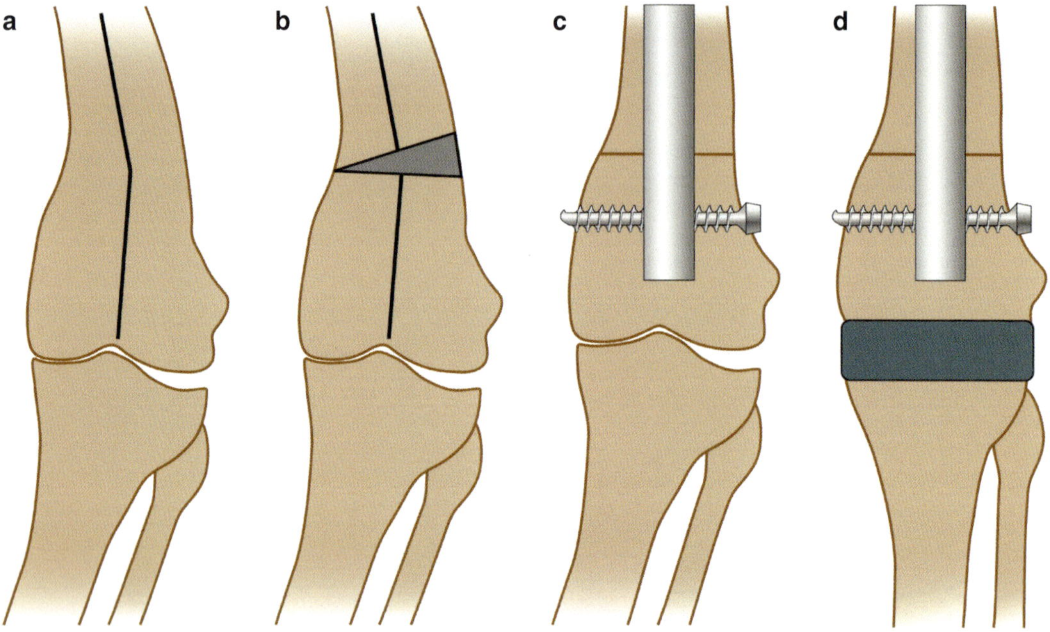

Fig. 11.7 Step-by-step technique of corrective osteotomy for femoral EAD during TKA. (**a**) Step 1 – The severity of femoral EAD is measured on preoperative standing knee radiograph. (**b**) Step 2 – The angle of wedge for the corrective osteotomy is determined on preoperative radiograph, and a lateral closing wedge osteotomy is performed to correct the EAD through a separate lateral incision. (**c**) Step 3 – The osteotomy is fixed using an intramedullary interlocking femoral nail. (**d**) Step 4 – The TKA is then performed in the routine manner in the same sitting

flexion and extension gaps. The alignment is then fully restored by performing a closing wedge corrective osteotomy (equal to the residual deformity present) at the apex of the tibial deformity. A long cementless stem for the tibial component ensures stability at the osteotomy site. The stem (which allows for compressive forces to act at the osteotomy site) along with adjuvant bone grafting (cancellous bone obtained from TKA bone cuts) hastens union at the osteotomy site. A step-by-step technique for corrective osteotomy in the tibia is illustrated in Fig. 11.8.

Precautions: The authors perform corrective osteotomy simultaneously with TKA. Proper planning on preoperative radiographs is important to decide the apex and amount of osteotomy required to correct the extra-articular deformity (see Chap. 8 for details). In cases with femoral extra-articular deformity, fixation at the osteotomy site is dictated by the anatomy of the femur and site of osteotomy; it should be rigid so that postoperative rehabilitation is not delayed or restricted after TKA. On the tibial side, a tibial component with a long stem helps in stabilising the osteotomy site without the need for additional fixation [5]. However, the surgeon should be careful while preparing the tibial medullary canal (to accommodate the long stem of the tibial component) to avoid inadvertent cortical penetration with the reamer tip or the tibial stem extender tip. Intraoperatively, the position of the trial tibial stem within the medullary canal should be verified with an image intensifier before final implantation.

Postoperative Care: Knee movements and partial weight-bearing ambulation in long-leg knee brace is commenced 48 h postoperatively. Patients are allowed full weight-bearing ambulation with a knee brace and stick if knee radiographs show satisfactory healing at 4–6 weeks. After 3 months, the brace and stick are discontinued once x-rays show that the osteotomy site had consolidated.

Tibial Tubercle Osteotomy (TTO)

Principle: The conventional medial parapatellar arthrotomy approach, although adequate in most

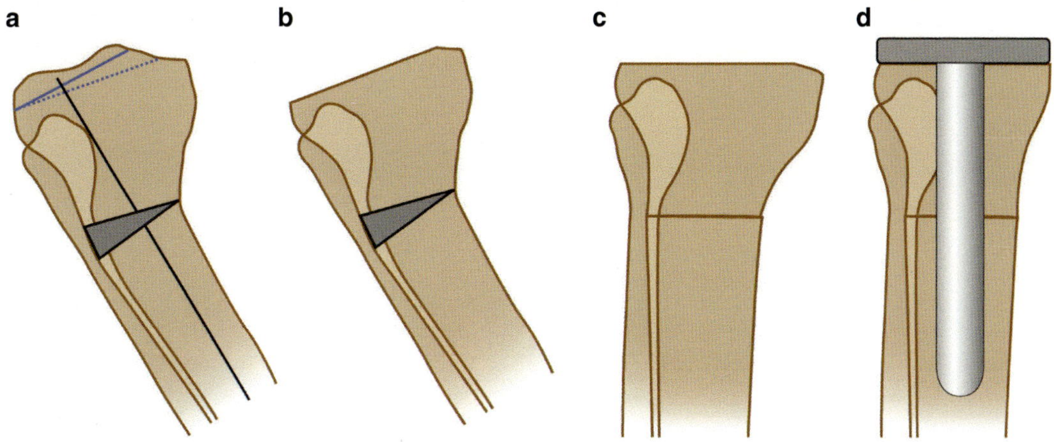

Fig. 11.8 Step-by-step technique of corrective osteotomy for tibial EAD during TKA. (**a**) Step 1 – The severity of tibial EAD is measured on preoperative standing knee radiograph. After performing the distal femoral cut, the tibial cut is performed at an angle equal to the tibial deformity (*dotted line*) ignoring the tibial EAD. *Solid line* indicates medullary axis of the tibia. (**b**) Step 2 – The angle of wedge for the corrective osteotomy is determined on preoperative radiograph, and a lateral closing wedge osteotomy is performed to correct the EAD through a separate lateral incision. (**c**) Step 3 – The osteotomy is gently closed using a valgus force, and limb alignment is checked for correction. The tibial canal is then reamed using progressive large reamers until endosteal "chatter" is felt. (**d**) Step 4 – The osteotomy site is now stabilised with a trial tibial tray with a long stem, the extension and flexion gaps are balanced, the femoral preparation is completed and the final alignment and balance are checked. During final implantation, only the tibial baseplate and metaphyseal part of stem are cemented, taking care no cement enters the osteotomy site

knees, may not be sufficient to achieve good exposure in stiff or ankylosed knees especially when associated with severe deformities. A tibial tubercle osteotomy (TTO) facilitates retraction of the quadriceps mechanism and allows adequate exposure in stiff, ankylosed knees undergoing TKA. The typical TTO involves detaching the patellar tendon with a block of the tibial tubercle and fixation of the block with either cortical screws or wires. The V-Y quadricepsplasty technique is an alternative to improving exposure in such difficult knees during TKA. However, this technique is associated with greater extensor lag and carries the risk of avascular necrosis of patella [10, 11].

Indications: Although frequently used in revision TKAs [11], the use of TTO in primary TKAs has not been universally accepted with doubts about its safety and reliability. Piedade et al. [12] in a comparison of 126 primary TKAs with TTO and 1,348 primary TKAs without TTO reported no significant difference in terms of postoperative pain and function and revision rates between the two groups. However, this technique may be associated with a higher rate of complications such as skin necrosis, proximal migration of the osteotomised tubercle, delayed or nonunion, persistent extensor lag and patellar fracture [12–14]. Young et al. [13] in a review of TTO done for primary and revision TKAs reported that there is an increased risk of patellar fracture when TTO is combined with a lateral retinacular release which may compromise the blood supply to the patella. Rarely, TTO may be combined with the lateral parapatellar arthrotomy in severe, fixed valgus deformity with associated patellar maltracking or patella baja [15] or may be used routinely for all primary TKAs in combination with an anterolateral approach [16, 17]. The rationale given for routine use of such an approach is that it provides better exposure, preservation of patellar blood supply, intact sensation over the saphenous nerve distribution and preserving the extensor mechanism [16, 17].

Technique: A more conservative modification of the TTO technique involves detaching the patellar tendon from the tibial tubercle with a thin layer of bone using a sharp osteotome, leaving the

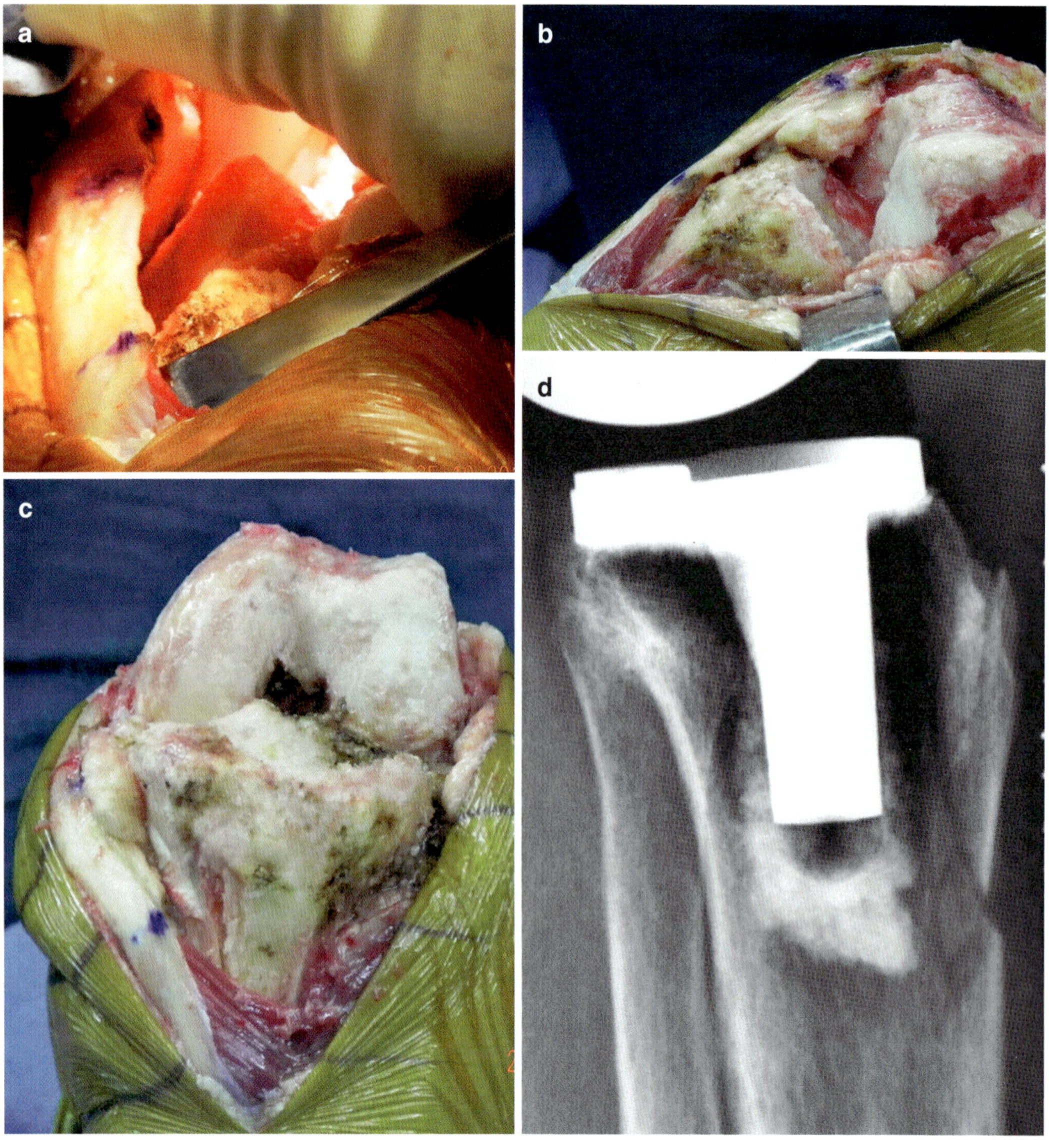

Fig. 11.9 Tibial tubercle osteotomy (TTO) during TKA. (**a**) The patellar tendon is detached with a thin layer of tubercular bone using a sharp osteotome. (**b**) Intraoperative photograph showing lateral view after detachment of the tibial tubercle showing continuity of the extensor mechanism. (**c**) Intraoperative photograph showing frontal view after detachment of the tibial tubercle. Note that the distal soft-tissue attachments of the tibial tubercle have been preserved. (**d**) Postoperative lateral knee radiograph of the same patient taken 2 days after surgery showing the repositioned tibial tubercle without any fixation

extensor mechanism intact distally and laterally. The authors use this technique in cases of stiff arthritic knees which undergo TKA as also when performing a lateral approach for a severe valgus deformity (Fig. 11.9). This technique has the advantage of being less traumatic, less painful and not requiring fixation. However, this approach may provide less access compared to the typical TTO and may have the risk of failure at its distal attachment if care is not taken intraoperatively. The layer of bone detached with the tendon facilitates healing without the need for fixation.

Postoperative Care: Postoperatively, the patient is allowed full weight-bearing ambulation in a long knee brace with static quadriceps exercises (although straight leg rising is discouraged)

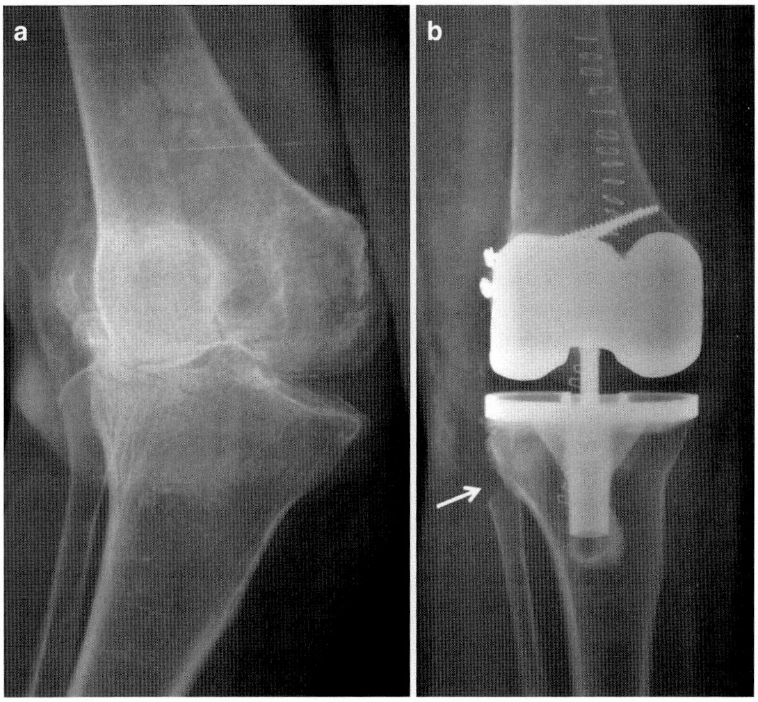

Fig. 11.10 Fibular head resection during TKA. (**a**) Preoperative standing knee radiograph of a patient showing severe valgus deformity with an associated flexion deformity. Acute correction during TKA may put this patient at risk for peroneal nerve palsy due to stretching of the nerve. (**b**) Postoperative standing knee radiograph of the same patient (a) showing a fibular head resection (*arrow*) done to facilitate full correction of valgus deformity and also to prevent excessive traction on the nerve during correction with TKA

on the day after surgery. Gentle, active knee flexion-extension is started 4 weeks after surgery with application of knee brace intermittently and knee flexion restricted up to 90° till the end of 8 weeks postoperatively. The brace is then discontinued and the patient encouraged to gradually increase flexion beyond 90° over the next 4 weeks.

Segmental Fibular Osteotomy

This may be indicated in cases of severe varus tibial extra-articular deformity where performing a closed wedge tibial osteotomy at the apex of the deformity may not afford full correction. Resecting 2 cm of fibula (subperiosteally) through a separate lateral approach is useful. A safe level at which to resect the fibula is four fingerbreadths above the lateral malleolus.

Fibular Head Resection

In severe valgus deformities with long-standing flexion contracture, there is a risk of peroneal nerve palsy from correcting the deformity at TKA. To minimise this risk, the authors subperiosteally resect the fibular head by osteotomising it at the neck of the fibula (Fig. 11.10). The attachments of the biceps tendon and LCL are preserved as the dissection is subperiosteal – similar to the manner in which medial tibial osteophytes are resected subperiosteally without damage to the MCL. Also in these cases, the knee is kept flexed 10°–15° over a pillow till the anaesthesia wears out and the patient is able to dorsiflex the foot and toes subsequently. The patient is encouraged to perform static quadriceps exercises to correct and maintain correction of the flexion contracture.

References

1. Mullaji AB, Shetty GM. Correction of varus deformity during TKA with reduction osteotomy. Clin Orthop Relat Res. 2014;472(1):126–32.
2. Dixon MC, Parsch D, Brown RR, Scott RD. The correction of severe varus deformity in total knee

arthroplasty by tibial component downsizing and resection of uncapped proximal medial bone. J Arthroplasty. 2004;19:19–22.
3. Mullaji AB, Shetty GM. Surgical technique: computer-assisted sliding medial condylar osteotomy to achieve gap balance in varus knees during TKA. Clin Orthop Relat Res. 2013;471:1484–91.
4. Mullaji AB, Shetty GM. Lateral epicondylar osteotomy using computer navigation in total knee arthroplasty for rigid valgus deformities. J Arthroplasty. 2010;25:166–9.
5. Mullaji A, Shetty GM. Computer-assisted total knee arthroplasty for arthritis with extra-articular deformity. J Arthroplasty. 2009;24:1164–9.
6. Mullaji AB, Padmanabhan V, Jindal G. Total knee arthroplasty for profound varus deformity: technique and radiological results in 173 knees with varus of more than 20 degrees. J Arthroplasty. 2005;20:550–61.
7. Mason JB, Fehring TK. Management of extra-articular deformity in total knee arthroplasty with navigation. In: Scott WN, editor. Insall & Scott surgery of the knee. Philadelphia: Elsevier Churchill Livingstone; 2012. p. 1234.
8. Engh GA, Ammeen D. Results of total knee arthroplasty with medial epicondylar osteotomy to correct varus deformity. Clin Orthop Relat Res. 1999;367:141–8.
9. Wang JW, Wang CJ. Total knee arthroplasty for arthritis of the knee with extra-articular deformity. J Bone Joint Surg Am. 2002;84:1769–74.
10. Hsu CH, Lin PC, Chen WS, Wang JW. Total knee arthroplasty in patients with stiff knees. J Arthroplasty. 2012;27:286–92.
11. Della Valle CJ, Berger RA, Rosenberg AG. Surgical exposures in revision total knee arthroplasty. Clin Orthop Relat Res. 2006;446:59–68.
12. Piedade SR, Pinaroli A, Servien E, Neyret P. Tibial tubercle osteotomy in primary total knee arthroplasty: a safe procedure or not? Knee. 2008;15:439–46.
13. Young CF, Bourne RB, Rorabeck CH. Tibial tubercle osteotomy in total knee arthroplasty surgery. J Arthroplasty. 2008;23:371–5.
14. Zonnenberg CB, Lisowski LA, van den Bekerom MP, Nolte PA. Tuberositas osteotomy for total knee arthroplasty: a review of the literature. J Knee Surg. 2010;23:121–9.
15. Apostolopoulos AP, Nikolopoulos DD, Polyzois I, Nakos A, Liarokapis S, Stefanakis G, Michos IV. Total knee arthroplasty in severe valgus deformity: interest of combining a lateral approach with a tibial tubercle osteotomy. Orthop Traumatol Surg Res. 2010;96:777–84.
16. Hirschmann MT, Hoffmann M, Krause R, Jenabzadeh RA, Arnold MP, Friederich NF. Anterolateral approach with tibial tubercle osteotomy versus standard medial approach for primary total knee arthroplasty: does it matter? BMC Musculoskelet Disord. 2010;11:167.
17. Hay GC, Kampshoff J, Kuster MS. Lateral subvastus approach with osteotomy of the tibial tubercle for total knee replacement: a two-year prospective, randomised, blinded controlled trial. J Bone Joint Surg Br. 2010;92:862–6.

12 Postoperative Pain Management and Rehabilitation

Introduction

Patients undergo TKA to gain relief from arthritic pain, to regain function and to improve their quality of life. However, the patient needs to deal with significant pain during the early postoperative period after TKA. Postoperative outcome and satisfaction after TKA depend to a large extent on optimal pain control [1–3]. Suboptimal pain management after TKA has severe consequences. It may not only lead to physical and emotional distress and dissatisfaction in the patient and relatives but often leads to longer hospital stay, delay in functional recovery and non-compliance of patients with rehabilitation programme. Delay in mobilisation due to excessive pain may also put the patient at increased risk for systemic complications such as deep vein thrombosis, pneumonia and thromboembolism [4, 5] or local complications such as residual knee deformity (usually fixed flexion deformity), limited knee ROM (typically flexion beyond 100°) and chronic pain at the surgical site [6–8]. Therefore, the importance of optimal pain control after TKA cannot be emphasised enough given the consequences.

Postoperative physical rehabilitation after TKA is equally important to help the patient achieve full functional recovery as soon as possible. Rehabilitation and pain control go hand in hand, and optimal pain control is necessary to initiate early mobilisation and ambulation and achieve functional recovery. This chapter aims to discuss the postoperative pain control and rehabilitation protocol being followed by the authors.

Pain After TKA

Postoperative pain is a complex phenomenon and the aetiology of acute postoperative pain in TKA is still unclear. However, both systemic and local factors are known to play a role in it [9]. Patient-specific factors such as age, gender, aetiology of arthritis, prior experience, expectations and the psychological make-up all have been reported to play a part in how postoperative pain is perceived and experienced after TKA [10, 11]. Intraoperatively, local factors such as the amount and depth of soft-tissue dissection or release, optimum limb alignment, component alignment and rotation and the soft-tissue balance achieved may have an association with recovery from acute postoperative pain and the risk of chronic persistent pain after TKA [9, 12–14]. Postoperatively, it has been reported that control of the local rather than systemic inflammatory response may be more important for early postoperative functional recovery [15].

In view of various systemic and local factors involved in acute postoperative pain, a multimodal approach to pain control has now become standard practice in patients undergoing TKA [16, 17]. The principle of this multimodal approach is to deploy various techniques and pharmacological agents which will act synergistically at different levels to achieve optimal pain control after TKA. The authors use a similar multimodal pain control protocol involving preoperative patient education, pre-emptive analgesia, optimal anaesthesia and surgical technique and postoperative analgesia in order to minimise pain

A.B. Mullaji, G.M. Shetty, *Deformity Correction in Total Knee Arthroplasty*,
DOI 10.1007/978-1-4939-0566-9_12,

and facilitate early functional recovery of the patient after TKA.

Multimodal Pain Management Protocol

Preoperative Patient Education

This involves educating the patient about the surgical procedure and postoperative recovery course after TKA. The patient is appraised about what to expect in terms of pain, complications and the time to reach a pain-free, fully functional joint after TKA. Patients are also encouraged to contact and discuss with patients who have already undergone TKA and have now fully recovered.

Pre-emptive Analgesia

After admission (previous night at 10 p.m.) – Tab etoricoxib 60 mg and tab gabapentin 300 mg
Morning of surgery (at 6 a.m.) – Tab etoricoxib 60 mg and tab gabapentin 100 mg

Anaesthesia

Spinal anaesthesia (unilateral TKA) or combined spinal + epidural (for bilateral TKA)

Surgical Technique

Skin incision only as much as required (usually extending from the upper pole of the patella to the tibial tuberosity)

Minimise soft-tissue release by excision of osteophytes before any soft-tissue release, graduated stepwise soft-tissue release and reduction osteotomy before any substantial release in case of varus deformity

Full correction of knee deformity in both coronal and sagittal planes, optimum component alignment and soft-tissue balance

Complete homeostasis and airtight closure to minimise chances of a postoperative haematoma and facilitate proper wound healing

Intraoperative Local Infiltration

What to infiltrate?

The periarticular infiltration "cocktail" contains the following constituents diluted to a total volume of 50 ml with 0.9 % normal saline:

Bupivacaine 0.25 % (2.5 mg/kg)
Fentanyl 200 mcg (50 mcg/ml)
Cefuroxime 750 mg
Triamcinolone 40 mg
Ketorolac 30 mg
Clonidine (1 mcg/kg)

The corticosteroid is excluded in patients with diabetes, rheumatoid arthritis, previous knee surgery and any immunodeficiency disease.

Where to infiltrate?

Edges of the arthrotomy, medial collateral ligament, lateral retinaculum and posteromedial soft-tissue sleeve

When to infiltrate?

After the components have been implanted and while the cement is setting

Postoperative Analgesia

First 48 h

Tab paracetamol 650 mg 8 hourly + tab ibuprofen 400 mg 12 hourly + diclofenac suppository 12.5 mg, one at night + tab etoricoxib 60 mg, one in the morning + tab gabapentin 300 mg, one at night

Local ice fomentation every 6–8 h

After 48 h till suture removal (2 weeks)

Tab paracetamol 650 mg 8 hourly + diclofenac suppository 12.5 mg, one at night + tab etoricoxib 60 mg, one in the morning + tab gabapentin 300 mg, one at night

Tab ibuprofen 400 mg 12 h or as and when needed

Local ice fomentation every 6–8 h

After suture removal till 1 month

Tab paracetamol 650 mg 8 hourly + tab meloxicam 15 mg, one in the morning + tab etoricoxib 60 mg, one at night + tab gabapentin 300 mg, one at night

Tab ibuprofen 400 mg as and when needed

Local ice fomentation every 6–8 h

Rehabilitation Protocol

All our patients are instructed and trained in five basic, simple exercises (Fig. 12.1) which need to be performed regularly throughout the day (10– 20 repetitions each, in 3–4 sessions per day). The patients are made familiar with these five exercises preoperatively using an illustrated instruction booklet which the patient can refer to from time to time postoperatively, and a resident/fellow/therapist demonstrates these exercises on day 1 postoperatively. Subsequently, till the time

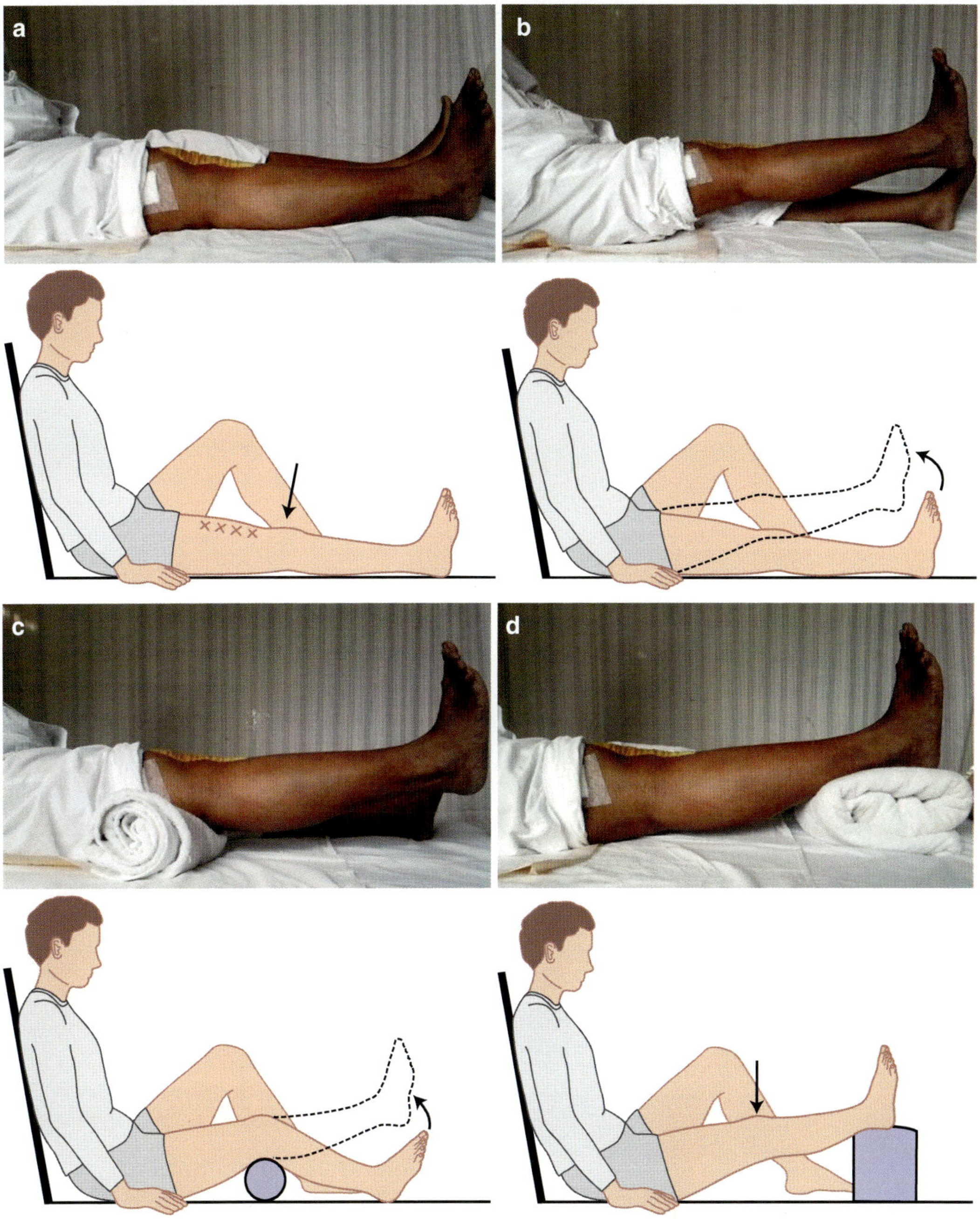

Fig. 12.1 The five basic exercises used in rehabilitation after TKA. (**a**) Static quadriceps contraction. (**b**) Seated straight leg raising. (**c**) Short arm knee extension. (**d**) Gravity-assisted active knee stretching. (**e**) Seated knee extension and flexion

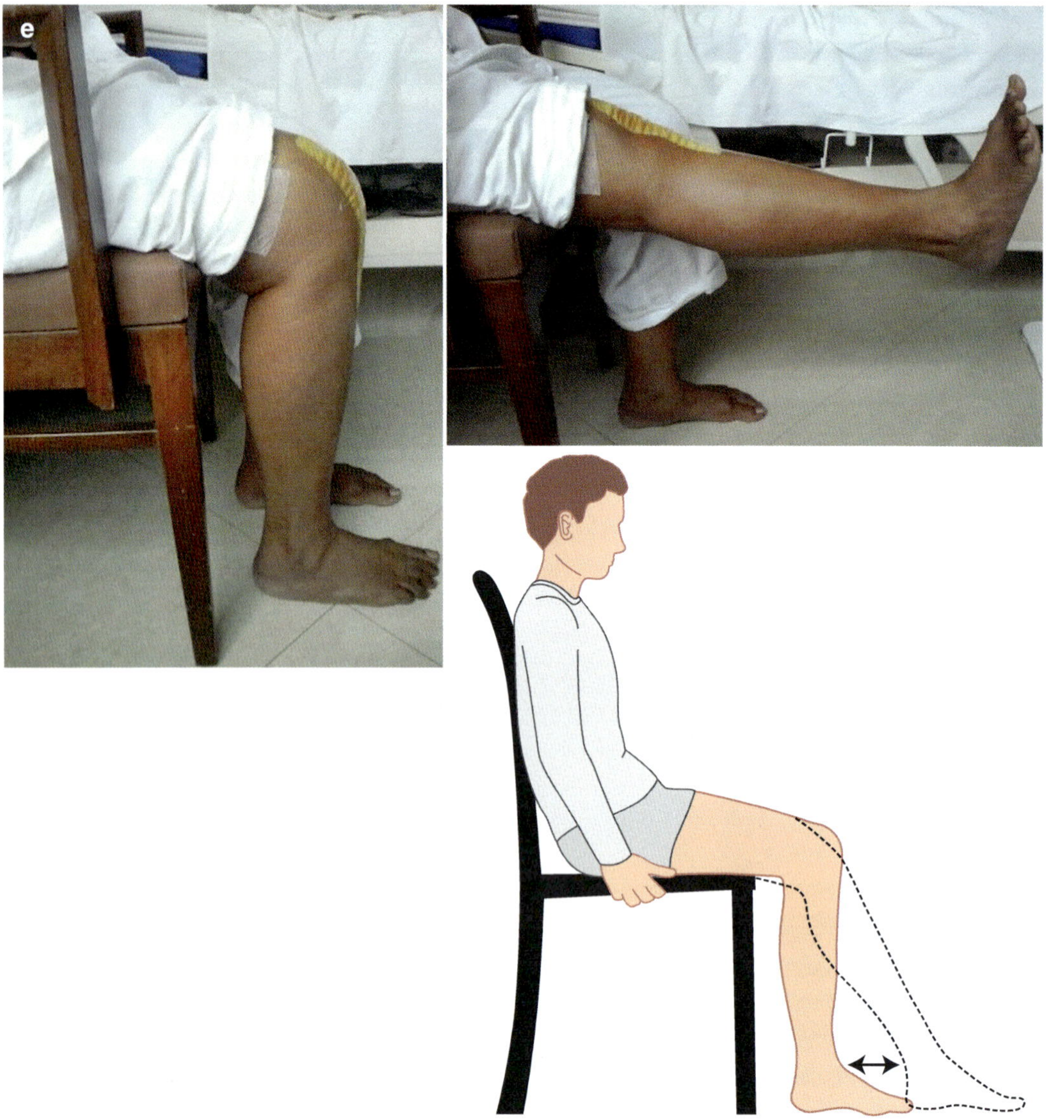

Fig. 12.1 (continued)

of discharge, the patient is assessed everyday by the surgeon for progress in knee motion and functional ability. A physiotherapist is asked to intervene only in special cases with excessive quadriceps weakness, slow improvement in knee flexion or gait abnormality.

Goals of Rehabilitation

1. Prevent wasting of the muscles and improve tone and strength of the muscles without increasing pain
2. Improve knee range of motion
3. Correct any residual flexion deformity or extensor lag if present
4. Improve gait
5. Be able to perform activities of daily living independently

Postoperative Rehabilitation

First 24 h

On returning to room after surgery – in bed, ankle and toe movements, log rolling of both lower limbs, static quadriceps contractions and turning on sides, 10 repetitions every hour

Next day morning – static quadriceps contraction, short arm knee extension, seated knee extension and flexion, straight leg raising and gravity-assisted active knee stretching (10 repetitions every 6 h). Standing and short walk with walker. Sitting on a chair

24–48 h

Static quadriceps contraction, short arm knee extension, seated knee extension and flexion, straight leg raising and gravity-assisted active knee stretching (10 repetitions every 6 h).

Walk with walker or stick (Fig. 12.2). Sitting on a chair and commode chair

48–72 h (discharge)

Static quadriceps contraction, short arm knee extension, seated knee extension and flexion, straight leg raising and gravity-assisted active knee stretching (10 repetitions every 6 h).

Walk with stick. Sitting on a commode

Stair climbing (Fig. 12.3), parallel bar walking and hip abductor strengthening in case of gait abnormality (waddling gait)

Faradic stimulation two to three times a day in case of significant quadriceps weakness and extensor lag

What should be achieved at the time of discharge?

Knee flexion of at least 100° in the sitting position

Extensor lag or residual flexion deformity of less than 10°

Getting out of bed and getting up from a chair without assistance

Walking with or without a stick

Ability to use commode

Stair climbing with a stick

72 h (discharge) to 2 weeks (suture removal)

Static quadriceps contraction, short arm knee extension, seated knee extension and flexion, straight leg raising and gravity-assisted active knee stretching (10 repetitions every 6 h).

Walk with stick. Sitting on a commode

After 2 weeks

Patients are clinically assessed at the end of 2 weeks postoperatively (during suture removal) for muscle strength (quadriceps/hamstrings), residual deformity (flexion or extension lag), knee flexion and gait, and specific exercises are prescribed. Quadriceps is strengthened by Thera-Band resistance exercises and knee extension using weight cuffs in cases with extensor lag. Knee flexion is increased by graduated active knee flexion and recumbent cycling (Fig. 12.4). Residual flexion deformity is corrected by gravity-assisted active knee stretching and use of a push-knee splint. Gait is improved with parallel bar walking, gait training and coordinated quadriceps and hamstring training (Fig. 12.5).

Special Cases

Bracing – Braces are usually avoided after TKA. Exceptionally, a long knee brace may be used in patients with long-standing quadriceps weakness to avoid sudden buckling of the knee and falls till the quadriceps have regained strength. A long knee brace may also be indicated in cases with long-standing hyperextension deformity of the knee and in cases where additional procedures such as a corrective osteotomy, lateral epicondylar or medial condylar osteotomy has been performed. A push-knee splint may be indicated in cases with any residual flexion deformity to achieve gradual full correction postoperatively.

Flexion Deformity – Although the authors achieve full correction of flexion deformity in most cases intraoperatively, some patients with long-standing, severe preoperative flexion deformity are at higher risk for recurrence. In such cases a push-knee splint is applied to be used while walking and for 40 min every 3–4 h at rest. The splint is then gradually weaned off over 3–4 weeks.

Hyperextension Deformity – Some patients with long-standing, severe preoperative hyperextension deformity are at higher risk for recurrence. Such patients are encouraged to keep a pillow under their knee at rest for 2 weeks after surgery, and gravity-assisted quadriceps tightening is avoided. A long knee splint is applied to be used while walking which is then gradually weaned off over 2–3 weeks.

Lateral Epicondylar or Medial Condylar Osteotomy – In cases where a lateral epicondylar or medial condylar osteotomy has been performed, the patient is allowed full weight-bearing ambulation with a long knee brace on the first postoperative day. Knee movement is

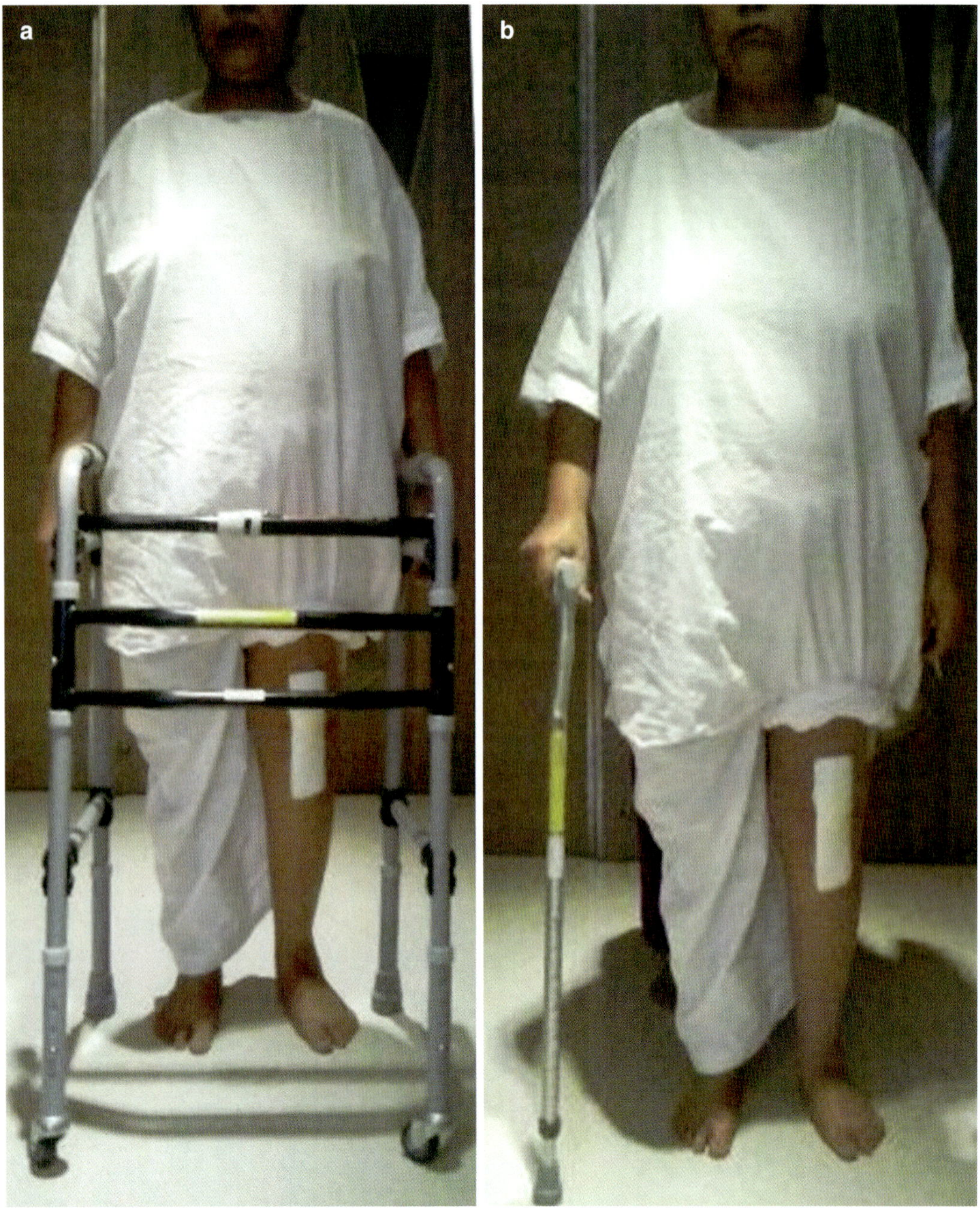

Fig. 12.2 Walking after TKA, 24–48 h postoperatively. (**a**) All patients can walk with a walker within 24 h of TKA. (**b**) Most patients are able to walk with a stick by 48 postoperatively

not allowed for 2 weeks after which the patient is advised to remove the brace three to four times a day and perform gentle, active knee flexion and extension. Knee brace is discontinued at 4 weeks and patient allowed full activity.

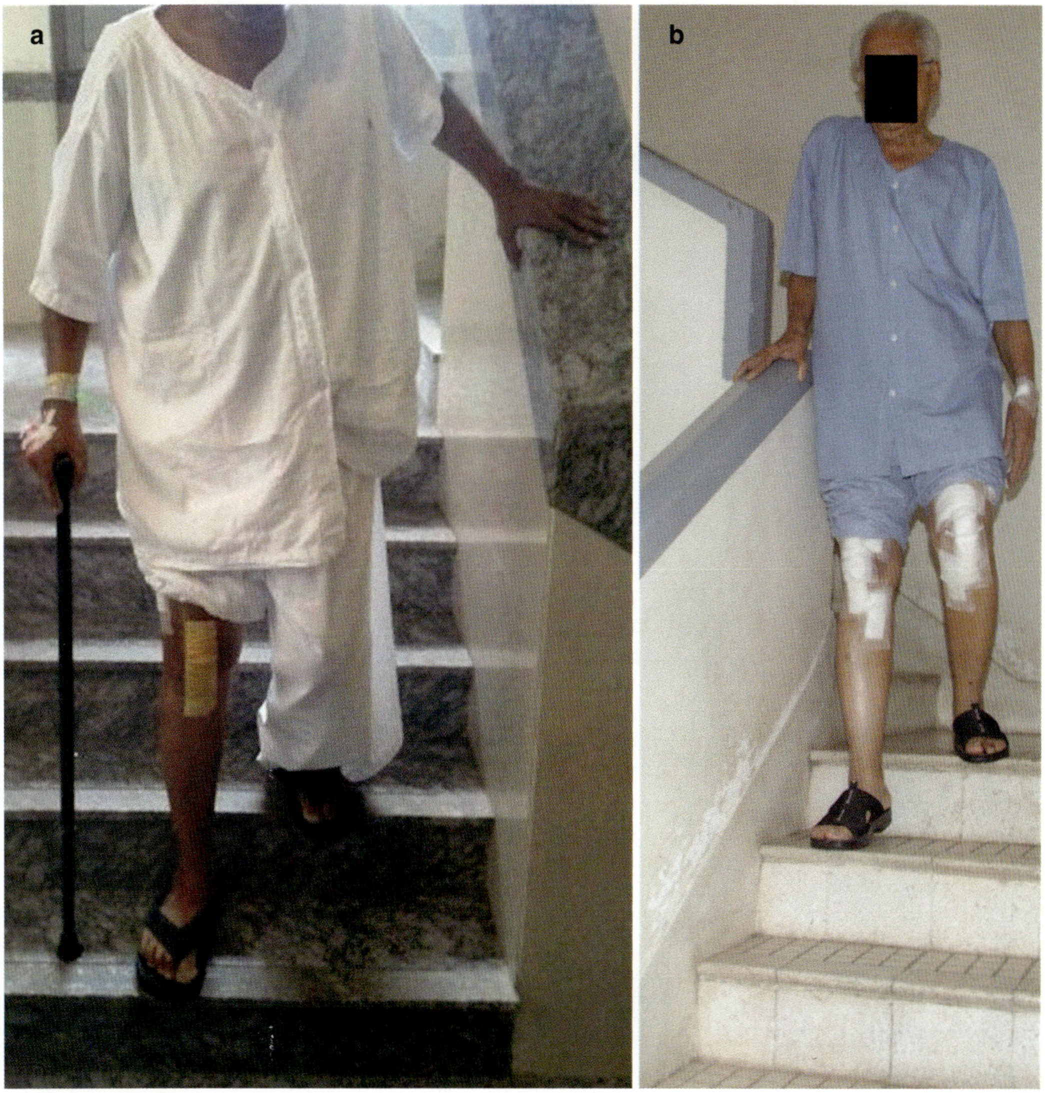

Fig. 12.3 Stair climbing after TKA, 48–72 h postoperatively. (**a**) All patients can climb steps by 72 h of TKA with the help of a walking stick. (**b**) Most patients can climb steps by 72 h of TKA without the help of a walking aid

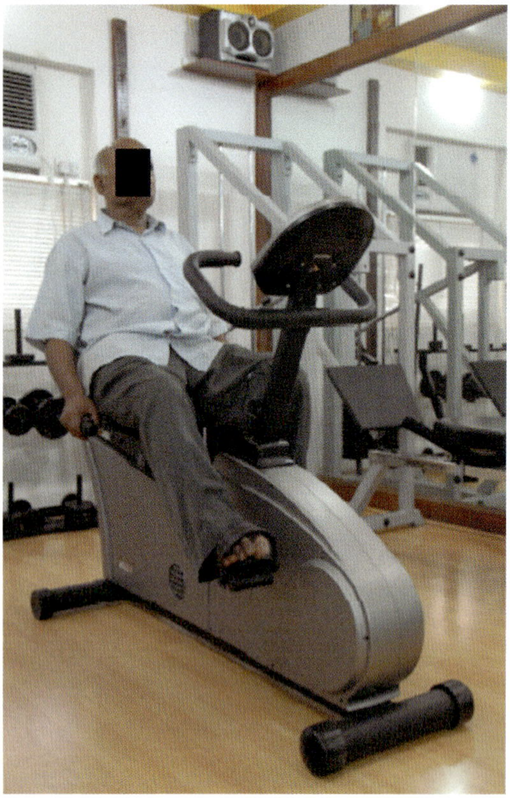

Fig. 12.4 Recumbent cycling to improve knee flexion and flexibility after suture removal

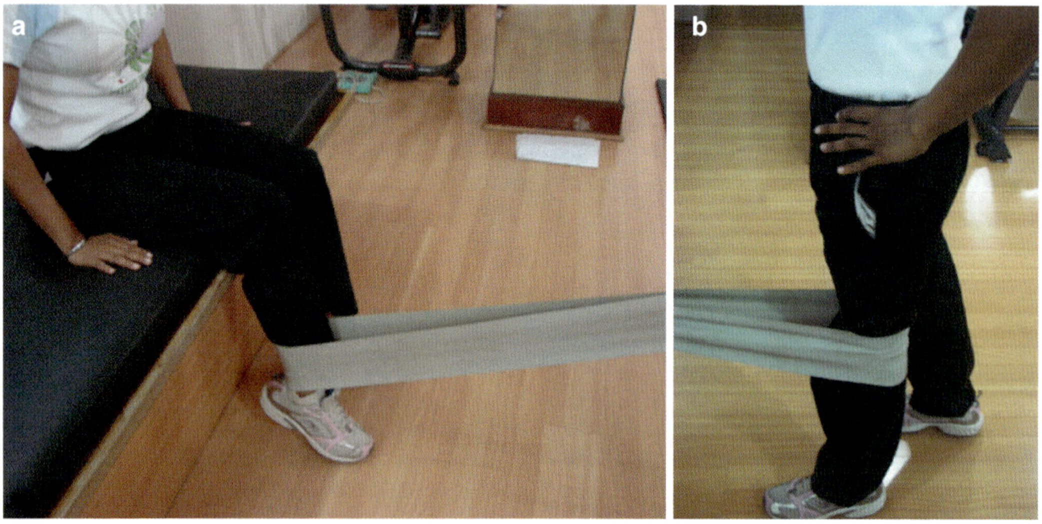

Fig. 12.5 Knee flexors strengthening with Thera-Band resistance exercises in both sitting (**a**) and standing (**b**) positions. To improve gait after TKA, knee extensors and flexors along with hip extensors and abductors need strengthening

References

1. Hamilton DF, Lane JV, Gaston P, Patton JT, Macdonald D, Simpson AH, Howie CR. What determines patient satisfaction with surgery? A prospective cohort study of 4709 patients following total joint replacement. BMJ Open. 2013;3:1–7.
2. Scott CE, Howie CR, MacDonald D, Biant LC. Predicting dissatisfaction following total knee replacement: a prospective study of 1217 patients. J Bone Joint Surg Br. 2010;92:1253–8.
3. Drexler M, Dwyer T, Chakravertty R, Farno A, Backstein D. Assuring the happy total knee replacement patient. Bone Joint J. 2013;95-B(11 Suppl A):120–3.
4. Husted H, Otte KS, Kristensen BB, Ørsnes T, Wong C, Kehlet H. Low risk of thromboembolic complications after fast-track hip and knee arthroplasty. Acta Orthop. 2010;81:599–605.
5. Xing KH, Morrison G, Lim W, Douketis J, Odueyungbo A, Crowther M. Has the incidence of deep vein thrombosis in patients undergoing total hip/knee arthroplasty changed over time? A systematic review of randomized controlled trials. Thromb Res. 2008;123:24–34.
6. Vince KG. The stiff total knee arthroplasty: causes and cures. J Bone Joint Surg Br. 2012;94(11 Suppl A):103–11.
7. Dennis DA, Komistek RD, Scuderi GR, Zingde S. Factors affecting flexion after total knee arthroplasty. Clin Orthop Relat Res. 2007;464:53–60.
8. Vilardo L, Shah M. Chronic pain after hip and knee replacement. Tech Reg Anesth Pain Med. 2011;15:110–15.
9. Brennan TJ. Pathophysiology of postoperative pain. Pain. 2011;152(3 Suppl):S33–40.
10. Desmeules F, Dionne CE, Belzile EL, Bourbonnais R, Champagne F, Frémont P. Determinants of pain, functional limitations and health-related quality of life six months after total knee arthroplasty: results from a prospective cohort study. BMC Sports Sci Med Rehabil. 2013;5:1–11.
11. Bonnin MP, Basiglini L, Archbold HA. What are the factors of residual pain after uncomplicated TKA? Knee Surg Sports Traumatol Arthrosc. 2011;19:1411–17.
12. Babazadeh S, Stoney JD, Lim K, Choong PF. The relevance of ligament balancing in total knee arthroplasty: how important is it? A systematic review of the literature. Orthop Rev (Pavia). 2009;1:70–8.
13. Huang NF, Dowsey MM, Ee E, Stoney JD, Babazadeh S, Choong PF. Coronal alignment correlates with outcome after total knee arthroplasty: five-year follow-up of a randomized controlled trial. J Arthroplasty. 2012;27:1737–41.
14. Nicoll D, Rowley DI. Internal rotational error of the tibial component is a major cause of pain after total knee replacement. J Bone Joint Surg Br. 2010;92:1238–44.
15. Ugraş AA, Kural C, Kural A, Demirez F, Koldaş M, Cetinus E. Which is more important after total knee arthroplasty: local inflammatory response or systemic inflammatory response? Knee. 2011;18:113–16.
16. Parvataneni HK, Ranawat AS, Ranawat CS. The use of local periarticular injections in the management of postoperative pain after total hip and knee replacement: a multimodal approach. Instr Course Lect. 2007;56:125–31.
17. Parvizi J, Miller AG, Gandhi K. Multimodal pain management after total joint arthroplasty. J Bone Joint Surg Am. 2011;93:1075–84.

Index

A.B. Mullaji, G.M. Shetty, *Deformity Correction in Total Knee Arthroplasty*,
DOI 10.1007/978-1-4939-0566-9, © Springer Science+Business Media New York 2014

Printed by Printforce, the Netherlands